Health Literacy From A Health Ethnology Perspective

Uwe H. Bittlingmayer • Zeynep Islertas •
Elias Sahrai • Stefanie Harsch •
Isabella Bertschi • Diana Sahrai

Health Literacy From A Health Ethnology Perspective

An Analysis of Everyday Health Practices of Migrant Youth and Families

Springer

Uwe H. Bittlingmayer
Institute of Sociology
University of Education Freiburg
Freiburg im Breisgau, Germany

Zeynep Islertas
Institute of Sociology
University of Education Freiburg
Freiburg im Breisgau, Germany

Elias Sahrai
Institute of Sociology
University of Education Freiburg
Freiburg im Breisgau, Germany

Stefanie Harsch
Center for Medicine and Society
Albert-Ludwigs-University Freiburg
Freiburg im Breisgau, Germany

Isabella Bertschi
Institute of Psychology
University Zürich
Zürich, Switzerland

Diana Sahrai
Institute of Educational Sciences
University of Education Freiburg
Freiburg im Breisgau, Germany

ISBN 978-3-658-42347-6 ISBN 978-3-658-42348-3 (eBook)
https://doi.org/10.1007/978-3-658-42348-3

This book is a translation of the original German edition „Health Literacy aus gesundheitsethnologischer Perspektive" by Bittlingmayer, Uwe H., published by Springer Fachmedien Wiesbaden GmbH in 2020. The translation was done with the help of artificial intelligence (machine translation by the service DeepL.com). A subsequent human revision was done primarily in terms of content, so that the book will read stylistically differently from a conventional translation. Springer Nature works continuously to further the development of tools for the production of books and on the related technologies to support the authors.

This Springer imprint is published by the registered company Springer Fachmedien Wiesbaden GmbH, part of Springer Nature.
The registered company address is: Abraham-Lincoln-Str. 46, 65189 Wiesbaden, Germany

Paper in this product is recyclable.

In memory of Peter-Ernst Schnabel, a
pioneer of German health science

Preface

This book was originally written for a German audience. In contrast to Anglo-American public health research, German public health research is characterised by the fact that ethnography is a method with little legitimacy and in need of justification. In this respect, many remarks, self-assurances and legitimation strategies are aimed at convincing the readership that ethnological or ethnographic research on everyday health behaviour is useful. Hopefully, this is much less the case with an English-speaking audience.

The reasons why we accepted the publisher's invitation to use a translation programme to present the book to an English-speaking audience more receptive to this method are based on three key considerations and observations.

First, for about two decades, health literacy research around the world has been very much focused on the idea of health literacy as a distinct individual competency. The idea that health literacy is a social practice, which we believe is much more plausible and sociologically grounded, and which has been developed through the pioneering work of Ulla Papen and more recently Silja Samerski, is still largely absent from mainstream health literacy research, which is dominated by social epidemiology. Recent developments towards research on organisational health literacy as a corrective and relief to health literacy that has been theoretically reduced as individualistic is not really helpful here because it simply shifts the level of the social to the organisation without understanding how the social embeddedness of individual health action works.

Second, by focusing qualitative health literacy research on ethnic minority children and young people, we aim to present analyses that are also comparatively marginalised in the dominant Anglo-American debate. In addition, we draw on the concept of family health literacy, which has been little developed internationally, to address the unequal distribution of opportunities to develop health literacy skills.

Third, the theoretical underpinning of health literacy (and public health in general) is weak. In contrast, our study is theory-driven. The theoretical considerations in our study are comparatively elaborate, which means that the positivist concepts of health literacy cannot keep up. In a way, this is calculated and represents an idea of public health that normatively points far beyond the conditions that empirical research currently has to catch up with.

We hope that native speakers will overlook the linguistic shortcomings and abbreviations that are certainly present, always on the lookout for the argument that might be hidden behind the cryptic explanations in German.

Our thanks go to Katrin Emmerich for initiating and supporting this project, which is largely harmless to us German researchers, and to Infancia Immaculate, who never lost patience. We would also like to thank Konrad Jocksch, who proof-read the files provided by the publisher with his usual sovereign manner.

We look forward with great anticipation to the publication of our book in English.

Freiburg im Breisgau, Germany — Uwe H. Bittlingmayer
Freiburg im Breisgau, Germany — Zeynep Islertas
Freiburg im Breisgau, Germany — Elias Sahrai
Freiburg im Breisgau, Germany — Stefanie Harsch
Zürich, Switzerland — Isabella Bertschi
Freiburg im Breisgau, Germany — Diana Sahrai
January 2023

Contents

1 Introduction: On the Necessity and Meaningfulness of a Health Ethnology Perspective in Health Literacy Research

Abstract

This book aims to make a theoretical and empirical contribution to health ethnology-inspired health literacy research in particular and public health research in general. Whenever an interdisciplinary approach to a field of research is chosen within established sciences, in our case public health, sociology of health and medicine, and medical anthropology, which does not necessarily seem to be compatible with the basic disciplinary self-understandings, then such an approach, from the very outset, is more clearly in need of legitimation than the recourse to the usual procedures would ever be. We want to take this into account briefly in the introduction and point out the limits and some fundamental problems of conventional health literacy research.

This book aims to make a theoretical and empirical contribution to health ethnology-inspired health literacy research in particular and public health research in general. Whenever an interdisciplinary approach to a field of research is chosen within established sciences, in our case public health, sociology of health and medicine, and medical anthropology, which does not necessarily seem to be compatible with the basic disciplinary self-understandings, then such an approach, from the very outset, is more clearly in need of legitimation than recourse to the usual procedures would ever be. We want to take this into account briefly in the introduction, pointing out limitations and some problems of principle in conventional health literacy research. In the further course of the book, we will then explore these weaknesses in greater depth through an analysis of the state of research, followed by a more immanent exploration of the health ethnology approach through case studies. It should be emphasised at the outset that this is explicitly not a matter

U. H. Bittlingmayer et al., *Health Literacy From A Health Ethnology Perspective*, https://doi.org/10.1007/978-3-658-42348-3_1

of replacing classical health literacy research, with its orientation towards basic socio-epidemiological arguments, with a health ethnology perspective, but it is about claiming a systematic complementarity, which becomes particularly virulent when it is a matter of establishing interventions for health promotion or prevention.

In the last decade, the amount of research literature on health literacy has exploded. In German-speaking countries, large-scale surveys have been conducted documenting the (poor) health literacy levels of the population in Germany, Austria, and Switzerland. For Switzerland, the results of a Switzerland-wide survey from 2015 state that more than half of the population has problematic (45%) or even insufficient (9%) health literacy (Schweizerische Akademie der Medizinischen Wissenschaften 2015). Similar figures are provided by the European Health Literacy Survey led by Jürgen Pelikan, which puts the group of people with problematic health literacy in Austria at 38.2% and the group of people with insufficient health literacy at 18.2%. The figures for Germany are similar (although here only data from North Rhine-Westphalia were initially collected): here 33.3% were found to have problematic health literacy and 12.4% to have inadequate health literacy (Pelikan et al. 2012a). Analogous figures are provided by more recent surveys in the environment of Bielefeld University as well: Eva-Maria Berens et al. show that more than half of the population do not have adequate health literacy, identifying a clear age gradient: the younger, the higher the health literacy on average (Berens et al. 2016; Schaeffer et al. 2016).

Overall, these quantitative studies for highly industrialised societies (with a few exceptions such as the Netherlands) identify about half of the adult population as deficient in terms of individual health literacy.

The implementation of such comprehensive population-based health literacy studies is a comparatively recent phenomenon and is related to large literacy studies that are designed to measure the literacy skills of the adult population and are complementary to the famous PISA studies. As the WHO, for example, prominently stated in its Nairobi Declaration, the first sentence under the heading of health literacy is: "Basic literacy is an essential building block for development and health promotion" (WHO 2009). The direct transfer of literacy to the health sector is momentous, because here a considerable need for (health policy) action can be claimed to strengthen the health literacy of the respective populations; this direct transfer can be traced not only in Germany or other industrialised nations, but meanwhile also in countries of the global South (cf. for example Haghdoost et al. 2015). Although the term health literacy was already used in Anglo-American health care research in the 1970s and was restricted to the health care actions of patients, *the current, now global health literacy discourse in 2000 is, in a sense, starting from scratch and exerting a noticeable influence on health policy concepts*

(WHO Europe 2013; Sørensen 2016, in press; van der Heide et al. 2019; Trezona et al. 2019). In Germany, the recent proclamation of a National Action Plan on Health Literacy, sponsored by the AOK and Doris Schaeffer, Klaus Hurrelmann and Ullrich Bauer, who are all relevantly known in public health, signals the highest level of public attention and policy relevance to date (Schaeffer et al. 2018). However, this enormously broad impact of health literacy research had a longer run-up.

In 2000, Don Nutbeam published a text on the subject and the concept of health literacy that has become a modern classic and is still constantly cited today. Since Nutbeam published his text, health literacy has been understood as the primarily cognitive ability of the individual to *make health-promoting decisions in everyday life*. To this end, a person should have the skills to search for and find, assess and apply health information (Sørensen et al. 2012a). In this context, Nutbeam distinguished three different health literacy levels, ranging from functional to interactive to critical, which according to Nutbeam are directly dependent on the literacy and numeracy level, that is, in a narrower sense, on the available written language and mathematical skills (Nutbeam 2000, 2008). The basic idea here, widely accepted into contemporary health literacy research, is that, according to Nutbeam, *literacy levels and health literacy levels can be analogized.* "The different levels [of health literacy; author's note.] are distinguished by the higher levels of knowledge and skills that progressively support greater autonomy and personal empowerment in health-related decision-making, as well as engagement with a wider range of health knowledge that extends from personal health management to the social determinants of health. These skills can be developed both through formal health education and other less formal exposure to health knowledge and practices" (Nutbeam 2009, p. 304).

With this approach, which has been decisively pursued and advanced by Don Nutbeam (cf. Nutbeam 1998, 2000, 2009) and Ilona Kickbusch (cf. Kickbusch 2001, 2002; WHO Europe 2013), health literacy – in German-language publications, especially in Switzerland synonymous with the term health competencies (Kickbusch and Hartung 2014, pp. 95–100) – is taken out of the narrow corset of immediate care actions and related to everyday health actions in the social spaces and lifeworlds of social actors. Health literacy then no longer exclusively denotes the orientation towards increasingly complex medical and nursing care systems, but also includes aspects of preventive action and the orientation towards and practice of health promotion – i.e., elements of everyday life outside of care activities are also included in the health literacy concept.

This successive expansion of the subject matter has not been without consequences for the underlying definitions and conceptual models of health literacy. One of the most important definitions developed in recent years is part of a very comprehensive model of health literacy, originated from the HLS-EU project (Health Literacy Survey of the European Union; Pelikan et al. 2012b) and was developed primarily by Kristine Sørensen. According to Sørensen, health literacy is "linked to literacy and entails people's knowledge, motivation and competences to access, understand, appraise, and apply health information in order to make judgments and take decisions in everyday life concerning healthcare, disease prevention and health promotion to maintain or improve quality of life during the life course" (Sørensen et al. 2012a, p. 3).

However, the expansion and extension of the health literacy concept does *not represent a radical new beginning for health literacy research,* because the majority of research is still conducted in a medicine-oriented manner and still refers to a narrow, care-related concept of health literacy. "The large majority of empirical HL research has used the Rapid Estimate of Adult Literacy in Medicine (REALM) and the Test of Functional Health Literacy in Adults (TOFHLA), or some variant of these tools [. . .]. The REALM is a word pronunciation test that uses medical words, an extremely narrow lens through [. . .]. Alternatively, the full TOFHLA includes reading, numeracy, and document literacy, and the modified cloze approach to ensure that the TOFHLA tests a person's understanding" (Nguyen et al. 2017, p. 190).

Operationalizations of person-related health literacy that, like REALM or TOFHLA, establish a direct link between individual written language skills and health literacy are rightly criticised as being far too narrow for a more comprehensive understanding of health literacy (see, among others, Nutbeam 2009, p. 304; O Neill et al. 2014, p. 2). However, they have long become standard practice in care and rehabilitation settings.[1] It is clear, however, that an expanded understanding of health literacy, which aims to take account of life-world contexts and (routinised) decision-making situations, must also be accompanied by survey methods other than word recognition tests or tasks to determine core mathematical skills. First, because even experts in medical health literacy research concede that the test fairness of care-oriented standard test procedures is limited, for example because ethnic minorities or people whose written language skills are limited only in the language of the majority society are systematically impaired and disadvantaged in

[1] In a short but all the more heretical statement that is worth reading, Vanessa Kronzer asks whether the time needed first to explain the questionnaire to patients and then to determine the health literacy level could not be more usefully spent on explaining things to patients calmly and talking to them: Kronzer (2016).

these tests (Nguyen et al. 2015, 2017; cf. also Nielsen-Bohlman et al. 2004a; Kiechle et al. 2015). Second, because the direct link between competencies based on written language in the narrower sense and health decisions relevant to everyday life and health-related behavioural routines remains a matter of speculation.

The more comprehensive models and their health literacy instruments, such as the health literacy scale used in the European Health Literacy Survey, comprise a total of 47 items and *cover the three areas of health care provision, prevention and health promotion in equal measure.* This is also intended to capture health-relevant life-world dimensions (Pelikan et al. 2012b). These self-report measures of health literacy primarily map attitudinal patterns of individuals, which conceptually say as little about *everyday health-related practices* as do the health literacy measures used in medical care. It is true that stable correlations can repeatedly be found between attitudinal measures of health literacy and health-related outcomes such as the use of preventive health services. But even in the more complex measurements, the *question* remains *open as to what exactly the relationship between attitudes is, general action resources (such as education, personality traits such as self-confidence or generalised resistance resources) and health-related everyday actions, including health-promoting decisions.*

This fundamentally complex issue, however, proves to be far too large to be dealt with within a single research project and should rather be part of an overarching research network. In the last 10 years, health literacy research has not only grown extremely quantitatively through the implementation of surveys more or less worldwide – with a simultaneous continuous dominance of the publication rate in the Anglo-American area -, but it has also become much more diverse. This diversification has occurred both conceptually and in terms of the target group specificity of health literacy. On the basis of these two differentiating developments, feasible qualitative research projects can be carried out that are somewhat narrower in their research questions. In the *ELMi* and *ELiS* projects presented in this book, which are part of the *overarching Health Literacy in Childhood and Adolescence project network,* we focus on three aspects in particular: on the one hand, an *age restriction of the target group (ELMi project) or specific family constellations (ELiS),* on the other hand, membership of an *ethnic minority,* and finally, the *connection between general action and health literacy.* In doing so, we pursue a micro-sociological, health-ethnological perspective that narrows down the research object of health literacy in several respects in order to gain more precise insights into the contexts of application and opportunity structures of health literacy at the level of the everyday behaviour of adolescents and families with children. In the following, the scope of our study will be narrowed down more systematically to children, adolescents and families (I) as well as to migrants (II).

(I) Children and adolescents have come late to the fore as a target group in health literacy research. Until well into the 2000s, complaints about research desiderata on health literacy among children and adolescents were the norm (Zamora et al. 2015). Early texts on children's and adolescents' health literacy largely remained within the framework of the care-oriented paradigm. In 2008, for example, Jennifer Manganello mapped out a framework and an agenda for research on adolescent health literacy, justifying the need for such an agenda in terms of rising rates of chronic disease among adolescents and poor literacy skills (Manganello 2008). Other publications have been devoted to adolescents in special risk settings, showing that a quarter to a third of adolescents living in borstals/institutions have limited health literacy skills in terms of responding to the REALM test (Trout et al. 2014). Only recently has work emerged that points to the particularities of model development and conceptualization of health literacy in children and adolescents and that argues for participatory approaches in health literacy research (see, among others, Bond and Rawlings 2019; Bröder and Carvalho 2019; Zamora et al. 2015; Broeder et al. 2017). Furthermore, more systematic reviews analysing concepts and models as well as measurement tools of health literacy in children and adolescents have emerged in recent years (Bröder et al. 2017; Okan et al. 2017b; Orkan et al. 2018) – (a detailed account of the state of research is provided below). With a view to health competencies in childhood and adolescence, which in an overall biographical perspective can (on average) be characterised as particularly healthy life phases (cf. for example Richter 2005), the focus is directed away from the provision of care towards the subject areas of disease prevention and health promotion. This is because health-related life course research assumes, for example, that behavioural routines, eating and exercise habits and fundamental attitude patterns and lifestyle orientations acquired in youth are decisive for the entire further course of life (cf. e.g., Telama et al. 1997; Richter 2005; Davey Smith 2008; Degenhardt et al. 2013; Levin-Zamir et al. 2017, pp. 134–135).

A second major continuous line with regard to general health literacy research in recent years is the evidence that socially underprivileged and disadvantaged groups generally have less health literacy – here considered as a hinge point for explaining unequal health outcomes – than middle-class or upper-class people (Quenzel et al. 2015; Pelikan et al. 2012b; Schweizerische Akademie der Medizinischen Wissenschaften 2015; Schweizerische Eidgenossenschaft 2016). This is generally assumed to be directly related to educational success and educational performance, which also correlates with social origin or social status – and in Germany this correlation is particularly clear in an international comparison. However, more complex studies show that economic situation and educational status – which in childhood and adolescence can only be represented to a limited extent on the basis of school attendance and school grades – each have an independent effect in explaining different health literacy levels (Pelikan et al. 2012a).

In addition to the health literacy research's turn towards adolescents being rather hesitant so far, a second target group is surprisingly little present, or has been excluded from the analyses by the specifically individualistic or individualising operationalization of health literacy: Families with young children. When it comes to the health literacy of children, parents or other guardians can hardly be left out, because – with the exceptions of institutionalised day-care and school breakfasts or nutrition-conscious school canteens – almost *the entire health behavior is mediated by the parents.* Consequently, parents are also blamed if, for example, specific groups of parents go less frequently to preventive check-ups with their children (Sahrai 2010b) or have lower rates of club sport. *In this context, the family, as the primary mediator of children's health competencies, should be considered above all as a provider of resources in the socialisation process* (Schnabel 2001a). Peter-Ernst Schnabel was one of the few to point out that health promotion should start with intact families, and the same can be said for the teaching of health literacy. This is where a supra-individual concept of *family health literacy* could lead further, which will be presented and discussed in the course of the third chapter and whose conceptualization we want to advance with our research (ELiS) (cf. Chap. 8).

(II) Migrants with and without their own migration history or members of ethnic minorities are named as a further group who are said to have limited health competences, irrespective of their economic resources for action and their available educational resources. The question of health competences of migrants becomes particularly relevant and explosive in the context of the social inclusion of refugees (Wångdahl et al. 2015). The overall difficulty here is that the available qualitative and quantitative approaches can hardly reflect the available resources for action of ethnic minorities. To a certain extent, the health outcomes of members of ethnic minorities oscillate back and forth between more positive effects on average compared to autochthones – which are usually associated with the so-called Healthy Migrant Effect (Sahrai 2009) or the Salmon Bias (Turra and Elo 2009) – and worse outcomes on average (RKI 2008). However, it is noteworthy – and we will return to this in more detail later in Chap. 3 – that children and adolescents from ethnic minorities are largely attributed negatively in the context of health behaviour (e.g. increased prevalence rates of obesity, poorer dental health, lower kindergarten attendance rates, lower attendance of U8 and U9 screening examinations; cf. on this Sahrai 2010c). These findings are often associated with an indictment of specific migrant parenting styles and parents are accused of not assimilating sensibly to mainstream society and its values and norms.

In quantitative measurement, the disadvantage of ethnic minorities in testing is acknowledged by renowned representatives themselves (Nguyen et al. 2017). But the limited test fairness so far only leads to the plea to use even more complex quantitative measurement methods (abandoning classical test theory in favour of item response theory or Rasch modelling), which cannot do justice to the possible, even if not necessarily existing or relevant, cultural differences of members of ethnic minorities (Nguyen et al. 2017). However, attitudinal measures with regard to health literacy, such as the European Health Literacy Scale, also contain possible biases if literacy and language levels are not sufficient for understanding the sometimes complex questions, or if there are different underlying understandings of health and illness which are made invisible by the questions.[2] In this respect, full test fairness cannot be assumed for attitude measurements in the sense of indirect measurement of health competencies. In this sense, the Israeli-American sociologist and health scientist Diane Levin-Zamir, who has long been established in health literacy research, also pleads: “More research should be carried out to explore the impact of culture on health decision making and health behaviors” (Levin-Zamir et al. 2017, p. 141).

From our perspective, it is precisely here that an ethnological approach can make a significant contribution to exploring health literacy among ethnic minorities. In doing so, we take very seriously positions that emphasise the lifeworld embedding of health. Faltermeier et al. wrote already more than 20 years ago that “health [. . .] is thus a topic [that] cannot be talked about in isolation from other aspects of lifestyle; therefore, health beliefs must be considered in their biographical and social context” (Faltermaier et al. 1998a, p. 323). Analogous considerations obviously apply to health literacy research. However, the ethnological perspective adopted here is once again particularly distinguished by the fact that action-guiding beliefs and resulting practices that may deviate from common notions of normality are examined with considerably lessened normative standards in place (on this, see the instructive text by Hehlmann et al. 2018). They are thus (Levin-Zamir et al. 2017) not a priori constructed as deficient. Rather, the epistemological goal is to understand these practices and underlying logics of action from their context and to recognise them as equally legitimate and inherently logical systems of meaning-making. So far, such a perspective has hardly been applied in health literacy research. This is explained in

[2] A positive development in this respect is that the European Health Literacy Scale has now been translated into many languages – in addition to the seven different European languages of the countries participating in the survey, e.g. Persian/Dari; cf. e.g. Harsch et al. 2021; Duong et al. (2017).

part by its proximity to health education, which is strongly tied to normative, expert-defined assumptions through the transmission of knowledge about health-promoting behaviours to improve the health of its target groups.[3] Similarly, as explained earlier, the discourse is still strongly committed to application in clinical settings. There, health literacy screenings primarily aim to identify those patients who, due to their low health literacy, require special care by medical staff.

An ethnological perspective on health literacy and health action, especially among minorities, distances itself from prior normative assumptions and the assumption that in the context of health literacy there is a right and a wrong or an "appropriate" or "insufficient/problematic" level of health literacy. Instead, the aim is to use a methodology that is close to everyday life and oriented towards the lifeworld of those being studied to work out which competences for maintaining health and caring for health are present among members of different cultural groups – even if these do not appear in the conventional questionnaire measurements or are devalued (Nguyen et al. 2017).

In addition to a perspective oriented towards difference rather than deficit, the embedding of health literacy in everyday life also plays an important role. The fact that 'objective' explanatory models developed by experts are not exclusively – and probably not even primarily – decisive for health and illness is shown, for example, in research on subjective health perceptions (cf. e.g., Faltermaier et al. 1998a; Flick 1998; Becker 2006; Eichler 2008; Huber et al. 2011). The shift in focus in health literacy research away from clinical-medical settings of health care towards studies close to everyday life is by no means new and is flanked in health policy terms by the WHO: "Health literacy initiatives work best when they customize approaches based on understanding the diversity of how individuals and communities approach health" (WHO Europe 2013, p. 23) and further "initiatives to build health literacy are best grounded in settings of everyday life" (ibid., p. 90). In our view, a health anthropological foundation as a primary research strategy offers the best access to comprehending the perspectives of those studied and thus make visible the inherent logic of the respective health action. Particularly in the context of programmatic WHO statements, we are of the opinion that a health ethnology approach can be seen as the royal road to implementing a salutogenetic perspective (Antonovsky 1987); *firstly,* because the naming of individual action resources, in contrast to deficiencies and deficits, can best be done through qualitative procedures of

[3] Faltermaier et al. (1998c), for example, distinguish a lay understanding of health from an expert understanding of health, a distinction that is problematic from the point of view represented here.

understanding and reconstructing meaning, and *secondly,* Antonovsky's health focus works on the same universal assumption of competence and recognition of the subjectivity of people as does the health ethnology understanding of actions.

The *research desideratum* formulated above as to *how attitudinal patterns and general action resources* are *related to health-related everyday actions and health literacy* can thus also be maintained with regard to the more specific target group of adolescents and families with young children on the one hand, while taking into account social disadvantage and the inclusion of cultural heterogeneities in national societies on the other. In our opinion, it can therefore be said that especially with regard to migrant youths and families, sensitive research gaps must be admitted existing within health literacy research, which cannot be adequately closed without further ado using the research approaches available to date.

For the micro-sociological-ethnic health perspective favoured here and, in our projects, all limiting contextual conditions have thus been named in order to specify the general research question in such a way that, from our point of view, it can be meaningfully addressed within the methodological approach we have chosen. *We are interested in empirical research on the interplay between general action competences and health competences among young people with a migration background and families with a migration background in everyday situations embedded in the life world.*

The fact that such research could be financed by third-party funds is a great rarity in Germany, but also in Switzerland. We were fortunate to be part of a research network for the study of health literacy in children and adolescents led by Ullrich Bauer, Orkan Okan and Paulo Pinheiro, and based at the Universities of Bielefeld, Paderborn, Duisburg-Essen, the Robert Koch Institute and the Freiburg University of Education (funded by the BMBF, funding code: 01EL1824E; duration 01.04.2015–31.03.2018). The Swiss subproject was financed by internal funds of the University of Teacher Education of the University of Applied Sciences and Arts Northwestern Switzerland. Without going deeply into the details of this research network (see Fig. 1.1 for an overview and the network homepage www.hlca-consortium.de for more details), we would like to briefly introduce the network in this introduction.

The primary objective of the overall collaborative project was to gain basic knowledge about health literacy, mental health literacy and eHealth literacy among children and adolescents.

In three work blocks (AB), health literacy was explored in three subprojects, namely basic research on health literacy (AB1), research on mental health literacy (AB2) and eHealth literacy (AB3). The focus of the overall collaborative was to assess the existing research on health literacy in children and young people, to

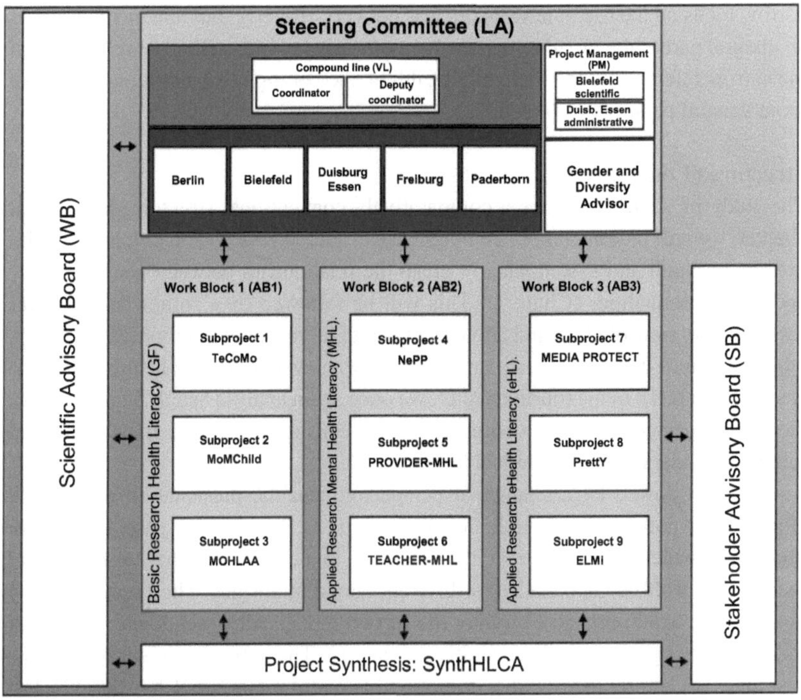

Fig. 1.1 HLCA research network

develop age-specific explanatory models, and to use this as a basis for designing evidence-based interventions (Zamora et al. 2015). In addition to children and adolescents, adults who work with adolescents, such as teachers, social workers or day-care assistants, were also the focus of the research activities of the network. The aim of the HLCA project network is to develop and provide measures for prevention and health promotion.

This book presents the results of the two research projects “ELMi – E-health literacy and minority health. An ethnographic study on the health-related use of new media among disadvantaged young people with a Turkish and Afghan migration background” and “ELiS – Health Literacy of migrants in Switzerland. An ethnological approach”, which was directly associated with the HLCA research network and located at the University of Teacher Education of the University of Applied Sciences and Arts Northwestern Switzerland under the direction of Diana Sahrai. In the course of the two projects ELMi and ELiS, it became increasingly clear that a narrow focus on the use of new media was not very effective, but that media use was an integral part of the broader management of everyday life, so that we reformulated the narrow reference to the topic of e-health literacy or digital health literacy under a more general perspective of action.

Structure of the Book

The study presented here has a comparatively conventional structure. In the next chapter, we will present a more comprehensive state of research on empirical health literacy research and systematically grasp the relationship between health literacy and health inequalities (Chap. 2). This will be followed by a somewhat narrower research overview of child and adolescent health literacy and family health literacy, which becomes directly relevant and virulent whenever children's health literacy is at stake (Chap. 3). In the fourth chapter, we once again analyse health literacy from a theoretical perspective and identify what we consider to be the most important research desiderata and theoretical bottlenecks.

This is followed by a change of perspective and the presentation of a health ethnological approach to health literacy (Chap. 5). Next, three case studies are presented, which are located at the interface to health inequality research and reconstruct health competencies of different ethnic minorities. The first case study analyses the health-related everyday life of two female adolescents with a Turkish migration background (third generation; Chap. 6). The second case study explores two male Afghan refugees with a migration history of their own (Chap. 7). The last case study refers to Latin American families with young children from Switzerland (Chap. 8). In the ninth and final chapter, the performance of a health anthropology-inspired approach and some overarching and central results are then presented once again, and an overarching conclusion is formulated (Chap. 9).

Part I

State of Research and the Need for a Health Ethnology Perspective

Health Literacy in the Context of Health Inequalities: A Framing and a Research Review

2

Abstract

In this chapter, we provide a general overview of the current state of health literacy research. In doing so, we take the liberty of proceeding more selectively and more broadly than is now the case with the systematic literature reviews based on the PRISMA standard that are customary in professional journals. On the one hand, because the subject area of health literacy is presented much more comprehensively than in a methodologically meaningful approach of a meta-analysis, which usually involves a compilation of the efficacy of specific active substances or interventions.

> What I hear far too rarely and far too little in discussions about health literacy – or more generally – about the chances of health promotion strategies, is that in almost all European countries poverty and social inequality are increasing faster or more than the best health promotion policies and primary prevention can compensate for. [. . .] Thus, the most important prerequisites for health literacy are consistently violated, and even if we cannot change this, we must say so. (Rosenbrock 2015b, p. 1)

In this chapter, we provide a general overview of the current state of health literacy research. In doing so, we take the liberty of proceeding more selectively and, at the same time, more broadly than is now the case with the systematic literature reviews based on the PRISMA standard that are customary in professional journals. On the one hand, because the subject area of health literacy is presented much more comprehensively than is the case with the methodologically meaningful meta-analysis approach, which usually involves a compilation of the efficacy of specific chemical agents or interventions. Rather, for our purposes, a more systematic treatment of the relationship between general health inequalities on the one hand and the role of health literacy on the other is relevant. In this respect, the framing is

U. H. Bittlingmayer et al., *Health Literacy From A Health Ethnology Perspective*, https://doi.org/10.1007/978-3-658-42348-3_2

broader in this body of research. The selection of literature used remains necessarily selective simply because we are unable to represent the entire international empirical state of knowledge here – because that would also mean discussing in more detail the current results of health literacy studies from Taiwan, Mongolia, Brazil, Australia, Kenya or Nigeria, for example – nor can we follow the health literacy concepts in all their small-scale differentiations – such as food literacy or diabetes literacy; nor are we in a position to conclusively discuss all the available measurement instruments. In this respect, this chapter does not aim to present an all-encompassing overview of health literacy research, but rather, more modestly, to formulate a research overview of the state of health literacy research, with a particular focus on health inequalities, as we see it.

In the last 10–15 years, a catching-up discourse on health inequalities has begun in the German-speaking world, which has been established for at least a decade longer in the Anglo-American world (cf. among others Black and Whitehead 1992; Blaxter 1983; Wilkinson 1996; Wilkinson and Marmot 2003). Via social epidemiological pioneers such as Andreas Mielck, Uwe Helmert or Thomas Elkeles, the realisation has gradually gained acceptance in Germany, Austria and Switzerland that scandalous health inequalities exist in these very rich countries with regard to the dependence of (multi-)morbidity and mortality on socio-demographic characteristics as well as healthcare inequalities (cf. Elkeles and Mielck 1997; Mielck 2000; Helmert 2003; Jungbauer-Gans and Kriwy 2004; Mielck 2005; Richter and Hurrelmann 2006a; Bauer et al. 2008; Lampert 2016; for the German discussion on health inequalities see Tiesmeyer et al. 2008; Bauer and Büscher 2008; Slotala 2011; Simon 2016). Even if the evidence is not entirely clear, it can be assumed that health inequalities have at least remained stable over the last 15 years. The life expectancy gap, the strongest indicator in terms of inequalities, was just under 9 years between the poor and wealthy population for men – according to data from the Socio-Economic Panel (SOEP) from 2001 to 2004 (Lauterbach et al. 2006). With Thomas Lampert et al. it is 10.8 based on an evaluation of SOEP data between 1995 and 2005 (Lampert et al. 2007). In a more recent WZB study, the life expectancy difference between rich and poor men is also just under 11 years (Habich 2013). The majority of studies assume a limited increase in health inequalities, such as those by Lars Kroll or Katharina Rathmann, who, however, link health inequalities more strongly to comparative international welfare state research (Kroll 2010; Rathmann 2015). Moreover, Habich's study puts the life expectancy gap for women at 8 years, which would be a reduction of almost 1 year compared to Lauterbach's study, which puts it at 8.9 years. The state of research on the dynamics of health inequalities must therefore be described as unclear and inconsistent overall in the German-speaking world; that there are massive health inequalities in Germany, Austria and Switzerland can, however, already be determined as a consensus reached as early as 2006 (Richter and Hurrelmann 2006b) and has no longer been seriously disputed to this day. As Thomas Lampert, one of the leading experts on health inequality research from the Robert Koch Institute, sums it up with regard to the development dynamics: "The present results, which were obtained primarily on the basis of the health surveys of the Robert Koch Institute and the SOEP, indicate that the observed health inequality has proven to be extremely stable over time and has even increased in part". (Lampert 2016, p. 131).

Now that the existence of health inequalities is no longer disputed, there are increasing efforts to determine the explanatory and causal factors. The following list is not intended to suggest completeness, but to hint at the great variety of different approaches: In recent years, a great variety of different explanatory approaches have been developed that can be associated with health inequalities. On the one hand, general models have been constructed to guide complex (multivariate) statistical testing (Mielck 2000, 2005; Klocke and Lipsmeier 2008; Klocke 2006) (see Fig. 2.1).

Studies have also been conducted to outline the contribution of individual factors such as individual or aggregate social capital (Kawachi et al. 1997; Siegrist et al. 2006; Hartung 2014), the influence of regional differences (when controlling for socio-demographic characteristics) (Bittlingmayer et al. 2009; Hoffmann et al.

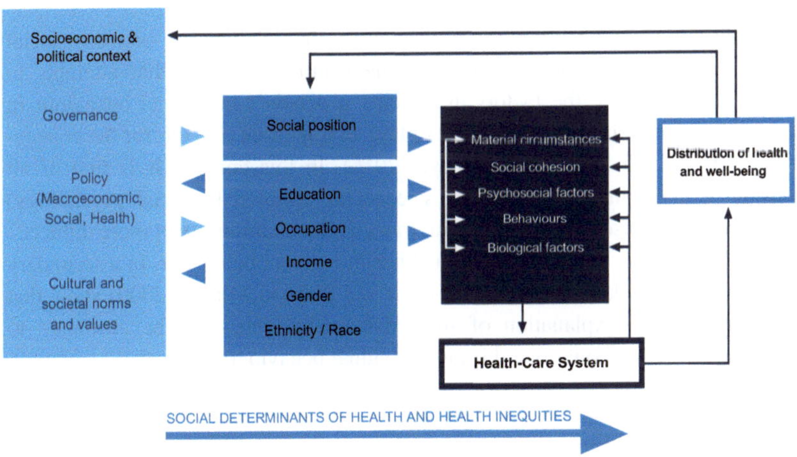

Fig. 2.1 Conceptual framework of the WHO Commission "Social Determinants of Health following Solar & Irwin 2007 and the Final Report of the WHO 2008." (Quoted from Lampert 2016, p. 130)

2014; Sundmacher 2016) or more general income inequalities (Wilkinson and Marmot 2003; Wilkinson 2005; Wilkinson and Pickett 2010). In a more recent paper, Kate Pickett and Richard Wilkinson argue that income inequalities exert a real causal effect on a range of unequal health outcomes (Pickett and Wilkinson 2015). Finally, the more fundamental link between broader social inequalities and health inequalities is also coming into focus (see e.g., Hradil 2006; Jungbauer-Gans and Gross 2006; Marmot and Wilkinson 2006; Vester 2009; Kroll 2010; Bittlingmayer 2016). Most studies attempted to determine the concrete extent of health inequalities, especially by focusing on specific target groups such as the poverty population (or, similarly, the unemployed, Hartz IV – welfare/dole – recipients), groups of ethnic minorities or people with a migration background or refugee experience (Razum 2006; Jungbauer-Gans and Gross 2006; Marmot and Wilkinson 2006; Vester 2009; Kroll 2010; Bittlingmayer 2016; Razum 2006; RKI 2008; Sahrai 2009) or women (Kolip 2000; Kuhlmann and Kolip 2008; Babitsch 2009; Kuhlmann 2016), children and adolescents (Richter 2005; Richter et al. 2008; Kolip et al. 2013; Rathmann 2015) or elderly people (Jahrbuch Kritische Medizin und Gesundheitswissenschaften 2013). With regard to the object dimensions of migration, ethnicity, gender, youth or age, it quickly becomes clear that health inequalities cannot be operationalized exclusively as social-epidemiological distribution measures, because social symbolism, devaluations and disregard play an important role in these areas (this is made very clear in Kolip 2000) – we will return to this in detail in Chap. 4 below.[1]

Finally, in the context of questions about the relationship between social determinants, health literacy and health inequalities, research that attempts to empirically determine the factors influencing a person's individual behaviour in relation to overarching social structures plays an important role (cf. for the conceptual level Sperlich 2016; Bittlingmayer 2016). In this context, it is first of all considered undisputed within social science (as opposed to social psychology) health inequality research that structural framework conditions exert more influence on health inequality than does individual health-relevant behaviour. In a secondary analysis of SOEP data, Johannes Giesecke and Stephan Müters (2009) show that two thirds of the explanation of subjective health status can be attributed to structural causes and only one third to individual behavioural aspects.

[1] The literature on the state of research reported here does not claim to be exhaustive. It would certainly be possible to draw on considerably more relevant studies. Nevertheless, the works cited provide a reasonable impression of the subject areas and basic motives of health inequality research.

Nevertheless, from the *analysis of social practices* perspective adopted here, the separation between social structures and individual behaviour can only be an *analytical* one, as the two interact inseparably in the everyday practices of real subjects. This is evident in the debate about so-called Healthy Lifestyles, often regarded as a guarantee for maximising a person's healthy life years. In a study dealing with health inequalities, William C. Cockerham et al. show on the basis of Russian data that social class, age, gender, milieu, and living conditions have the power of determining health-related individual behaviours in one direction or the other: "The analysis shows that variables in each of the categories were associated with particular health lifestyle practices and self-rated health." (Cockerham et al. 2006, p. 195).

Such analyses also exist for Germany: "The present empirical analysis of the relationship between class affiliation and three important characteristics of individual health behaviour (smoking, obesity, sporting activity) can sustainably confirm that socio-structural conditions (material situation, educational resources and occupational position) in Germany continue to shape individual health behaviour to a great degree". (Helmert and Schorb 2006, p. 137). Health-promoting individual decisions, which are made in the lifeworlds of social actors and which, taken together, constitute a health-promoting lifestyle, are neither the product of a conscious decision, nor can individual actions simply be subtracted from social structures. Rather, individual actions – and this also applies to any competencies – are indissolubly permeated by social structural frameworks and opportunity structures (Sperlich and Mielck 2003; Nideröst 2007; Vester 2009), as well as by social relations of recognition and power (Foucault 1983; Kühn 1993; Brunnett 2009).

Even if the importance of societal inequality structures for individual health in general and for health inequality relationships in particular is hardly in doubt, an increased popularity of behavioural approaches to dealing with such inequality relationships can be observed in recent years. This turn towards health behaviour is fuelled by role models staged in the mass media, such as the "sovereign subject as self-provider of his/her health" (Schmidt 2017, p. 158). After all, avoiding behaviours that are detrimental to health seems to be an attractive and implementable health policy strategy, at least to counter rising costs in the health sector or rising obesity rates (already in childhood and adolescence) and also to be considered successful in the context of smoking rates that have been declining for years. It is from this point of reconstruction and argumentation that the health literacy discourse and approach gains its particular relevance. For on the one hand, as will be shown, it provides a substantive explanatory perspective at the interface between structure and individual behaviour, especially for adolescents

(Paakkari et al. 2019a), and secondly, it is particularly amenable to the current neoliberal health policy line, which prioritises behavioural change (Schmidt 2008; Simon 2011; Schmidt 2017; cf. Lessenich 2013 on this, going beyond and across the health field), because structural inequalities can be transformed into individual skills deficits (Bauer 2019a). Moreover, health literacy is also associated with cost reductions across the health care sector: "Overall, the long-held promise of health literacy is that improved health literacy will produce improvements in health status – ideally at lower costs." (Pleasant et al. 2018, p. 2).

In any case, there is a large consensus in current public health research and practice that health literacy is a promising approach that can make inequality-generating differences in care provision, prevention or health promotion tangible in ways other than the socio-epidemiological presentation of significant correlations pointing to social inequalities, but also that health literacy is closely linked to the issue of health inequalities (a strong overview is provided by Mantwill et al. 2015). Furthermore, the concept increasingly serves as a promising starting point for prevention and health promotion. For example, the National Action Plan for Health Literacy in Germany was recently presented in Berlin, highlighting the importance of the health literacy concept for prevention and health promotion, in addition to its proximity to health policy (Schaeffer et al. 2018). Furthermore, the Center for Health Literacy was opened at Bielefeld University in 2019. Due to the proven association between low health literacy and various negative health outcomes such as lower self-rated health, more frequent use of health services and difficulties in interacting with health professionals, health policies based on population-wide health literacy strengthening are trusted to contribute significantly to health equity. In this sense, the WHO Shanghai Declaration was formulated in 2016 as a call on all relevant parties involved to strengthen health literacy (see Box 2.1).

Box 2.1: WHO Shanghai Declaration (Extract)

Health literacy empowers and drives equity

Health literacy empowers individual citizens and enables their engagement in collective health promotion action. A high health literacy of decision-makers and investors supports their commitment to health impact, co-benefits and effective action on the determinants of health. Health literacy is founded on inclusive and equitable access to quality education and life-long learning. It must be an integral part of the skills, and competencies developed over a lifetime, first and foremost through the school curriculum.

(continued)

Box 2.1 (continued)

We commit to

- recognize health literacy as a critical determinant of health and invest in its development;
- develop, implement and monitor intersectoral national and local strategies for strengthening health literacy in all populations and in all educational settings;
- increase citizens' control of their own health and its determinants, through harnessing the potential of digital technology;
- Ensure that consumer environments support healthy choices through pricing policies, transparent information and clear labelling.

2.1 Definitional Approaches to Health Literacy

Despite this large consensus on the importance of health literacy, consensus is nowhere near in sight when it comes to precisely defining health literacy; on the contrary, the debate on the correct definition of health literacy has been described as contested terrain (cf. e.g., Pleasant and McKinney 2011; Mackert et al. 2015; Pleasant et al. 2018). And despite the strong growth in research interest in health literacy, there is a great deal of ambiguity about the dimensions it includes. To date, there is no universally accepted definition of health literacy; rather, there are different approaches to describing the concept (Abel 2008; McCormack et al. 2010; Kickbusch 2009; Frisch et al. 2012; Wills 2009; Pleasant 2014). For example, in the words of one of the most renowned researchers* Diane Levin-Zamir, health literacy research continues to be described as a "work in progress" and a dynamic construct (Levin-Zamir et al. 2017, p. 133). Therefore, no gold standard has been established to date with regard to methodological issues and measurements of health literacy (Nguyen et al. 2017, p. 190). Currently, more than 150 different measurement methods for health literacy are said to exist (Orkan et al. 2018 an overview of existing health literacy instruments can be found at https://healthliteracy.bu.edu/). In view of the large number of health literacy operationalizations, we therefore only want to trace important developments in the definitional approaches to the concept of health literacy in a little more detail.

An early definition from the relevant journal *Das Gesundheitswesen* describes health literacy as "the degree to which individuals have the capacity to obtain, process, and understand basic health information and services needed to make appropriate health decisions" (Parker et al. 2003, p. 147). Health literacy is seen here as a set of individual skills in medical word recognition, text comprehension and numeracy that enable a person to acquire and use new information from the health context. This definition has been widely criticised as it conceptualises health literacy more or less exclusively as an individual-level construct (Berkman et al. 2010). This gives rise to the danger of locating low health literacy levels as a deficit on the part of the patient and in this way placing the responsibility for corrective actions in the case of low health literacy exclusively on the person (Bernhardt et al. 2005; Freedman et al. 2009).

The Shanghai Declaration attempts to counter this problem, for example, by making the health literacy of professionals a health system dimension in its own right (see Box 2.1 above; for non-individual health literacy perspectives, see (Dodson et al. 2015; Bruland et al. 2017), among others).

A modified version of Parker and colleagues' definition was proposed by Nancy Berkman's team at the Agency for Health Care Research and Quality: according to them, health literacy is "[t]he degree to which individuals can obtain, process, understand, and communicate about health-related information needed to make informed health decisions" (Berkman et al. 2010, p. 16). Oral communication is explicitly emphasised here as a critical component of health literacy. The reformulation of "have the capacity to" to "can" is intended to counter the criticism outlined above of understanding health literacy as an exclusively individual construct. The emphasis is to be placed on know-how that individuals can acquire, instead of speaking of a more or less primordial ability in the sense of cognitive dispositions. This is intended to lead to a more dynamic understanding of health literacy. Similar approaches, such as the one by David Baker (2006), understand health literacy as a variable construct depending on the medical problem in hand, the medical professional(s) in charge, and the health care system. In this conception, health literacy refers only to a specific treatment situation and may find a different expression in the same person under different conditions. A similar formulation emphasises the potential for change by defining health literacy as "the wide range of skills and competencies that people *develop* to seek out, comprehend, evaluate and use health information and concepts to make informed choices, reduce health risks and increase quality of life" (Zarcadoolas et al. 2005, pp. 196–197). An important aspect of this approach is the link between health literacy and quality of life. This dimension takes health literacy out of the care-related setting and connects it at least loosely with motives for everyday lifestyles. However, the extension to life-world dimensions of health literacy was already laid out earlier, but closely linked back to individual educational competencies and written language performance. Nutbeam's

(2000) influential proposal, already briefly touched upon in the introduction, conceptualises health literacy as a hierarchical construct and distinguishes three levels: (1) *functional/basal health literacy* as sufficient literacy skills to function in everyday situations, (2) *interactive/communicative health literacy* as a combination of literacy and social skills that enables information acquisition from different communication channels, and (3) *critical health literacy* as elaborate cognitive and social skills that enable critical analysis of health information and thus increased control over one's life. By clearly hierarchizing these three levels, both quantitative and qualitative assessment of health literacy become possible. In addition, this conception underlines the possibility of expanding competencies in the area of health literacy and the associated gain in autonomy (Tones 2002; Nutbeam 2009).

The close connection between educational competencies and health literacy at first appears to be extremely obvious, because a large number of empirical studies show a high correlation between formal education and health literacy in very different countries. For example, a Japanese representative study from 2006 found that people with low levels of formal education were more likely to have limited communicative and critical health literacy skills in the sense of Nutbeam (Furuya et al. 2013). In a recent representative study in Switzerland, it was shown that people with lower formal education have lower health literacy on average (Schweizerische Akademie der Medizinischen Wissenschaften 2015). Finally, the Robert Koch Institute also presented a representative study in 2013 that found the proportion of people with inadequate health literacy within the group of people with low formal education almost twice as high as the proportion found in the group of people with high formal education status (Jordan and Hoebel 2015). However, the close linkage between health literacy and formal education implied by Nutbeam's model is less self-evident than it seems at first glance (for a detailed discussion, see Bittlingmayer and Sahrai 2019). To use a somewhat polemical example, it is not mandatory for a person with a low level of schooling who uses tobacco on a daily basis to first obtain a high school diploma in order to arrive at the decision to quit smoking. We will return to this point in more detail in Chap. 4.

A definition which, going beyond formal educational qualifications, links health literacy to skills for promoting and maintaining health comes from the World Health Organization (WHO): "Health literacy represents the cognitive and social skills which determine the motivation and ability of individuals to gain access to, understand and use information in ways that promote and maintain good health" (WHO 1998, p. 10). This is the only definition that includes the aspect of motivation to maintain health. However, the formulation that health literacy is a prerequisite for the motivation to promote and maintain personal health is clumsy and demonstrably inaccurate (Powell et al. 2007).

The largest recent research project in the field of health literacy was the *European Health Literacy Survey (HLS-EU),* which involved research teams from eight European countries (Pelikan et al. 2012b). Based on a systematic review of definitions and concepts in the field of health literacy, the HLS-EU consortium defines health literacy very comprehensively as

> people's knowledge, motivation and competences to access, understand, appraise, and apply health information in order to make judgments and take decisions in everyday life concerning healthcare, disease prevention and health promotion to maintain or improve quality of life during the life course. (Sørensen et al. 2012a, p. 3)

This conceptual model relates health literacy to a person's health status or quality of life. It also relates health literacy to health care in the institutional sense, to disease prevention and to health promotion. It conceptualises health literacy as a multi-layered concept that goes well beyond mere medical word understanding (Pelikan et al. 2012b; Sørensen et al. 2012a). A similar definition comes from Switzerland:

> Health literacy is the ability to translate knowledge about the maintenance and recovery of physical, mental and social well-being into personal and collective decisions and actions in a way that has a positive impact on one's own health and the health of others, as well as on living and environmental conditions. (Netzwerk Bildung + Gesundheit Schweiz 2019)

As can be seen from the two extensive formulations, efforts are being made to combine the different definitions and to propose as uniform a solution as possible (Sørensen et al. 2012a). However, there is scepticism as to whether this is possible at all, as research contexts and objectives in the different application areas of health literacy are hardly comparable (e.g., Chinn 2011).

If, as in the variant of the European Health *Literacy* Survey, *health literacy* is *freed from the care-related corset* and a definition is chosen that *seeks to cover* the *areas of prevention and health promotion* in *addition* to informed action *in* care-relevant settings, then *the health literacy concept* is *necessarily associated with lifeworld action references, which brings the concept close to an everyday life sociology of health actions.* This conceptual closeness between day-to-day competencies, subjective relevance decisions and lifeworld practices on the one hand, and an expanded health literacy concept that is not reduced to health care actions is not, however, reflected – as will become clear in the following – in the attempts to operationalize health literacy.

2.2 Measurement or Recording of Health Literacy

As there is no single definition of health literacy to date, there are also widely varying approaches to measuring the construct (Mackert et al. 2015; Pleasant et al. 2018; Canadian Council on Learning 2007; Abel 2008).

Initially, literacy, and thus indirectly health literacy as well, were seen as a direct consequence of school education, which is why the number of years of education was chosen as an indicator (Berkman et al. 2010). However, as it soon became apparent that literacy skills correlate only to a limited extent with the length of education, schooling was discarded as a direct indicator of literacy. A strong focus on reading and writing and basal numerical skills long characterised the efforts to measure health literacy (Kutner et al. 2007).[2] Following several American literacy studies as well as the International Adult Literacy Survey (IALS) from 1994 to 1998 (Murray et al. 1998), items to measure health literacy were systematically collected and classified for the first time. This resulted in the Health Activities Literacy Scale (HALS) (Rudd et al. 2004). However, due to its length, the HALS was not suitable for examinations in a clinical-medical context, so shorter tests of written-language-based comprehension were devised in this area. The first test is the Rapid Estimate of Adult Literacy in Medicine (REALM) (Davis et al. 1993; Murphy et al. 1993). It involves 66 words from a medical context that the person being tested must read out aloud. Scoring is based on the number of words correctly read aloud and provides an assessment of reading skills by grade level. In addition, a version has been developed for adolescents, the REALM-Teen (Davis et al. 2006). The second instrument, used primarily in clinical settings, is the Test of Functional Health Literacy in Adults (TOFHLA) (Parker et al. 1995). It contains three text passages with 50 reading comprehension tasks and 17 items on numerical skills. There is also a short form, the S-TOFHLA (Baker et al. 1999), which contains only two text passages and four numeracy items. Both forms of the TOFHLA report three levels of deficient, borderline, and adequate health literacy by way of assessment. The reading comprehension tasks have been validated for use with adolescents (Chisolm and Buchanan 2007). In addition, the Brief Health Literacy Screen (BHLS) (Chew et al. 2004; Wallston et al. 2014), which contains only three items, and the Newest

[2] It should at least be mentioned in passing that the Social Literacy or New Literacy Studies approach (cf. Street 1984, 2003), which takes a different view of written language competencies than is common in the now dominant PISA competency tradition, has hardly been utilised in health literacy research to date; how fruitful such a perspective can be for health literacy research becomes clear in Papen (2005, 2008, 2009). More recent connections can be found in Samerski (2019), Pinheiro (2019), Bauer (2019a), Pinheiro et al. (2021).

Vital Sign (NVS) (Weiss et al. 2005), with six questions, are very brief indeed. These two tests are intended for use as screening instruments in medical settings and, according to Nutbeam (2009), measure "health-related literacy in clinical settings" (p. 304), which calls into question their use in contexts other than medical.

It is clear from the measurement methods presented that they all measure very narrowly defined skills that do not do justice to today's broad theoretical understanding of health literacy (Pleasant and McKinney 2011; Levin-Zamir et al. 2017). Also, most of them focus on measuring functional health literacy (critically, for example, Sørensen et al. 2012a). In an effort to capture health literacy as a multi-layered concept, the HLS-EU consortium developed the European Health-Literacy-Study-Questionnaire (HLS-EU-Q) for its study. It contains 47 questions that assess subjectively perceived difficulty in performing certain health-related tasks. On a scale of 0 to 50 points, four levels of health literacy are distinguished: inadequate, problematic, sufficient, and excellent, with the two lowest levels collectively referred to as "limited health literacy" (Pelikan et al. 2012a, b, 2019). An important difference to the other measurement instruments presented is that they are designed as self-report questionnaires. Thus, the measurement is subjective compared to the assessments by tests of functional health literacy, which are classified as objective (Sørensen et al. 2012a).[3] Here, too, an abridged version was developed that is intended to map the three dimensions of health literacy with 16 items (HLS-EU 16), although it is no longer able to distinguish between the three factors on the basis of factor analysis.

All instruments presented so far measure health literacy quantitatively and have mostly been developed in a clinical-medical setting. The aim of the measurements is to obtain an estimate of the existing skills of the person examined, usually patients, within the shortest possible time. This runs counter to the effort to adequately reflect the complexity of health literacy within the measurement instruments (Jordan et al. 2010). What is lacking to date are measurement methods that take into account the evolution of health literacy definitions toward more of a social science perspective. Josephine M. Mancuso rightly states in this regard:

> Many constraints exist to the assessment of health literacy. (...) Health literacy includes more than word recognition, reading comprehension, and numeracy. The existing measures and screenings do not fully grasp the concept of health literacy in terms of language, context, culture, communication, or technology. Thus, we do not

[3]We are very sceptical here as to whether the concept of objectivity in performance measurements is tenable from a scientific and epistemological point of view, but we do not wish to go into this aspect in any further detail here – see Chap. 4.

> yet possess a measure that takes into account the full set of skills and knowledge associated with health literacy. (Mancuso 2009, p. 87)

This statement identifies several criticisms of the instruments commonly used to measure health literacy:

- Many current conceptions of health literacy, and thus the measurement tools based on them, exhibit an individualistic and a cognitivist bias. They focus (too) strongly on literacy skills and notions of health action as rational and calculated decision-making (van der Vaart et al. 2011; Pleasant et al. 2018; Bittlingmayer and Sahrai 2019; Sørensen and Pleasant 2017; Pitt et al. 2019; Sentell et al. 2017).
- Existing tools are not sufficiently culturally sensitive. This point must also be considered in translations (Levin-Zamir et al. 2017; Nguyen et al. 2017).
- The context of a health-related *action* is not sufficiently taken into account. As mentioned several times, most instruments explicitly refer to clinical medical settings (Nguyen et al. 2015; Papen 2009, 2008; Samerski 2019; Pitt et al. 2019; Bauer 2019a).
- The potential of different technologies to support health communication is not used. The current test procedures are largely limited to paper-pencil questionnaires, although digital media in particular are said to have very great potential in the area of health literacy (Mancuso 2009; Pleasant et al. 2018).
- The communicative context in which (the application of) health literacy is mostly embedded is not taken into account enough. Whether a patient with little knowledge of the national language actually asks critical questions about his treatment plan during the two-minute visit by the chief physician is primarily determined by the social situation: The power asymmetry between doctor and patient, but also, for example, the trust in a person with more knowledge in the field related to health, significantly influence the patient's behaviour (Papen 2008, 2009; Bauer 2019a).
- Existing measurement tools are deficit-oriented due to their history of being developed as screening tools for inadequate health literacy. The primary goal is to identify insufficient competencies (Nguyen et al. 2015; Pleasant and Rikard 2013; Pleasant et al. 2018). A resource-oriented perspective that aims to make existing health-related competencies visible and usable has been neglected so far (Bittlingmayer and Sahrai 2019; Saboga-Nunes et al. 2019).

The more complex definitions of health literacy here presented, which are influential within the current discourse (Nutbeam 2009; Sørensen et al. 2012a; Bröder et al.

2017), have in common that they have taken the health literacy concept out of its original care-specific context and moved it conceptually closer to everyday action competencies and lifeworld embeddings. Thus, there has been a methodological shift outside of the clinical setting from the direct measurement of written language competencies to the indirect measurement of self-attributed health literacy skills.

2.3 The Relationship Between Health Literacy and Health Outcomes

As has already been explained in detail, the definition and, to a lesser extent, the recording of health literacy have been subject to some significant changes in recent years. As a result, the validity of studies that establish links between one variety of health literacy and health status is also limited to a certain extent. It is difficult to arrive at reliable comparable statements on the basis of the different definitions used (Mackert et al. 2015). Nevertheless, the available studies provide valuable clues as to how a possible link between social inequalities and health inequalities could be established. The findings presented in the following underline the importance attributed to health literacy in the context of health inequalities, personal responsibility and health-related prevention.

The improvement of health literacy is considered an important political and societal goal, as numerous studies have shown a connection between low health literacy and poorer health outcomes (cf. e.g., Berkman et al. 2004; DeWalt and Hink 2009). A review that considered studies from 1980 to 2003 was able to show that patients with low health literacy had on average 1.5 to 3 times as high a chance of showing a specific negative outcome as did patients with at least sufficient health literacy (DeWalt et al. 2004). Among other things, low health literacy is associated with poorer general health, greater use of health services and higher health care costs (Canadian Council on Learning 2007; Nielsen-Bohlman et al. 2004b; Statistics Canada and OECD 2005; Weiss 2005). According to findings of the Adult Literacy and Life Skills Survey (ALLS), there are associations between, among other things, low health literacy skills and low life satisfaction or health-related limitations in activities of daily living and social activities. Other studies show that low health literacy is consistently associated with higher prevalence of chronic diseases and lower coping skills (DeWalt et al. 2004; Rothman et al. 2009; Williams et al. 1995; Zarcadoolas et al. 2006; Sarkar et al. 2006). Other correlations exist between low health literacy and more frequent hospitalizations (Baker et al. 1997; Baker et al. 2002; Cimasi et al. 2013; Fleisher et al. 2014; SCHILLINGER et al.

2002), repeated and serious use of emergency services (Griffey et al. 2014; Mancuso and Rincon 2006), lower participation in preventive measures (Bennett et al. 2009; Cho et al. 2008), poorer understanding of package inserts and general health messages (Wolf et al. 2007), and poorer adherence to self-administered medication (Lin et al. 2014; Rothman et al. 2009; Weiss 1999; Zhang et al. 2014). Basically, at least for Germany, older people show lower health literacy (Berens et al. 2016). Moreover, there is a negative association between health literacy and mortality rates in older people (Baker et al. 2008; Bostock and Steptoe 2012; Sudore et al. 2006), as well as in patients in outpatient treatment after heart failure (Peterson et al. 2011). In an Australian cohort study, low health literacy was associated with high blood pressure, smoking, diabetes and physical inactivity, as well as depression (Appleton et al. 2015). Low health literacy is not only associated with factors of reduced physical health but can also be linked to poorer mental health (Lee et al. 2010). Negative psychological correlates of low health literacy include lower psychological well-being (Tokuda et al. 2009), low self-efficacy (Como 2014; Sarkar et al. 2006), lower perceived quality of life (Mancuso and Rincon 2006; Song et al. 2012), and increased depressive symptoms (Lincoln et al. 2006). Low health literacy is manifested by difficulties in filling out forms in medical contexts, in following medication prescriptions, and especially in doctor-patient interactions (SCHILLINGER et al. 2004; Seurer and Vogt 2013), for example, by not asking questions (Katz et al. 2007). To make matters worse, it has been shown that individuals with low health literacy feel shame for their low competencies in this regard (Chew et al. 2004; Mancuso 2009). This can lead to attempts to hide reading or vocabulary difficulties (Parikh et al. 1996). Other research has also shown that individuals with low health literacy are less likely to ask clarifying questions due to embarrassment or even fear, which can hinder accurate diagnosis of an individual's health problem (Vernon et al. 2007). In order to ensure access to health care and to increase equity in this context, a sensitive assessment of health literacy is therefore crucial. Now that the importance of health literacy for different health outcomes has become clear, the following section shows how health literacy is specifically distributed in relation to the population.

2.4 Distribution of Health Literacy in the Population

Low health literacy is – despite different paradigms in measurement and theoretical conceptualization – by no means a marginal phenomenon. According to several studies, there is a significant proportion of people with low health literacy even in

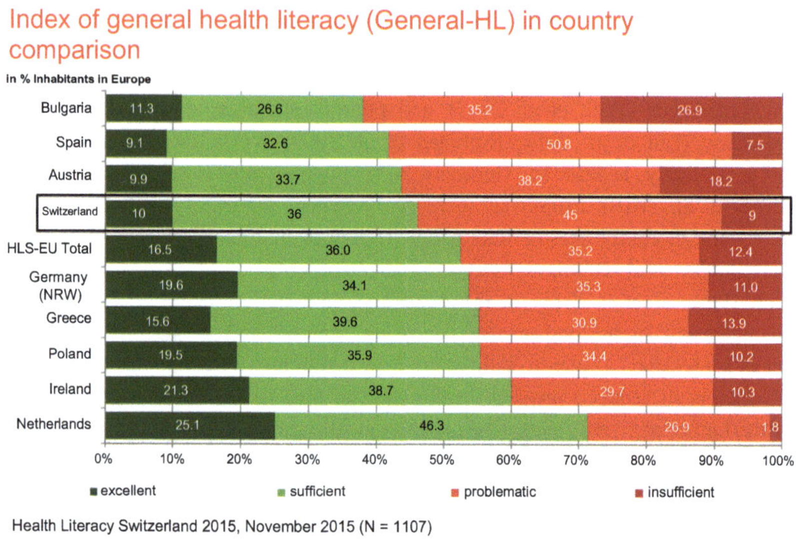

Fig. 2.2 Health literacy in European comparison, plus Switzerland

countries with high income levels. The Institute of Medicine, for example, in its somewhat overly optimistically titled report *Health Literacy: A Prescription to End Confusion,* concluded that more than 90 million adults in the United States lack the skills necessary to use the American healthcare system effectively (Nielsen-Bohlman et al. 2004b). The Adult Literacy and Life Skills Survey (ALLS) showed that in many high-income countries, less than half of the population achieves adequate health literacy levels (Soricone et al. 2007). Current figures on the prevalence of low or adequate health literacy in Europe are provided by the European Health Literacy Survey (HLS-EU), which was conducted between 2010 and 2012 (see Fig. 2.2).

Across all eight participating countries or regions, just under half of the population has limited health literacy. The highest rate of limited health literacy is found in Spain at 58.3 %, the lowest in the Netherlands at 28.7% (Pelikan et al. 2012b). The results for Germany (North Rhine-Westphalia) show that 45.9% of the population have limited health literacy (Pelikan et al. 2012b; Mensing 2012).

For Switzerland, a study is available according to which the German-speaking population of Switzerland has a very high level of health literacy: according to this study, 93.6% of the people examined have an adequate level of health literacy. The differences to the other two language regions are striking: in the French-speaking part of Switzerland, the proportion of people with an adequate level of health literacy is 83.2%, while in the Italian-speaking part of Switzerland it is 66.7%. Health literacy was measured here with the S-TOFHLA, which is why only functional health literacy in the narrow sense can be depicted (Connor et al. 2013). In addition, there is a study that uses the HLS-EU-47 instrument and provides comparative figures for Switzerland, showing that Switzerland is in the middle of the field among European countries (see Fig. 2.2).

Another large-scale representative survey for Germany delivers similarly alarming findings. In this study, too, for which Doris Schaeffer and Klaus Hurrelmann were responsible, less than half of the German population have sufficient health literacy on average, while the other half have limited health literacy (cf. Table 2.1). Health literacy was measured here as a self-report using the HLS-EU 47 instrument. The results are even worse than those of the European survey, in which Germany was only represented by participants from North Rhine-Westphalia.

After we have been able to clarify the problem dimension of lacking health literacy, measured with standardised instruments, in the following we have to ask more precisely about possible social determinants of low health literacy and the general connection with social and health inequalities.

2.5 Social Determinants of Health Literacy

Consistently, all the studies cited show correlations between health literacy and various sociodemographic variables. This inevitably raises questions about social and health inequalities in the healthcare system, which fall directly into the area of health policy (cf. explicitly WHO 2016; cf. as national examples, among others, Canadian Council on Learning 2008; The Scottish Government 2014; Schaeffer et al. 2019), but also point clearly beyond this, for example to the education system. Among other things, health literacy appears to decline the lower the level of education. In Canada, for example, the ALLS showed a positive correlation between the level of education and the health literacy score (Canadian Council on Learning 2007). This relationship was confirmed in the HLS-EU study, which also found that a lower health literacy level was associated with lower social class and income (Pelikan et al. 2012b).

As age increases, health literacy decreases (Australian Bureau of Statistics 2006; Rudd et al. 2007; Statistics Canada and OECD 2005; Berens et al. 2016). Age even amplifies disparities based on educational attainment (Canadian Council on

Table 2.1 Health literacy scores* stratified by age groups

		15–29		30–45		46–64		65–99	
		%	(n)	%	(n)	%	(n)	%	(n)
Limited	Inadequate	6.8	(25)	7.0	(34)	9.4	(58)	15.2	(70)
	Problematic	40.5	(152)	40.2	(197)	45.8	(283)	51.1	(236)
Not limited	Sufficient	42.5	(159)	44.3	(217)	37.1	(229)	30.7	(142)
	Excellent	10.3	(39)	8.5	(42)	7.8	(48)	3.0	(14)
Mean**	(SD)	33.8	(6.3)	34.0	(6.0)	32.8	(6.1)	30.7	(6.0)

Source: Berens et al. 2016, p. 4

*Measured as perceived difficulty to perform health information tasks

**p-value from one way ANOVA: $p < 0.001$

Learning 2007). Children and adolescents are comparatively rarely examined in health literacy studies; a fact that has been widely criticised (DeWalt and Hink 2009; Manganello 2008; Zamora et al. 2015; Bröder and Carvalho 2019; Broeder et al. 2017; Wolf et al. 2009; Yin et al. 2007). The few studies are usually limited to non-representative samples. According to their findings, between one-tenth to one-third of adolescents exhibit limited to insufficient health literacy. Alexandra S. Trout and colleagues tested adolescents from an American residential institution and concluded that almost one third (31%) had difficulty understanding basic patient information due to their limited health literacy (Trout et al. 2014). In a study of HIV-infected adolescents from the US, 20% were found to have limited health literacy (Navarra et al. 2014). A Taiwanese sample of adolescents showed a much lower proportion (9.7%) with low health literacy. At the same time, this study confirmed the socio-demographic risk factors for low health literacy: If the adolescents came from families that belonged to an ethnic minority, had a low income or the parents had no tertiary education, the children were significantly more likely to have a low health literacy level (Chang et al. 2015).

A direct correlation between ethnicity and health literacy levels can also be statistically demonstrated in many studies. Ethnic minority groups are disproportionately affected by low health literacy in the US (Kutner et al. 2007; Vernon et al. 2007). Individuals with an immigrant background tend to have lower health literacy scores than those without an immigrant background (Abrams et al. 2009), although the association is not clearly demonstrable in all studies (Pelikan et al. 2012b). If a connection between migration status and health literacy can be proven, migrants with a mother tongue other than the national language are particularly affected. This can be explained, at least in part, by the focus of measurement instruments on written language comprehension, which are offered in the official language of the country (Australian Bureau of Statistics 2006). Within the migrant population in Switzerland, people from Kosovo, people with low levels of education, men and older people tend to have lower knowledge of what symptoms indicate a visit to the doctor (Ackermann Rau et al. 2014). In Germany, a representative survey to determine the health literacy level of the adult population refrained from specifically identifying people with a migration background or migrant history (Jordan and Hoebel 2015).

A review of findings on health literacy and migration or cultural differences found much evidence that a migration background is associated with lower compliance, poorer outcomes for chronic diseases and less frequent participation in preventive measures such as breast cancer screening. Low health literacy is cited as an explanation in most studies. This is explained, among other things, by very different health perceptions and practices in the countries of origin and language barriers (Shaw et al. 2009; Levin-Zamir et al. 2017). A recent study from the USA was able to show that women from low-income minority groups with low literacy and numeracy skills report great difficulties in dealing with contraception. As a result, this population has a high rate of unintended pregnancies (Yee and Simon 2014). In Switzerland, increased rates of abortion among migrant women have been documented on several occasions (Merten and Gari 2013). Among others, a study among undocumented (so-called "sans papiers", formerly pejoratively called "illegals") but well-educated migrant women, mostly from Latin American cultural backgrounds, showed that 40% of the respondents had experienced at least one unwanted pregnancy and almost half of them had had an abortion (Sebo et al. 2011). A Swedish study assessed the health literacy of refugees and their health status. It showed that among refugees, a high proportion had low to insufficient health literacy (Wångdahl et al. 2015). A systematic literature review showed a correlation between migration status and the omission of various preventive health measures such as vaccinations and screenings. Low health literacy, among other things, is used as the main factor to explain this (Kowalski et al. 2014). Contrary to the previous correlations, a study from Canada shows that among immigrants there is a negative correlation between health literacy level and self-reported health status. Subsequently, the authors hypothesise that improving immigrants' health literacy could achieve two goals: An improvement in health as well as an improvement in local language skills (Ng and Omariba 2010).

Many of the findings presented support the hypothesis that a migration background can be seen as a risk factor for lower competencies in the area of health literacy. According to Ingleby, however, this view is insufficient (Ingleby 2012). He argues that the integration of migrant populations into Western health systems should also include their active participation. The values and idea systems of those affected should be consistently taken into account in the development and expansion of disease care, curative care, rehabilitation, prevention and health promotion, rather than pushing migrants into mere assimilation into existing structures with target-group-specific programmes. Zou and Perry or Mergenthal argue similarly: it is not enough to state that migrants are difficult to reach for health promotion due to low health literacy and cultural, linguistic and socioeconomic barriers (Mergenthal 2014; Zou and Parry 2012). These factors must be consciously taken into account in the planning of health strategies and programmes. In Switzerland, efforts are being made in this regard as part of the National Programme Migration and Health. Among other things, the Federal Office of Public Health, in collaboration with Health Promotion Switzerland (2008), issued a guide to *migration-oriented prevention and health promotion.* Overall, studies on the health and health literacy of migrants should conduct balanced surveys and consciously examine the sometimes contradictory findings. There is a great deal of ambivalence due to findings that underline the "healthy-migrant effect" and those that identify migration as a health risk factor, while it has still not been conclusively clarified to what extent these different results are also due to statistical artefacts (Razum and Spallek 2009; Spallek and Razum 2008a). It should also be pointed out here once again that the migrant population is by no means a homogeneous population group in itself. As has already been noted, there are major health and socio-demographic differences between migrants of different origins. Important factors influencing the relationship between migration and health include the motives for migration, the personal experience of the migration process, the legal and social situation in the host country, educational success and specific ethnicity (for example, as an ethnic minority oppressed by a national majority (Kurds, Alevis, Hazara, etc.) (Schenk 2007)).

In this chapter, we have first discussed the definitional difficulties in adequately defining health literacy and reported on measurement problems, some of which are considerable. We have then presented the importance of health literacy for a range of health outcomes and traced the considerable quantitative dimensions of limited health literacy. Finally, we have identified a number of social determinants that significantly influence individual health literacy – always measured by literacy tests or self-reports.

In the following chapter we want to narrow down the state of research on health literacy to the two target groups that are of particular interest to us in the ELMi and ELiS projects: migrant adolescents and migrant families with young children.

Health Literacy in Childhood and Adolescence and the Need for Family Health Literacy

3

Abstract

Childhood and adolescence are generally and on average considered to be the healthiest periods of life in the overall biography. Nevertheless, in recent years there has been an increased attention to the topic of childhood and adolescent health in science and practice, because, also on the basis of better data, there is more and more evidence that overall social and health inequality has an effect even in childhood and adolescence: "Since about 10–15 years, there has been a stronger focus on childhood and adolescence, because it has become more and more clear that the influence of social status on health is already apparent at a young age."

An Overview of the Quantitative Research Situation

Childhood and adolescence are generally and on average considered to be the healthiest periods of life in the overall biography. Nevertheless, in recent years there has been an increased attention to the topic of childhood and adolescent health in science and practice, because, also on the basis of better data, there is more and more evidence that the overall social and health inequality has an impact even in childhood and adolescence (cf. on this, for example, Inchley et al. 2016; Okan et al. 2019b): "For about 10–15 years, there has been a greater focus on childhood and adolescence, as it has become more and more clear that the influence of social status on health is already apparent at a young age." (Lampert 2016, p. 131). The social inheritance of health risks alluded to here is particularly sensitive from a normative point of view, as it obviously contradicts the idea of equality of all individuals enshrined in the German constitution. However, if children at a very young age are significantly more likely to be affected by various diseases and/or risk factors or to have their health potential curtailed due to specific conditions of growing up, such

U. H. Bittlingmayer et al., *Health Literacy From A Health Ethnology Perspective*, https://doi.org/10.1007/978-3-658-42348-3_3

as a lack of resources in households, a poor housing situation, and few local opportunities for individual development (RKI 2009; Ravens-Sieberer et al. 2018; Lampert and Schenk 2004; Lampert et al. 2010), these findings are contrary to the equality ideals of highly industrialised societies and they are at least as much a challenge to the idea of health promotion and prevention in the reference discipline of public health. It becomes clear in the subject area of childhood and adolescent health that health cannot, without further ado, be defined as an individual good (Bauer 2019a) that is exclusively dependent on one's own health-oriented lifestyle, but is always embedded in intergenerational relations on the one hand (Schnabel 1988, 2001a; Okan et al. 2019b), and in normative notions of health on the other (Kühn 1993; Bittlingmayer et al. 2008; Schmidt 2014, 2017). The connections between social inequalities, families, children and adolescents, and health literacy will be traced in more detail in the following. In doing so, we will trace the state of research and repeatedly point out limitations and gaps in the field of research, which is dominated by quantitative studies.

In the first section, the relationship between health inequalities and their consequences in childhood and adolescence is discussed in more detail and recent findings from health reporting are compiled (Sect. 3.1). In a second step, the health literacy of adolescents is discussed (Sect. 3.2). In the further course of the chapter, we will also discuss the comparatively very limited state of research on health literacy among children and relate this to the intergenerational relationships that are particularly complex in childhood and which can hardly be ignored in the analysis of children's health literacy (Sect. 3.3). In this section, we will also use our own data on the quantitative distribution of health literacy among 11- to 15-year-old children to demonstrate the extent to which such a standardised approach to the health literacy of children and adolescents is valid. Finally, we devote a separate section to the topic of digital health literacy among children, adolescents and parents, on the *one hand* because it is currently being discussed very widely and, on the other hand, because digital health literacy is associated with significant promises that are supposed to lead to a reduction in unequal health literacy and health inequalities (Sect. 3.4).

3.1 Child and Adolescent Health in the Context of Family Social Inequality

The topic of social inequality in childhood and adolescence continues to make waves. For example, the public is scandalised by children living in poverty, who – directly relevant to health – have to go to school without breakfast, are overweight, rarely engage in sports and therefore have low motor skills, or whose everyday media consumption is already considered to be significantly too high in childhood. These findings are then associated with a lack of educational competencies – or even more dramatically: with a lack of educational interest – from which the (innocent) children and young people have to suffer. The fact that child poverty is, as a rule, embedded in family poverty is hardly sufficiently brought to bear in the scandalised discourses.

A public health perspective provides a more differentiated and empirically saturated picture. It is true that the topic of family health as a whole, at least in the German-speaking countries, has been dealt with surprisingly little within public health research in its entire breadth, measured against the paramount importance of family socialisation for a healthy upbringing (Schnabel 1988, 2001a). However, the fact that family socialisation has enormous consequences for individual health biographies and that it would therefore be negligent to isolate children and adolescents as victims of poverty, as it were, is confirmed by very different research perspectives within the health sciences: *Firstly,* social epidemiology points out that "in childhood, *family resources* are of particularly great importance. These include social support and backing from parents, as well as well-developed family cohesion and a positive family climate" (Ravens-Sieberer et al. 2018, p. 77). At the same time, however, the family is also determined here as a potential risk factor, a place of possible health risks which could be established as a place of prevention by improving parenting skills (Ravens-Sieberer et al. 2018, pp. 83–85). *Second,* in the health promotion perspective, the family is also described as a place "that gives people emotional support, where they can feel loved and accepted and are integrated into a supportive system that can also protect them in stressful situations.[. . .] [The] family as a 'primary socialisation instance' [determines] significantly the attitude and later health behaviour of children." (Geene 2018, p. 371).

It is well established that behavioural patterns, dispositions or attitudes acquired in childhood and adolescence are particularly difficult to change in the course of life because, according to French sociologist Pierre Bourdieu, the earliest experiences are extraordinarily comprehensive and formative and condense into an individual habitus (more on this in the following fourth chapter). For this reason, from the perspective of child and youth research, "an extension of the health patterns practiced in the family of origin into adulthood" (Klocke 2006, p. 201) is also to be expected (similarly Levin-Zamir et al. 2017, p. 135).

Furthermore, risk patterns or (chronic) disease symptoms that already appear in childhood and adolescence are considered more serious in their courses than those that only appear in adulthood. "Obesity developed in childhood poses the risk of permanent obesity that persists into adulthood. Often, the disease course is even more severe in adulthood if obesity developed in childhood and adolescence." (Krug et al. 2018, p. 4). Adolescent health research also notes that "the family [is] by far the most significant setting for health. The influence of the family environment not only persists during adolescence, but is evident almost throughout the life course – albeit to varying degrees." (Richter 2008, pp. 19–20). By the same token, research in the context of health reporting also emphasises: "The health behavior of children is [. . .] initially influenced primarily by the family of origin and the social environment in which they grow up. Parents, in their role model function – especially in the first years of life – are essential for the health behaviour of their children." (Kuntz et al. 2018, p. 46).

The emphasis on the importance of family socialisation for the entire health biography encounters a situation in society where massive social inequalities, in the form of scarcity of resources, can influence the health of future generations and drive families beyond the margins of everyday coping strategies. The fact that this always involves an intergenerational interplay of precarious resource endowments is emphasised from very different directions. For example, the Committee on Economic, Social and Cultural Rights of the United Nations Economic and Social Council, in its critical opinion on the sixth report of the Federal Republic of Germany of 2018, under the heading of child poverty, is particularly explicit about the link between child and family poverty, expressing concern that "19.7% of children under 18 (2.55 million) live in poverty, mostly with a single parent or in families with two or more siblings." (Vereinte Nationen. Wirtschafts- und Sozialrat 2018, p. 6). It directly links this finding to policy governance instruments designed to end child poverty and, most importantly, to benefit parents. In its recommendation, the UN body says:

> The Committee recommends that the State [meaning here and hereinafter the Federal Republic of Germany; author], with the aim of eradicating child poverty, continuously examine whether benefits for children, including child benefit, child supplement and the education and participation package, are adequate. It also recommends that the State collect data on benefits for children, including take-up, and take the necessary measures to address the difficulties faced by eligible households in accessing benefits. (Vereinte Nationen. Wirtschafts- und Sozialrat 2018, pp. 9–10)

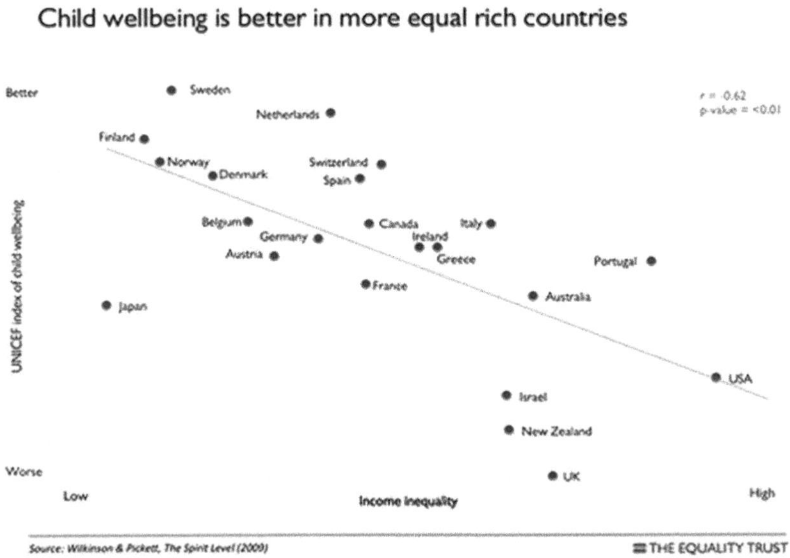

Fig. 3.1 Child well-being in relation to income inequality. (Source: www.equalitytrust.org.uk)

The direct link between inequalities in society as a whole and the health or morbidity of the next generation is impressively demonstrated – at a general and abstract level – by social epidemiology. According to Pickett and Wilkinson (2015), income inequality in a country can be determined as a causal factor for population health in all its aspects. The rule of thumb here can be: The more socially equal a highly industrialised society is, the healthier the population and the better opportunities for development the upcoming generation has. Finally, as illustrated in Fig. 3.1 below, Wilkinson and Pickett can show that *even children's well-being depends significantly on the extent of income inequality in a country.*

From our point of view, these empirical findings on the correlations between general social inequalities and health outcomes, which filter through to children's well-being, speak very clearly against a definition of the tasks of child and youth policy formulated in the Federal Government's fifth Poverty and Wealth Report: "Secondly, it is the task of child and youth and education policies to promote children and young people even better individually and as independently as possible of the resources in their parental home in order to improve social participation and advancement opportunities." (Bundesministerium für Arbeit und Soziales 2017,

III). In addition to the irritating absence of family policy from the list of relevant policy fields, the health, educational, and life opportunities of children and adolescents cannot be separated from the familial and social conditions in which they grow up (Okan et al. 2019b), as studies from education and public health research have been showing for 15 years now.

This is exactly what the specific childhood- and youth-related social epidemiology for Germany clearly shows: In a general assessment of the immediate consequences of family poverty to children based on empirical surveys, the health reporting of the Robert Koch Institute supports the positions of the UN Social Council and those of Wilkinson and Pickett cited above:

> Income poverty can not only lead to restrictions in the consumption and leisure behaviour of children and adolescents but can also have an unfavourable influence on the family climate and parenting behaviour. The resulting psychosocial stresses can have a lasting negative impact on adolescents. Education as a characteristic of the social situation is relevant not only for placing individuals in the social structure but also for the development of health-related attitudes and behaviour patterns. Coming from resource-poor families, children and adolescents often experience not only poverty but also social exclusion, which can subsequently lead to emotional instability, impaired cognitive and linguistic development as well as school performance and behavioural problems. Further consequences of poverty arise in relation to the well-being and health of adolescents: Socially disadvantaged children and adolescents are less likely to rate these as very good; they are more likely to have health impairments, accidental injuries and dental problems. (RKI 2009, P. 17)

The empirically based assessment of the Robert Koch Institute, which has so far at least been unsuspected of left-wing radicalism or hasty scandalisation, thus points to the fact that income poverty influences interactions, educational opportunities, experiences of discrimination, impaired development and mental and physical health. Therefore, there is an obvious need to address income poverty in order to minimise the consequences that arise from it. In the following section, health inequalities among children and adolescents are outlined more clearly.

3.1.1 Findings of German Health Reporting on Unequal Child and Youth Health

Health reporting, which has been greatly expanded in Germany over the last 20 years and for which the Robert Koch Institute in particular is responsible, provides a large number of individual indicators showing that the social background of children and adolescents exerts huge influence on the overwhelming majority of disease outcomes. For the *reference year 2008,* Ulrike Ravens-Sieberer and Michael Erhart summarise the state of research on the relationship between social inequality and health in childhood and adolescence as follows:

> Mortality and disease incidence is relatively highest among children from low socio-economic strata – with the exception of allergies, neurodermatitis and bronchitis [. . .]. Children and adolescents with low socio-economic status also partly practise less favourable health behaviour [. . .]. The children suffer injuries more frequently [. . .] and participate less in preventive medical check-ups [. . .].[. . .] Children from socially disadvantaged families – with the exception of allergic diseases – [are] more frequently physically and psychologically impaired, [. . .] [consume] psychoactive substances [. . .] more frequently, [show] poorer nutritional behaviour [. . .] and [are] more frequently overweight. (Ravens-Sieberer and Erhart 2008, pp. 43–44)

The situation of health inequality for children and adolescents from low social status *has not improved since then.* In the evaluation of the first wave (2009–2012) of the Children's Health Survey, for example, it was found that children and adolescents of low social status, compared with children and adolescents from middle and higher social status, bear an increased risk of describing themselves as having only limited health, being mentally abnormal, exhibiting a higher level of health-damaging behaviour and taking advantage of fewer early disease detection programmes (Lampert et al. 2015). In some cases, the inequalities are dramatic – for example, almost 30% of girls aged 3–17 from the lower social class are found to have mental health problems, compared to 15.7% of girls from the middle and 8% from the upper classes. Among boys aged 3–17 years, 37% with low social status, 22.1% with medium social status and 11.6% with high social status show mental abnormalities (Lampert et al. 2015, p. 19). The current evaluations of the second wave of KiGGS (2014–2017) show stable social inequalities in health behaviour and health risks: Children and adolescents with low social status exercise less, eat and drink less healthily, and are more frequently affected by overweight and obesity (Kuntz et al. 2018).

3.1.2 Health Inequalities and the Migration Background of Children and Adolescents

In the context of analysing the connection between social and health inequalities, it is striking in the overall view that an unequal health socialisation is not seriously denied by anyone, but that social epidemiology and health reporting do not take up the state of sociological inequality research, which in the last 20 years has increasingly dealt with the entanglement of different dimensions of domination. Multidimensional inequality theory, dealt with under the catchword of "intersectionality", attempts to fathom, for example, the complex, mediated ways in which gender, ethnicity and class interrelate (Winker and Degele 2010; Hormel 2012). This idea of *mediating* central structural dimensions has not yet fully penetrated public health and social epidemiological research (cf. in more detail farther below Chap. 4). An important indicator of this is, for example, the visible neglect of the ethnic dimension, particularly in the context of child and adolescent health (e.g., in Wallmann et al. 2012). If, as in the health reporting presented here, the effects of the social origin of children and adolescents are precisely recorded with regard to health risks and morbidity rates, then affiliations to ethnic minorities are left out; and vice versa, if migration, immigration history or migration background is examined with regard to effects beneficial or detrimental to health, then socio-economic positions are either completely disregarded or "modelled" as control variables or covariates in regression models.

When asking about the health effects of a one-sided or two-sided migration background, highly questionable groups of parents, children and adolescents are then formed, who only have the one characteristic in common of not being born in Germany or growing up under conditions in which one parent or both parents were not born in Germany. Consequently, in contrast to the clearer findings of the socio-economic health determinants, somewhat confused results are presented. Here is an example: "In the context of other predictors, low or medium family wealth increases the probability of low life satisfaction by a factor of 2.0 and 1.4, respectively. In contrast, under control of the other factors, if the mother was born in another country this has a protective effect. Under these conditions, the risk of low life satisfaction for the child drops to about a factor of 0.6. Interpreting this surprising finding is difficult." (Erhart et al. 2008b, p. 152).

The category of one-sided or two-sided migration background is extremely unsatisfactory from a theoretical point of view and, as an isolated variable and independent determinant, represents a highly controversial construction in sociological research. First of all, because the switch, common by now, in survey techniques from the legal category of citizenship or nationality to the category of migration background refers to cultural differences that are difficult to grasp, without knowing whether they can or must be overcome at all. In addition, the migration background category, which is primarily linked to cultural differences, runs the risk of essentialization (Emmerich and Hormel 2013; Scherr and Niermann 2012). Moreover, parts of educational research argue that social educational inequalities have nothing to do with children's migration background, but are either used as a posteriori legitimation for selection mechanisms internal to the school system (Gomolla and Radkte 2009; Gomolla and Radtke 2000; Hormel and Scherr 2004) or, in the context of quantitative empirical studies, it is shown that statistically significant differences in the educational success of children and adolescents with a migration background disappear significantly or completely when socio-economic status is controlled for (Kristen and Dollmann 2012; Becker and Beck 2012). From the perspective of public health and health promotion, the deconstructivist positions should be taken seriously that warn against statistically constructing large social groups and, on the basis of these constructions determining intervention programmes, target groups or general group characteristics, as the case might be (Emmerich and Hormel 2013). Incidentally, the same also applies to socio-economic constructions of large groups, which are initially, as Pierre Bourdieu put it, classes on paper that do not necessarily have anything to do with the attitudinal patterns and lifeworlds of the people themselves (Bourdieu 1985).

And yet the question of the interplay between migration background, cultural differences, gender and social class in the area of health arises in a way that is fundamentally different from the highly influential educational science or in pedagogical-psychological education research. This is because the outcome is much more concrete and directly related to one's own psycho-physio-socio-somatic existence, and cultural differences can have a more direct impact on somatic existence, for example in the form of dietary regulations, or even – in the case of the prohibition of alcohol in specific Muslim or Buddhist religious interpretations – themselves be oriented towards health promotion and prevention. Cultural differences do demonstrably exist, and they can have a direct effect on the health of children and adolescents (Bittlingmayer and Sahrai 2010; Sahrai 2009). In this respect, the socio-epidemiological findings should also be taken seriously that attest higher health risks to specific migrant groups, such as in the context of dental health, preventive care, obesity or impaired psychological well-being (Erhart et al. 2008b, p. 158) or, on the positive side, prove lower adolescent alcohol consumption (Erhart et al. 2008b, p. 149). And that is why the use of a migration background variable in the context of public health is appropriate, at least as long as the construction mechanisms of social groups are not ignored and the categories are not essentialized (for more on this see Chap. 4).

However, these factors and interrelationships then lead to the question of how everyday practices are shaped, of lifestyle patterns and behaviours that are beneficial or detrimental to health, and along which the abstract statistical structural categories materialise. The fact that the individual factors age, gender, ethnicity and social class each exert an independent influence with regard to health-promoting lifestyles has been clearly demonstrated for adults by William Cockerham et al. (Cockerham et al. 2006). The simultaneous dependence of health determinants on different structural dimensions, as postulated here, can also be traced in children and adolescents. Andreas Klocke and Gero Lipsmeier were able to show in complex empirical analyses, for example, that with regard to the "identification of social determinants of health and health behaviour [...] the variables of the internal family space (conversations with the mother, type of family, unemployment, wealth, nationality) all [prove] to be significant". (Klocke and Lipsmeier 2008, p. 252).

The findings presented so far point to a central consideration with regard to the health literacy of children and adolescents. The health literacy of children and adolescents *cannot* be determined *independently* of the overall family situation – the conceptualization of health literacy as an individually available competence must be clearly restricted at least for childhood and adolescence. This brings us to the state of research on health literacy, first among adolescents and then among children and families (Sect. 3.3) in the narrower sense.

3.2 Health Literacy of Young People

Even in 2015, after around 15 years of intensified international health literacy research, the consensus, at least in German-speaking public health, is that children and adolescents have been largely neglected as a target group of health literacy research (Zamora et al. 2015). The focus to date has clearly been on the adult population, "less is known about the health literacy of youth" (Trout et al. 2014, p. 37), and the main complaint is a lack of theoretical explanatory models and empirical data to analyse the specifics of child- and youth-specific health literacy (Zamora et al. 2015; Manganello 2008).[1] To date, there have been comparatively few studies of health literacy in children and adolescents, and the associations between health literacy and health outcomes in these age groups are also poorly understood (more on this below). The considerably expanded empirical research on child and adolescent health in the context of health reporting and social epidemiology presented above in the last decade thus does not correspond to similarly

[1] Orkan Okan, Janine Bröder and other colleagues from the Bielefeld health literacy research context around Ullrich Bauer and Paulo Pinheiro have recently formulated a five- or six-dimensional conceptual model with which the special characteristics of children and adolescents are to be taken into account when researching their health literacy. This is a promising approach, but one in which the different dimensions would have to be placed in a theoretical relationship more strongly than has been the case to date; cf. Bröder et al. (2017), Okan et al. (2019b, pp. 77–79).

expanded health literacy research in these age groups (Okan et al. 2017b). The special features of children and adolescents with regard to health literacy, which consist in both biomedical age-specific development risks, in the social dimension in the intergenerational dependency relationship with the – as a rule – parental caregivers, as well as in the ongoing and particularly intensive general competence development, are not represented by health literacy research focused on adults (Okan et al. 2017b, p. 16).

Although research into health literacy in childhood and adolescence is still considered a clear research desideratum, there are now a number of studies that analyse the age-specific relationships between health and illness and health literacy in these age groups, at least in some areas (Bröder and Carvalho 2019). The research on health literacy among adolescents is considerably more productive than that on children, especially younger children (more on this below).

In a US study that aims to determine the level of available health literacy among the special risk group of adolescents growing up outside their families in institutional care, the following distribution of health literacy is described on the basis of the Newest Vital Sign test: 23% of the approximately 250 adolescents surveyed have a high probability of limited health literacy, 42% have the possibility of limited health literacy and 35% have adequate health literacy (Trout et al. 2014, p. 39). In a smart German study, the health literacy of groups considered vulnerable – here: older people, (younger) people with low levels of education and socio-economic resources, and people with a migration background" (Quenzel et al. 2016b, p. 5) – were investigated within a theoretically pre-defined sample. The study is able to show that disadvantaged young people, defined here as being 15 to 25 years old (the age group usually addressed by youth sociology), with and without a migration background, have significantly lower health literacy than the average population from North Rhine-Westphalia (see Fig. 3.2).

Overall, according to the data collected by Gudrun Quenzel et al., almost three quarters (73.5%) of the disadvantaged groups show limited health competencies. Unfortunately, the young people under legal age are not presented separately in this study. Olli Paakkari and colleagues provide completely different data for Finland. Within the framework of the Health Behavior in School-Aged Children study initiated by the WHO, which for many years has included regular surveys of students in grades 5, 7 and 9, the authors documented a very high level of (self-reported) health literacy on average for the Finnish part of the study (for seventh and ninth graders). "Approximately one-third of the adolescents manifested a high level of HL, around 60% had a moderate level of HL, and about one-tenth had low HL. The HL level was lower for boys than for girls, and lower for 7th graders than for 9th graders. In the total sample, the strongest explanatory variables for HL were

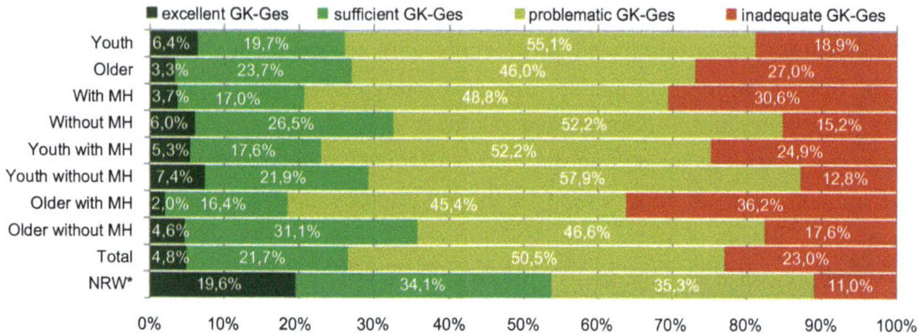

Fig. 3.2 Distribution of health literacy (comprehensive) in socially disadvantaged population groups compared to the general population (Source: Quenzel et al. 2016b, p. 24)

school achievement in the first language, and educational aspirations." (Paakkari et al. 2018).

The most comprehensive study to date comes from Austria and is based on a representative survey of 15-year-old Austrian adolescents (Röthlin et al. 2013). This work was directly related to the European Health Literacy Survey (Pelikan et al. 2012b) and used an only very slightly modified instrument (HLS-EU 47-Questionnaire) to measure adolescents' health literacy. Conceptually, the adolescent survey works with the same comprehensive theoretical health-literacy framework model developed in the main study (Sørensen et al. 2012a). The HLS-EU measurement instrument distinguishes between disease management or care behaviour, prevention behaviour and health promotion behaviour as the three relevant reference levels of health literacy (on the substantive distinction between prevention and health promotion, see Schnabel 2007b). The instrument allows both the distinction between the dimensions, i.e., disease coping, prevention and health promotion, and the construction of an overall index of health literacy. In the following Fig. 3.3, the results of the adolescent and adult surveys are presented both as an overall index of health literacy (in the first row of Fig. 3.6) and in the different dimensions (in rows 2 to 4 of Fig. 3.6). First of all, it becomes apparent that more than half of the adults and half of the adolescents have limited health literacy (combining the categories inadequate and problematic), according to the terminology of the author. Overall, however, there are *no significant differences in the extent of limited health literacy between Austrian adolescents and the adult population.*

However, *significantly more adults* are grouped in the *inadequate health literacy* category in the overall index than adolescents. With regard to the three health literacy dimensions, adolescents have significantly lower values in the areas of coping with illness and health promotion in the particularly sensitive *inadequate*

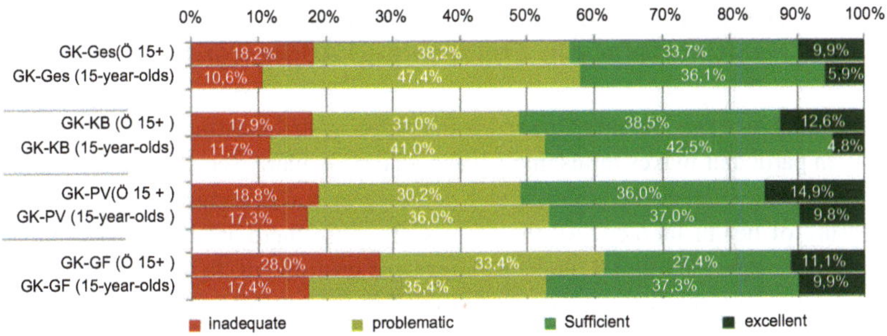

Fig. 3.3 Percentage distribution of the different levels of the four health literacy indices for the sample of 15-year-olds (N = 571) and the Austria (15+) sample (N = 1015). (Source: Röthlin et al. 2013, p. 40)

health literacy category than the adult reference group. This could mean that the finding of an age gradient in the context of health literacy is already evident at a much earlier age and not only in late adulthood or old age (Berens et al. 2016). However, the findings are not particularly consistent, but strongly depend on the measurement instrument used. In the Austrian study, the Newest Vital Sign Test (NVS) is also used to measure so-called functional health literacy. The NVS "assesses reading comprehension and numeracy by giving individuals a specially designed ice cream nutrition label and asking them six questions about the label (e.g., 'If you eat the entire container, how many calories will you eat?').[. . .] Scores range from 0 to 6, with each question being worth 1 point. Scores of 0–1 suggest high likelihood of limited literacy, 2–3 indicate the possibility of limited literacy, and 4–6 indicate adequate literacy." (Trout et al. 2014, p. 38). If the health literacy of adolescents and adults is now compared on the basis of the NVS and not the HLS-EU instrument, which was also the basis of the study by Berens et al., the findings in the Austrian study are reversed: "While the 15-year-olds achieve an average of 3.5 points, the Ö15 + sample achieves 4.1 points. This means that the average in the Austrian 15 + total population is more than 17% higher than in the 15-year-olds. Thus, adults perform significantly better on the NVS test than adolescents." (Röthlin et al. 2013, p. 41).

It becomes clear in the overall view of the international studies that the percentages of young people with low, limited, sufficient or excellent health literacy differ considerably in an international comparison. Obviously, this is largely due to the fact that health literacy is measured in very different ways, just as it is in the adult population.

3.2.1 The Heterogeneity of Instruments Used to Measure Health Literacy in Children and Adolescents

The question of the instruments used is therefore, as the Austrian study by Röthlin et al. in particular makes refreshingly clear, also particularly sensitive in the context of the health literacy of children and adolescents for determining the available measure of health literacy. All the more so because there are hardly any studies that use the same definitions, understandings and instruments. In a recent systematic review of instruments for measuring health literacy in children and adolescents, Orkan Okan and colleagues show how inconsistent the relationship between definitions, instrument development and measurement is, even in this limited field of research:

> Each instrument used a different, study-specific understanding of health literacy, and two instruments were underpinned with a health literacy definition that was specifically developed for the instrument. In the other 13 studies, the researchers referred to different existing definitions but did not make clear whether or not these definitions were underlying their instruments, and of these, six studies referred to the definition provided by Nutbeam. (Orkan et al. 2018, p. 9)

Another systematic review on definitions and theoretical models of child and adolescent health literacy comes to the same conclusion (Bröder et al. 2017). In a broad overview, three major dimensions of heterogeneity can be identified in the determination of children's and adolescents' health literacy. One of the more central lines of difference in the context of adolescents' health literacy is *firstly* – analogous to the models of adult health literacy – whether a narrow understanding of health literacy, i.e. only related to the disease care sector, prevails or whether other contexts and fields of action (such as prevention and health promotion) are included in the health literacy concept, as for example Don Nutbeam, Ilona Kickbusch, Doris Schaeffer and Kristine Sørensen suggest. This would be the *motive of* the *different objective scope of* health literacy.

A *second* important line of differentiation is whether health literacy is understood only as an individual competence and resource for action, or whether setting and community references are also directly incorporated into the concept (as in St Leger 2001; Paakkari and George 2018). This can be determined as a *motif of the action-theoretical grounding* of health literacy, i.e. as individual behaviour at the level of conscious deliberation and available information, or as the inclusion of contexts of action and organisational settings (the latter was, for example, the thrust of the "7th Global Conference on Health Promotion" in Nairobi in 2009 or the health literacy discussion of the World Health Organisation; cf. on this WHO 2009; WHO Europe 2013).

And *thirdly*, there are differences in the theoretical and empirical modelling of children's and adolescents' health literacy in that either only functional health literacy is considered or health literacy in its entire breadth of interactive and critical dimensions is included in the conceptualisations. This could be identified as the *dimension* of *normative anchoring*, which opens up a broad spectrum of health literacy approaches spanning between the poles of (behaviourist) behavioural regulation (for one's own good) in relation to the clinical setting, and questions about the relationship between health literacy and social justice (Bittlingmayer and Sahrai 2019; Paakkari and George 2018; Paakkari et al. 2019a, p. 1). All of these dimensions and distinguishing criteria are highly relevant even for determining child and adolescent health literacy. The table "Definitions of health literacy in children and adolescents" (Bröder et al. 2017, p. 5) (Table 3.1) illustrates precisely how wide the range of approaches is in terms of content.

3.2.2 Health Literacy of 11- to 15-Year-Old Adolescents in Germany

In order to get an overview for Germany as well (comparable with the Austrian one), we conducted our own study. For this purpose, we integrated the health literacy measurement into an ongoing evaluation study and attempted to survey the health literacy of sixth grade students.

Many studies point out that the school years are a particularly sensitive and relevant phase of life for acquiring life skills and health-related competencies (e.g., Wallmann et al. 2012, p. 5). Therefore, Lions Quest developed the non-target-group-specific, general life skills program 'Growing Up', which can be used in grammar schools as well as in the often ignored lower secondary schools and special schools. The program is sponsored by the non-profit relief organisation of the German Lions, has been used throughout Germany for more than 20 years by now, and can be considered one of the most widespread school-based life skills programs in the entire German-speaking world (see, among others, Kähnert 2003; Bauer 2005; Bittlingmayer and Sirch 2006; Hartung 2014; Gerdes et al. 2016, 2018; Matischek-Jauk et al. 2017). From 2015 to 2018, evaluation research measuring the effectiveness of the extracurricular teaching program "Lions Quest Growing Up", was conducted at the University of Education Freiburg by Jürgen Gerdes, Gözde Okcu, Igor Osipov, and Uwe H. Bittlingmayer (Gerdes et al. 2016, 2018; Osipov et al. 2017).

Table 3.1 "Definitions of health literacy in children and adolescents"

Definitions of children's and young people's health literacy		
Children and primary school students		
A	Fok and Wong (2002)	"The meaning of health literacy to children is defined as "to understand and act upon physical and psycho-social activities with appropriate standards, being able to interact with people and cope with necessary changes and demands reasonable autonomy so as to achieve complete physical, mental and social well-being."
B	Brown et al. (2007)	"For this study, health literacy was defined simply as the ability to understand health information and to understand that actions taken in youth affect health later in life, combined with the ability to access valid health information."
Young people and secondary school students		
C	Massey et al. (2012)	"We take an expanded perspective of health literacy and define it as a set of skills used to organize and apply health knowledge, attitudes and practices relevant when managing one's health environment."
D	Paakkari and Paakkari (2012)	"Health Literacy is defined in the following terms: Health literacy comprises a broad range of knowledge and competences that people seek to encompass, evaluate and use. Through health literacy competences people become able to understand themselves, others and the world in a way that will enable them to make sound health decisions, and to work on and change the factors that constitute their own and others' health chances."
E	Wu et al. (2010)	"Health literate individuals are able to understand and apply health information in ways that allow them to take more control over their health through for example appraising the credibility, accuracy and relevance of information and acting on that information to change their health behaviours or living conditions."
F	Gordon et al. (2011)	"Health literacy is the degree to which individual's have the capacity to obtain, access, process, and understand basic health information and services needed to take appropriate health decisions and involves an ongoing process of building individual and community capacity to understand the components of health."
Different age groups or considering a life course perspective		
G	Borzekowski (2009)	"Health literacy is not just the ability to read, rather, it is a set of skills that involve recognizing, processing, integrating and acting on information from a variety of platforms. Those between the ages of 3 and 18 can seek, comprehend, evaluate and use health information especially if materials are presented

(continued)

Table 3.1 (continued)

Definitions of children's and young people's health literacy		
		in ways that are age appropriate, culturally relevant, and socially supported. The development of health literacy among children and young people can empower the vulnerable and "marginalized" group to be more engaged, more productive and healthier."
H	Soellner et al. (2014)	[Translated] The working definition defines health competences as an accumulation of skills and capabilities that someone has at one's command to be able to act in daily life and in dealing with the health system, in such a way that positively affects one's health and well-being
I	Mancuso (2009)	"A process that evolves over one's lifetime and encompasses the attributes of capacity, comprehension, and communication The attributes of health literacy are integrated within and preceded by the skills, strategies, and abilities embedded within the competencies needed to attain health literacy. The outcomes of health literacy are dependent upon whether one has achieved adequate or inadequate health literacy and have the potential to influence individuals and society."
J	Nutbeam [35]	"The personal, cognitive and social skills which determine the ability of individuals to gain access to, understand, and use information to promote and maintain good health."
K	Sørensen et al. (2012a)	"Health literacy is linked to literacy and entails people's knowledge, motivation and competences to access, understand, appraise and apply health information in order to make judgments and take decisions in everyday life concerning healthcare, disease prevention and health promotion to maintain or improve quality of life during the life course."
L	Zarcadoolas et al. (2005)	"Health literacy evolves over one's life corse, starting at an early age and, like most complex human competences is impacted by health status as well as demographic, socio-political, psychosocial and cultural factors". "We define health literacy as the wide range of skills and competences that people develop to seek out, comprehend, evaluate and use health information and concepts to make informed choices, reduce health risks and increase quality of life."

Source: Bröder et al. 2017, p. 5

Within the framework of an evaluation study of the school-based life skills development program Lions-Quest 'Growing Up', students of the 5th and 6th grade level from the existing range of school types (from special schools to grammar schools) from six federal states were interviewed at three different points in time (before, during and

> after a one-and-a-half-year intervention phase). A total of 123 project classes were initially recruited (of which 111 project schools were still in the sample at the last survey date) and randomly assigned to the intervention and control groups. Accompanying the survey, the teachers of the participating project classes were interviewed about the program (intervention), just at three points in time. (Gerdes et al. 2018, p. 2)

A total of (N = 1672) students participated across all three measurement time points, of which N = 832 (50.1%) were boys and N = 831 (49.9%) were girls. During the 2017 data collection period, participating pupils* were on average 12.58 years old, i.e., 49.1% were 11 or 12 years old, 43.5% were 13 years old and 7.4% were 14 or 15 years old. Classes of all school types were included: Gymnasium (grammar schools) (38.7%), primary schools (in Berlin and Brandenburg primary schools go up to grade 6) and comprehensive schools (14.1%), Real-, Ober-, Sekundarschulen (29.9%), Hauptschulen (12.0%) (??) and Förderschulen (special schools) (5.3%) from the six federal states Lower Saxony, Brandenburg, Saxony-Anhalt, North Rhine-Westphalia, Hesse and Bavaria (one school from Mannheim was also included in the sample).

The proportion of pupils with a migration background was 31.5%, which is slightly below the national average in this age group. Only 5.1% (N = 84) of the students stated that they were born abroad. In our sample, the proportion of pupils whose father's or mother's place of birth was abroad was higher at 25.4% (N = 382) and at 24.5% (N = 389) respectively. 11.3% of the students (N = 224) in the total sample had a one-sided migration background and 20.2% (N = 407) of the students had a two-sided migration background.[2]

In addition to numerous demographic data, the availability and development of individual life skills were measured by using common psychometric scales (including general self-efficacy beliefs, empathy, communicative skills). In particular, the areas of social skills, self-esteem, empathy, emotion regulation and cultural heterogeneity acceptance were recorded (Gerdes et al. 2016), as well as *health literacy in the third wave.*

For the quantitative assessment of health literacy, an instrument was used that was developed in parallel within the framework of the Health Literacy in Childhood and Adolescents research network to determine health literacy in children. The MoMChild project was concerned with the development of a valid quantitative scale for measuring health literacy in children aged 9–10 years, using the HLS-EU

[2] In addition to the general variable of migration background, we also collected data on ethnicity. We were and are aware of the problem of essentialising very heterogeneous groups.

scale developed by Jürgen Pelikan and others as part of the European Health Literacy Survey, which has already been mentioned several times.[3] The instrument constructed in Bielefeld comprised a total of 26 items in the first version available to us at the time of the survey. This Bielefeld scale was then shortened to 15 items in its final version in an extensive pre-test (Bollweg et al. 2020a). Because the final information for the scale validation was not yet available and we did not have enough space in our questionnaire, we had decided at that time to shorten the scale to a total of 16 items and to delete the items that we considered the most difficult for children to assess. After the validation of the Bielefeld scale, the items we used only intersect with 10 items, so comparison with the Bielefeld study does not make much sense.

The remaining 16 items comprise – much like the Health Literacy Model of the HLS-EU-Q47 – questions on skills (finding, understanding, assessing and applying) as well as on health promotion, disease prevention, health care, supplemented by general questions. We document the instrument we used here once in full for the sake of transparency. Here, the health literacy scale consists in questions 3, 5, 7 and 8, while the other questions flank the scale.

Except for questions1 and 6, all questions in this scale are presented in a four-step response format: 1 for "very easy", 2 for "rather easy", 3 for "rather difficult" and 4 for "very difficult" plus the option "don't know", as shown in Fig. 3.4 of the overall questionnaire. The first question introduces the topic and its familiarity in general by asking the students to state whether they have ever tried to find out something about the topic of health with the gradation yes vs. no. Question 6 goes one step further and asks how often the student thinks about whether the health-related information he/she has heard is correct with the answer options "(almost) never", "rarely", "sometimes", "often", "(almost) always" and "don't know".

More than 60% of the surveyed students stated that they had already tried to find out something about the topic of health (61.5%) (N = 1012), with girls answering yes significantly more often. However, searching for health-related information alone is not an indication of health literacy; it is significant to assess the accuracy of health information and to question the content if necessary. To the question "when you hear something about health, how often do you think about whether it is true?" a quarter of the students answered "rarely" or "(almost) never".

[3]More detailed information on the MoMChild project, which was conducted at Bielefeld University under the direction of Paulo Pinheiro by Orkan Okan and Torsten Bollweg, can be found at www.hlca-consortium.de.

1) Have you ever tried to find out something about health? *Please mark with a cross!*

Yes	
No	

2) How easy or difficult is it for you to find out about health?

Tick please!

very simple	rather simple	rather difficult	Very difficult	don't know
❑	❑	❑	❑	❑

3) How easy or difficult is it for you to ...

Please make a cross in each line!

	very simple	rather simple	rather difficult	Very difficult	don't know
1. Find out how to get well quickly when you have a cold?	❑	❑	❑	❑	❑
2. figure out what you can do to keep from getting too fat or too thin?	❑	❑	❑	❑	❑
3. Find out what food is healthy for you?	❑	❑	❑	❑	❑

We now want to know from you <u>how well you understand the things</u> you hear or read about health!

4) Most of what I hear or read about health is....

Tick please!

very easy to understand	rather easy to understand	rather difficult to understand	very difficult to understand	don't know
❑	❑	❑	❑	❑

5) How easy or difficult is it for you to ...

Please make a cross in each line!

	very simple	rather simple	rather difficult	Very difficult	don't know
1. understand what the doctor is telling you	❑	❑	❑	❑	❑
2. to understand why you need vaccinations?	❑	❑	❑	❑	❑

Fig. 3.4 Question area health and health skills in the Life Skills Evaluation Study; third wave. (Adapted from Bollweg et al. 2020b, in press)

3. to understand what your parents tell you about your health?	❐	❐	❐	❐	❐
4. Understand why you also need to rest sometimes?	❐	❐	❐	❐	❐

Everywhere you can learn something about your health. But not everything you hear or read is true! So sometimes you have to judge for yourself what is right and what is perhaps rather wrong.

Judging, that is:

- **decide what is right or wrong**
- **decide who is right**
- **decide what is better**

6) When you hear something about health, how often do you think about whether it is true? *Please mark with a cross!*

(almost) never	rare	sometimes	often	(almost) always	don't know
❐	❐	❐	❐	❐	❐

7) How easy or difficult is it for you to ...

Please make a cross in each line!

	very simple	rather simple	rather difficult	Very difficult	don't know
1. To judge what is good and what is bad to get rid of a cold?	❐	❐	❐	❐	❐
2. to judge whether it is true what can happen to you later if you start smoking?	❐	❐	❐	❐	❐
3. assess how where you live (neighborhood, districts, street) relates to your health?	❐	❐	❐	❐	❐
4. assess how your behavior (exercise and diet) relates to your health?	❐	❐	❐	❐	❐

Often it is not enough just to know what is healthy. Some things have to be done! How is that with you?

Fig. 3.4 (continued)

8) How easy or difficult is it for you to ...

Please make a cross in each line!

	very simple	rather simple	rather difficult	Very difficult	don't know
1. to do what your parents tell you to do to get better?	❐	❐	❐	❐	❐
2. to call an ambulance in case of emergency?	❐	❐	❐	❐	❐
3. to stick to what you have learned in traffic lessons learned?	❐	❐	❐	❐	❐
4. to eat healthy?	❐	❐	❐	❐	❐
5. to have a say in whether or not School gives healthy food?	❐	❐	❐	❐	❐

Fig. 3.4 (continued)

Figure 3.5 shows the response distribution of the 18 items used for the health literacy scale. It can be seen here that more than 80% of the respondents usually consider the task to be very simple or simple. The overview of the response variance thus illustrates quite clearly that in Germany, too, 11- to 15-year-old children and adolescents *on average already have a high (self-assessed) level of health literacy.*

However, it should be noted in this distribution that for each of the 18 items between one third and just under half of the 6th graders opted for the category "don't know" not shown here. This means that a large number of cases drop out of the more complex calculations – in our view, the now common procedure of imputing missing values is only of limited use because the "don't know" category, unlike traditional "missing values", is to be regarded as a content-related statement that should not simply be replaced by one of the other content-related categories. However, it should be kept in mind *that the instrument used is subject to some uncertainty, which is no longer apparent from the figures.*

In order to determine the possible social factors in the development of adolescent health literacy more precisely, the individual items were first combined into an unweighted sum score. Because the procedure of Jürgen Pelikan and others from the HLS-EU context implies that those children and adolescents who had ticked the category "don't know" are to be excluded from the calculations, the number of cases is reduced to just over 900 children and adolescents (N = 913). However, the dropouts do not show any significant differences with regard to migration background, gender and age in comparison with the sample, so there is no systematic bias. Only the state of Hesse is more strongly represented because there were fewer

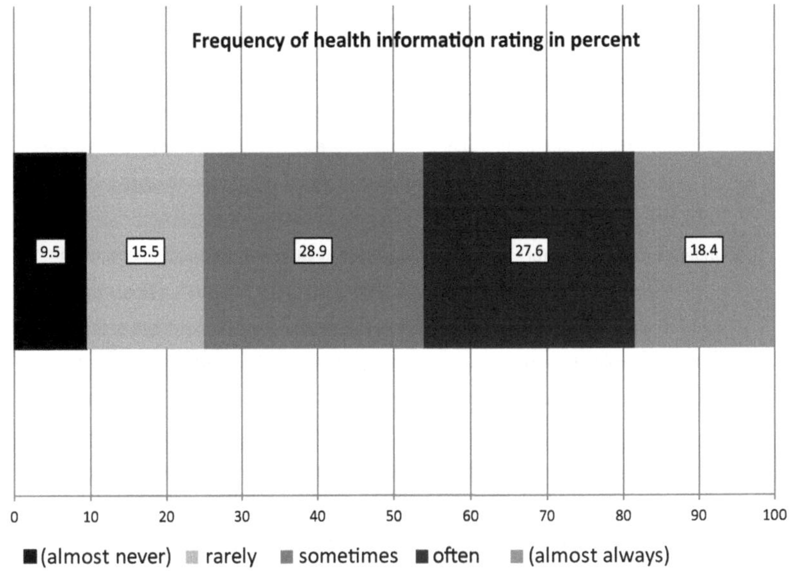

Fig. 3.5 Frequency of evaluation of health information N = 1012. (Own representation)

systematic dropouts in school participation here, and grammar schools are somewhat more frequent in the sub-sample (Fig. 3.6).

The calculated sum score was reversed by recoding so that high scores indicate high health literacy and can take values between 16 and 64, with 64 signifying the best score; this is the value achieved when an adolescent answers "very easy" to each of the questions shown above. Conversely, 16 is the score obtained when a person rates all questions as very difficult for him or her. The validity of the scale across the 16 items of the health literacy measurement (shown in Fig. 3.8) is comparatively high with a Cronbach's alpha of 0.877, so that a sum score can plausibly be formed here.

After compiling the sum score, we examined which social determinants for health literacy can be found at the individual level. We were guided by our analyses of the social determinants of the individual availability of life skills (Gerdes et al. 2016) and tested the virulent background variables, i.e., gender, federal state, age, migration background, school performance, parents' level of education and school type attendance, for their effects on individual health literacy, using a linear regression analysis. Some determinants for life skills also have a measurable effect on health literacy, while others such as the federal state (with the exception of

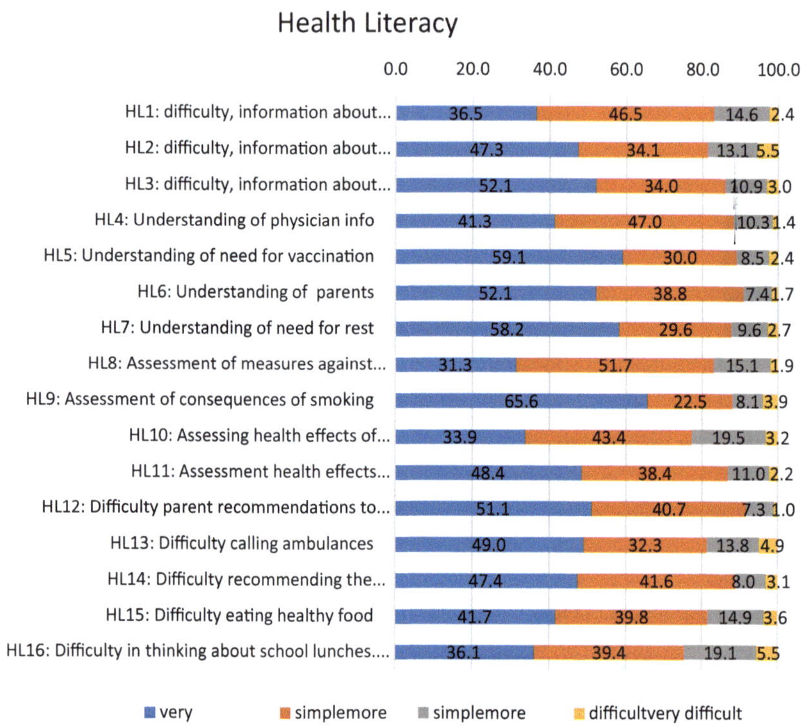

Fig. 3.6 Health literacy of 6th grade adolescents. On average, N = 1529 individuals participated per question, from N = 1353 (HL16) – N = 1614 (HL4). (Own representation)

Saxony-Anhalt, whose students have particularly low health literacy), but also age (11–15) do not play a role in the explanation. With regard to the significant determinants for child or adolescent health literacy frequently named in the literature, the following initially bivariate correlations are found in our data:

- Social background: based on the Family Affluence Scale, which is also widely used internationally in youth research (see e.g., Paakkari et al. 2018), there is a significant association between the social background of children and adolescents and self-reported health literacy (Anova, $p = 0.036$). Children and adolescents from the lowest wealth quartiles have the lowest scores on the health literacy scale, while children from the top quartile have the highest;
- Father's school education level: especially children and adolescents whose fathers have a high school diploma have higher scores on the health literacy

scale (Anova, $p = 0.05$; although the number of "don't know" answers is high here, so the correlations are hardly reliable);

- Mother's school education level: although the general trend of the distribution is similar to the father's school education, the significance level is not reached (Anova, $p = 0.130$; again, the number of "don't know" answers is very high);
- Own immigration history: Children and adolescents with own immigration history ($N = 51$), i.e., who were born abroad, do not differ significantly from those ($N = 861$) who were born in Germany (t-test, $p = 0.653$);
- Migration background: in our data, the unclear correlations known already from childhood- and adolescence-related health inequality research show up as well, which calls into question the generalised and undifferentiated use of the migration background variable as a whole. According to our data, children and adolescents with a unilateral migration background show significantly higher health literacy than children and adolescents with a bilateral or no migration background (Anova, $p = 0.033$);
- Gender: our sample also shows the oft-described gender difference with regard to (self-reported!) health literacy. Boys attribute higher health competencies to themselves than do girls (t-test, $p = 0.016$)
- School performance: Students with better school grades (measured as an index of Math, German, English, and Sports grades) achieve significantly higher scores on the sum score, even though the relation is not entirely linear (Anova, $p = 0.000$);
- School type attendance: Although pupils in special education have on average the lowest health literacy, the overall association between school type affiliation and health literacy is not significant (Anova, $p = 0.101$).

Examining bivariate associations with a linear regression, some effects cancel each other out, while others remain stable. According to our data, there are significant associations with gender, the birthplace of the father (but not the mother), school performance, and the wealth level of the family of origin; the other effects (e.g., one-sided migration background) disappear statistically or cancel each other out or are theoretically inconsistent.

It should also be noted that the explanatory power of the regression models we calculated is a very weak 2.4% (adjusted r-squared), so that we can assume there are further determinants that we did not get to see.[4] Because the large number of "don't

[4]However, in many studies the explained variance is relatively low. In a recent Lithuanian study, for example, an explained variance of 9% is achieved, a value that is not outstanding either but remains uncommented here. Cf. Sukys et al. (2019, p. 7).

know" responses limited the number of cases, we could not include an arbitrary number of variables in the regression model, but rather had to take a stepwise approach and sort out variables repeatedly. We document here only one of many models that we calculated, to illustrate the correlations that are – from our point of view – theoretically fairly convincing as well (cf. Table 3.2).

As can be seen in Table 3.2 above in the documentation of the coefficients, there is the gender difference already mentioned, according to which boys attribute to themselves higher health literacy than do girls. Pupils whose fathers were born abroad have lower health literacy – but there is no correlation with the mother's place of birth. This is not particularly plausible: it is unlikely that an explanation based on socialisation theory can be found that convincingly comments on these parental differences.

Furthermore, a significant difference can be found between very good students and good students with regard to self-reported health literacy. A significant difference in self-reported health literacy cannot be found between very good and average students but can be found between very good and poor students. These non-linear relationships cannot be very well interpreted because the notion of the relationship between health literacy and individual school performance is only convincing in the context of a continuous model. Finally, our data indicate significant differences between students' wealth levels and self-reported health literacy. Students from the lowest wealth quartile have the lowest scores compared to all other peers. As already clearly emphasised, these significant correlations are theoretically convincing – at least in part – but their significance is considerably limited by the fact that, on the one hand, the proportion of students excluded from the analysis due to "don't know" answers is large and that the explained variance of the regression model is very low. However, it is also clear in our study that the vast majority of students (at least those who did not even once tick "don't know") consider themselves to be health competent.

The predictors of health literacy that we found are also found in other studies. A recent Lithuanian study, for example, found comparable predictors, which are, however, operationalized differently, see below – of health competencies: "Analysis demonstrated that gender, grade, and family affluence were significant predictors of HL. School achievement was also significant predictor of HL." (Sukys et al. 2019, p. 7).[5]

[5] In addition, the Lithuanian research group, which was involved in the internationally recognized Health Behavior in School-Aged Children studies, also investigated whether health promotion and preventive measures implemented in schools have an impact on

Table 3.2 Linear regression sum score health literacy

Variables entered/removed[a]

Model	Variables entered	Variables removed	Method
1	FAS dummy lower vs. upper wealth level, gender, Very good vs. good school performance, Country of birth father, FAS dummy lower wealth level vs. lower wealth middle, Very good vs. (rather) poor school performance, FAS dummy lower wealth level vs. wealth middle, Very good vs. mediocre school performance, FAS dummy lower wealth level vs. upper wealth middle[b]		Enter

[a]Dependent variable: Health literacy sum score (16 items)

[b]All requested variables entered

Model Summary

Model	R	R square	Adjusted R square	Std. error of the estimate	Change statistics				
					R square change	F Change	df1	df2	Sig. F change
1	0.190[a]	0.036	0.024	6.822	0.036	2.926	9	705	0.002

[a]Predictors: (Constant), FAS dummy lower vs. upper wealth level, gender, Very good vs. good school performance, Country of birth father, FAS dummy lower wealth level vs. lower middle wealth level, Very good vs. (rather) poor school performance, FAS dummy lower wealth level vs. middle wealth level, Very good vs. mediocre school performance, FAS dummy lower wealth level vs. upper middle wealth level.

ANOVA[a]

Model		Sum of squares	df	Mean square	F	Sig
1	Regression	1225,653	9	136.184	2.926	0.002[b]
	Residual	32,812,073	705	46.542		
	Total	34,037,726	714			

[a]Dependent variable: Health literacy sum score (16 items)

[b]Predictors: (Constant), FAS dummy lower vs. upper wealth level, gender, Very good vs. good school performance, Country of birth father, FAS dummy lower wealth level vs. lower middle wealth level, Very good vs. (rather) poor school performance, FAS dummy lower wealth level vs. middle wealth level, Very good vs. mediocre school performance, FAS dummy lower wealth level vs. upper middle wealth level.

(continued)

Table 3.2 (continued)

Variables entered/removed[a]			
Model	Variables entered	Variables removed	Method

Coefficients[a]						
Model		Unstandardised coefficients		Standardised coefficients	t	Sig
		B	Std. Error	Beta		
1	(Constant)	48.975	1.558		31.434	0.000
	Gender	1.050	0.518	0.076	2.028	0.043
	Country of birth father	1.437	0.615	0.092	2.338	0.020
	Very good vs. good school performance	−1.530	0.707	−0.102	−2.165	0.031
	Very good vs. mediocre school performance	−0.678	0.728	−0.046	−0.931	0.352
	Very good vs. (rather) poor school performance	−1.892	0.923	−0.094	−2.050	0.041
	FAS dummy lower wealth niv vs. lower wealth middle.	2.825	1.047	0.149	2.699	0.007
	FAS dummy lower wealth level vs. middle wealth level.	1.918	0.994	0.119	1.929	0.054
	FAS dummy lower wealth level vs. upper middle wealth level.	2.524	0.988	0.167	2.554	0.011
	FAS dummy lower vs. upper wealth level	3.408	1.067	0.202	3.195	0.001

[a]Dependent variable: Health literacy sum score (16 items)

In a final step, for comparability with the Austrian study (Röthlin et al. 2013), which here follows the general approach of the EU Health Literacy Survey (Pelikan et al. 2012b), we dichotomized the abbreviated version of the health literacy scale of the MoMChild project and recorded the health literacy of adolescents in different fields. Following the Austrian reference study's division of the health literacy scale into three groups (Röthlin et al. 2013), according to our data:

- *79.5% of adolescents had adequate health literacy;*
- *16.4% had a problematic and*
- *only 4.1% had inadequate health literacy*

However, as should be made clear here, these findings should only be interpreted with caution, on the one hand, because of the high proportion of "don't knows" in the young people's answers and, on the other hand, in consideration of the measurement instrument used here. A recent Lithuanian study of seventh to tenth graders, for example, arrives at completely different assessments based on a short instrument developed by Lena Paakkari and colleagues (Paakkari et al. 2016). The instrument focuses on other areas, such as critical health literacy and democracy orientation, and is therefore considerably more demanding overall than the HLS-EU short version we used, despite containing only 10 items. "The HL instrument used contains ten items related to theoretical and practical knowledge, critical thinking, self-awareness, and citizenship." (Sukys et al. 2019, p. 5). In Lithuania, on this basis, across all age groups, about 12% of people are attested low health literacy, about 70% moderate health literacy, and about 17% high health literacy (Sukys et al. 2019).

There are massive shifts after the dichotomization of the items[6] with regard to significant differences in health literacy, which have to do with the lower differentiation and the overall very high values. An appropriately formed health literacy factor has the consequence that almost all correlations found on the health literacy quad scale fall below the significance level. Finally, we wanted to replicate the Austrian finding by Röthlin and colleagues that health literacy as measured by the

individual health literacy levels, with quite positive consequences: "Among variables related to a perceived school focus on healthy lifestyle promotion, only the prevention of bullying was a significant predictor of HL. School-based health promotion events held in the previous three months were also a significant predictor of HL." (Sukys et al. 2019, p. 7).

[6]We excluded the cases with white-not-answers and set 1 for a negative response and 2 for a positive response, so that higher scale scores are associated with higher self-reported health literacy. The range across all 16 items of the health literacy scale is thus from 16 to 32.

widely used instruments is dependent on the level of formal schooling.[7] Therefore, we first examined whether the school type is related to the individual health literacy level. Indeed, at first sight, the school type corresponds with the health literacy level of the students. The following table and figure illustrate the distribution of health literacy along the school type attendance (Fig. 3.7; Table 3.3).

If – as in the Austrian reference study – the correlation is presented along the three categories used to roughly determine individual health literacy, the following picture emerges (cf. Fig. 3.7). It is true that a – more or less – linear dependency can be established between the type of school and the respective proportions of sufficient, problematic or inadequate self-reported health literacy. Thus, for example, grammar school pupils and pupils of comprehensive schools[8] state with clearly more than 80% that they have sufficient health literacy, and this at an average age of 12 years. Although pupils in special schools fall significantly behind, even among them almost 70% state that they have sufficient health literacy skills, while the figure for pupils in lower secondary schools is just under three quarters.

Although the correlations are bivariate significant (Chi-Square: 16,107; df 8; $p = 0.041$), school type in multivariate calculations does not provide significant further clarification compared to the determinants already presented, and the effects disappear behind the other correlations. Thus, at the level of multivariate calculations, we cannot confirm the school type dependence of sixth graders' self-reported health competencies.

Finally, while in other studies health literacy is subdivided into the four skills (e.g., find, understand, assess, apply) and three domains (general, health promotion, disease prevention, disease treatment, here supplemented by 'general'), in our data only small correlations can be found between the items of the respective skill or domain. However, those students who stated that they had sought information about health showed significantly better health literacy than those who answered 'no'. (ρ

[7] In the study by Wallmann et al. (2012), in which the health knowledge ("factual knowledge about health in the sub-areas of nutrition, prevention, leisure and body knowledge) of North Rhine-Westphalian seventh graders was determined by means of a health quiz, there are also highly significant school type differences in the addressed areas of nutrition and body knowledge as well as prevention and leisure. Across all areas, grammar school pupils performed best and secondary modern school pupils worst (with one exception, where secondary modern school pupils were even worse; special schools were not taken into account). However, there were no gender differences at all, which is somewhat surprising in view of the rest of the health literacy research.

[8] We also surveyed Brandbenburg, a state that, alongside Berlin, has installed a 6-year primary school. Elementary schools are considered true comprehensive schools, so the categories are merged here.

Table 3.3 Anova – Dichotomised sum score health literacy in dependence on school type attendance

					95% Confidence interval for mean			
	N	Mean	Std. deviation	Std. Error	Lower bound	Upper bound	Minimum	Maximum
High School	377	30.20	2.423	0.125	29.96	30.45	16	32
Primary and comprehensive school	136	30.36	2.286	0.196	29.97	30.75	21	32
Middle school	253	29.62	2.614	0.164	29.29	29.94	20	32
Secondary modern school	123	29.85	2.322	0.209	29.43	30.26	23	32
Special needs school	29	28.72	3.250	0.604	27.49	29.96	19	32
Total	918	29.97	2.495	0.082	29.81	30.13	16	32
	Sum of squares		df		Mean square	F	Sig	
Between groups	119,453		4		29,863	4879	0.001	
Within groups	5587,693		913		6120			
Total	5707,146		917					

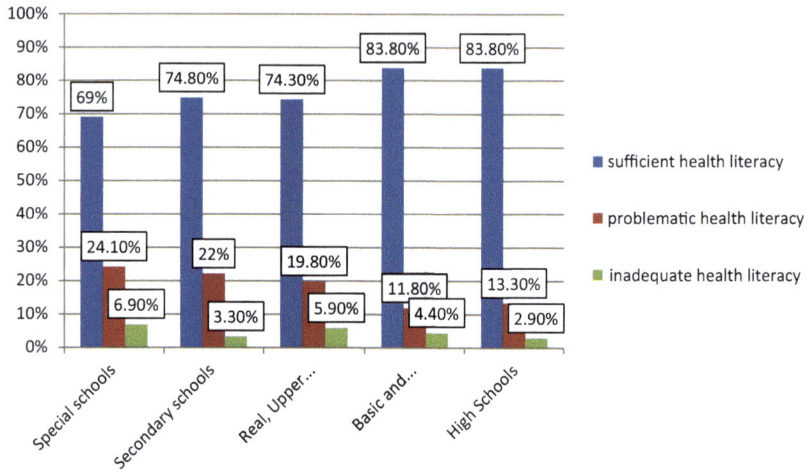

Fig. 3.7 Health literacy by school type; N = 918. (Own representation)

= 0.122, $p < 0.001$). In contrast, the frequency of (critical) evaluation of health information was not related to health literacy.

Overall, our study replicates the Austrian finding (Röthlin et al. 2013) that students assess themselves to be very health competent in the context of a self-report. In our study, this seemed to go for even younger children as well. However, we will discuss in more detail in the further course to what extent much is gained with this on average extremely positive self-assessment.

3.2.3 Effects of Adolescent Health Literacy

Because health literacy was not the focus of the main study, we did not collect a battery of possible outcome variables on which health literacy in adolescence could have a positive influence. We simply wanted to examine whether self-reported health literacy was related to self-assessed health status – with response options of "very good," "good," "fair," "poor," "very poor," and "don't know." After excluding the "don't know" answers, a comparison of means reveals highly significant differences in the assumed direction: the better the reported health status, the higher the mean score on the health literacy scale, i.e., the higher the individual health literacy (see Table 3.4). An S-N-K post hoc test revealed significant mean differences across all three categories of self-reported health literacy.[9]

However, it should be noted that we cannot say anything about the direction of the effects: whether better health leads to higher health literacy or vice versa, higher health literacy leads to better health must remain open on the basis of our data. The ambiguities in theoretical conceptualization are also highlighted by a strong study by Leena Paakkari and colleagues (Paakkari et al. 2019b). Using representative data on 11-, 13- and 15-year-old Finnish students collected and analysed in the Health Behavior in School-Aged Children-Study, Leena Paakkari and colleagues used pathway models to test whether adolescents' health literacy functions as an independent determinant of individual health outcomes or as a mediator of underlying structural inequalities. According to their calculations, both are the case:

> We tested whether among adolescents HL [meaning health literacy; d. V.] is an *independent* factor explaining health outcomes, and also whether it *mediates* the association between the structural stratifiers and the health outcomes. Both hypotheses were confirmed. HL was found to be an independent factor explaining disparities in health. Thus, higher HL was related to positive health outcomes, and its role persisted after the structural stratifiers (school achievement, educational aspiration, family affluence scale, age and gender) were added to the model. HL also served as a partial mediator. The role of HL as a mediator seemed to be stronger in relation to the perceived health indicators (i.e. self-rated health, alertness, self-esteem, life-satisfaction and multiple health complaints) than it was to health behaviors.[. . .] The mediating role was clearest in relation to school-related factors (i.e. school achievement and educational aspiration), and to all the other health indicators except smoking. Poor school achievement is connected to a lower level of HL, and hence to poorer health outcomes. (Paakkari et al. 2019a, p. 4).

The simultaneity of determination and mediation of health literacy effects on health attitudes and health behaviour is empirically well determined but cannot satisfy from a theoretical point of view. This inconsistency in the relationships between health literacy and health-related outcomes is fairly frequent for the age groups of children and adolescents and more or less independent of the measurement methods. In a large representative study of students from Taiwan, there are associations between individual health literacy and overweight or underweight in 11- and 12-year-old children even after controlling for socio-demographic variables, but the statistically significant associations do not follow a clear direction:

[9] Without being able to pursue this further at this point, an analysis of the relationship between general life skills and self-reported health skills would be promising.

Table 3.4 Relationship between health literacy and general health status

Current state of health

	N	Mean	Std. deviation	Std. Error	95% Confidence interval for mean		Minimum – very good	Maximum – very poor
					Lower bound	Upper bound		
Inadequate health skills	35	2.77	0.973	0.164	2.44	3.11	1	5
Problematic health skills	147	2.16	0.836	0.069	2.03	2.30	1	4
Sufficient health skills	715	1.82	0.882	0.033	1.76	1.89	1	5
Total	897	1.92	0.903	0.030	1.86	1.98	1	5

ANOVA

Current state of health

	Sum of squares	df	Mean square	F	Sig
Between groups	40,680	2	20,340	26,352	0.000
Within groups	690,049	894	0.772		
Total	730,729	896			

"After controlling for sex, ethnicity, self-rated health status and health behaviors, being in the highest quartile of health literacy was associated with lower likelihood of being either underweight or obese. However, higher health literacy was associated with higher likelihood of being overweight than having normal weight." (Shih et al. 2016, p. 4).

The particular strength of the study by Paakkari and colleagues, however, lies in pointing out that the theoretical understanding of health literacy does not yet go very far and is still rather empirical-inductive. Overall, most studies concentrate on determining the impact of unequal individual health literacy on health behaviour or direct health outcomes.

Studies show that the extent of health literacy could be relevant for the personal health biography already at an early age. A systematic review has shown that low health literacy among adolescents is associated with increased risk behaviour and is associated with an overall increase in unhealthy behaviour (DeWalt and Hink 2009). By the same token, a Taiwanese study has shown that among sixth grade students, as health literacy levels increase, risk-taking decreases and reinforcement of health-promoting behaviours are observable (Liu et al. 2014: cited from the abstract available online). Furthermore, an intervention study demonstrated a positive effect of improved health literacy on self-efficacy in adolescents (Nutbeam 2000). Health literacy thus has a protective weight that could make it a key concept in health promotion, especially in childhood and adolescence. (Okan et al. 2017b).

To summarise the state of quantitative research, the available studies on health literacy in adolescence identify on the one hand higher self-reported health literacy among adolescents than among adults – this is shown by our own data as well as by the data from Austria. We are, for the time being, inclined to interpret these high values as a high level of *health self-confidence among* adolescents, especially if it is taken into account that adults score better when health literacy gets measured by other instruments. The influence of adolescent health literacy on various health-related behavioural characteristics (especially nutrition or risk behaviour), person-related competencies and life skills (e.g., self-efficacy) and at least partially on health outcomes can be described as assured. After the state of research on health literacy in adolescence has been presented, the following section looks in more detail at health literacy in children and their families.

3.3 Health Literacy of Children and Family Health Literacy

With regard to research on child health literacy, there is a large consensus in public health, medical research and social epidemiology: the state of research on children is extremely poor (Maier and Felder-Puig 2017). The aetiology, genesis and individual expression of child health literacy are poorly understood (Okan et al. 2015, p. 930). As mentioned several times before, this is quite surprising, considering the importance of especially very early behavioural manifestations for later health-related lifestyle, which after all follows the general rule that the earlier a behaviour or disease detrimental to health is established, the worse the consequences (Okan 2019b). Health-related attitudes and health behaviours "formed during childhood greatly predict adult health patterns. For example, children's food preferences and media behaviors are significantly related to being overweight or at risk for obesity in adulthood." (Borzekowski 2009, p. 287).

However, the fact that health literacy, not only in adolescents but also in children and young children is addressed at all, *directly* and not only indirectly via their parents, in itself requires explanation, since part of the classic image of childhood is the massive dependence on older reference persons, above all on parents and guardians, to whom an overriding influence on the health of children is attributed. Especially in the context of health-damaging behaviour during pregnancy, this motive becomes virulent, for example, when the mother smokes or drinks alcohol, or another close caregiver (father, stepfather/adoptive/foster father, cohabitant, uncle, aunt, etc.) consumes tobacco in the vicinity of the mother, thus condemning the mother (and the foetus) to passive smoking. This conceptualization of childhood follows the idea that children are very special beings worthy of protection and very special vulnerable beings who are best served by adults behaving in their best interests – which of course includes enforcing the prohibition of things that lead or could lead (in the medium and long term) to conditions detrimental to health, such as excessive consumption of sugary drinks or sweets.

Nevertheless, the concept of child health literacy conveys more than the paternalistic perspectives on childhood briefly alluded to here, which define the child as a comparatively passive receptor of surrounding socialisation conditions. Childhood and also early childhood health literacy conveys at least one further meaning that goes hand in hand with the fact that notions of childhood have gained significant momentum in the social sciences and simple models of conditioning/imprinting, as classically spelled out by Talcott Parsons in socialisation research, have receded into the background (Bröder and Carvalho 2019). Instead, children are theoretically conceptualised as active shapers of their own environment – in contrast to incompetent, incomplete adult social actors – in childhood research (Alanen 1988; Bründel and Hurrelmann 1996; Bühler-Niederberger 2010; Andresen and Möller 2019). This subjective, individual-oriented understanding of early childhood is directly transferred to health literacy research in the German-speaking context, for example, in the Bielefeld Research Group on Health Literacy (cf. e.g., Okan 2019b; Bröder and Carvalho 2019; Okan et al. 2015; Pinheiro et al. 2021). This active understanding of childhood makes itself felt when very young children are attributed the ability to make their own health beneficial decisions (Rubene et al. 2015): 'Health literacy skills should be encouraged at a very young age [. . .] even the youngest child is able to gain the necessary skills on a path towards health literacy. Those between the ages of 3 and 18 can seek, comprehend, evaluate, and use health information, especially if materials are presented in ways that are appropriate, culturally relevant, and socially supported." (Borzekowski 2009, pp. 287, 288).[10]

Moreover, the notion of child health literacy is consistently linked to the dimension of empowerment (Rubene et al. 2015, pp. 334–335). This linking of health literacy and empowerment was already introduced and unfolded by Don Nutbeam in his classic contribution (Nutbeam 2000). But in the context of child health literacy, this research strand refers to a balancing, compensatory effect – Lena Paakkari and colleagues attribute an actual moral dimension to health literacy because, at least potentially, the compensatory dimension of health literacy can lead to social equality being significantly strengthened (Paakkari and George 2018, p. 3; Paakkari et al. 2019a, p. 1).

These considerations, which are based more on equity theory and the sociology of childhood, are extremely plausible, but have the flaw that it is hardly possible to measure the level of individual health literacy in 2-, 3- or 4-year-old children at all, let alone precisely. There is great disagreement about "at what point children and adolescents can take responsibility for their health, or at what point health-related learning starts." (Maier and Felder-Puig 2017, p. 9). A very ambitious project under the title MoMChild, which we have already presented in the previous chapter, has adapted the Health Literacy Scale of the European Health Literacy Survey for 9- to

[10]More recently, the concept of Child Well-Being has been developed and empirically pursued more comprehensively. The explicit aim here is to explore the individual spaces of action of adolescents and children in greater detail. In this research, "child and youth theoretical assumptions on the subject status of adolescents, critical debates on the social positioning of children and adolescents as well as [. . .] power imbalances between children and adults" are linked to Andresen and Möller (2019, p. 16). A future merging of this research strand with child-, youth- and family-related health literacy research seems promising.

10-year-old children and presented a validated instrument that is currently being tested in a larger-scale study (Bollweg et al. 2020a, in press; Bollweg et al. 2020b, in press). According to our own study, however, at least one third of pupils (12 years old on average (see Sect. 3.2) were unable to answer the questions. The KiGGS study of the Robert Koch Institute also includes 3- to 10-year-old children. However, it is the parents of the children who fill out the questionnaires that are interviewed here, and it is only from the age of eleven that children or adolescents are expected to report on their own health. Overall, especially when children self-report on specific health issues such as aesthetic body image, there is always the danger that general self-confidence and self-esteem are measured rather than health literacy in the narrower sense, without this being adequately reported. There is, however, one finding in the research literature that directly links children's health literacy with disease outcome: Low health literacy in children appears to be associated with higher body mass index (BMI) (Sharif and Blank 2010).

However, addressing child health literacy exclusively is not particularly plausible, because "in order to reach children, we had to engage with many different categories of adults – teachers, parents, school principals and administrators, educational officials and health professionals, and policy makers in local and national government" (Sijthoff 2014, p. 73). In this sense, *achieving high levels of (early) child health literacy is always a collaborative effort and a shared responsibility of family, educational institutions, healthcare system, mass media, or even religious prescriptions* (Rubene et al. 2015, p. 335). Analytically isolating children or their health literacy seems naive. Therefore, the determination of child health literacy cannot be achieved without considering parental caregivers. When dealing with the health and health literacy of children, therefore reference must always made to intergenerational relationships (cf. Brady et al. 2015).

However, the analysis of intergenerational relationships in particular is generally approached in the literature in such a way that the activity and autonomy theoretically attributed to children is again withdrawn and the measurable effects of parental health literacy on the outcomes of childhood disease factors are specified. First, high maternal educational attainment is generally considered an important predictor of high child health literacy (Okan et al. 2017b, p. 11). However, the focus is on the now well-documented relationship between low health literacy among parents – or, more precisely, mothers – and the health status or health behaviour of their children.

It has been shown, for example, that low health literacy in mothers is associated with a lower birth weight of their babies (Forbis et al. 2002; Yin et al. 2007). Mothers with low health literacy breastfeed their children less frequently and for a shorter period of time (Speer 2017, p. 16). Mothers with low health literacy are less likely to take advantage of preventive health services for themselves and their children and have difficulty correctly understanding and following instructions about their child's medication (Sanders et al. 2009; Yin 2017). If the parents of children with a chronic illness have low health literacy levels, this is often associated with poorer disease management in the child (Ross 2001; DeWalt et al. 2007). Children of parents with low health literacy are less likely to have health insurance,[11] more likely to have untreated health problems, and less likely to have a peadiatrician in charge (Sanders et al. 2005; Miller et al. 2010). At the same time, parents with low health literacy are significantly more likely to visit emergency medical facilities with their children without having an actual emergency present, at least in the United States. Michael Speer – as Don Nutbeam classically did – first points to the very close connection between reading/writing skills and health literacy, between literacy and health literacy. From this close connection, he describes the links between low maternal health literacy and new-born or infant care and draws the following broad conclusion: "Low parental literacy [as the most important predictor of health literacy in the care-oriented measurements; addition by the authors] affects almost every aspect of newborn and infant care, including breastfeeding, use of the emergency room, medication administration, and participation in social welfare programs." (Speer 2017, p. 16). On this basis, one of the common calls is to improve child health literacy by strengthening parental or, more commonly, maternal health literacy (Maier and Felder-Puig 2017, p. 38).[12]

However, it is precisely at this largely consensual interface of the significance of parental or maternal health literacy for child (health literacy) development that two difficulties arise. *First,* the question relevant to the theory and practice of socialisation of the actual health literacy transmission as it takes place in families on a daily basis remains largely in the dark. This assessment is widely accepted internationally: "There is a need for further research in this context […] to

[11] This connection refers to the U.S.A.; however, it is somewhat absurd in the context of health literacy, because it can surely be assumed that even (very) uneducated parents know that health insurance makes sense for themselves and their child(ren). If this connection is seriously argued, it is evidence of health literacy taking the place of the discussion about poverty and social inequality and transfiguring brutal deficits in health care in terms of competence theory.

[12] Of course, this is not entirely consistent argumentation, because the basis of the close correlation (in standardized measurements) of literacy and health literacy would first have to lead to a massive general education initiative and strengthening of the literacy level of mothers. However, this educational policy step is rarely taken explicitly. On the other hand, we will discuss in detail in the next chapter how problematic this education-based argumentation is.

determine how exactly health literacy is transmitted from parents to their children in order to develop effective programs and interventions." (Maier and Felder-Puig 2017, p. 38). And further, "The impact of parental health literacy and the health outcomes of young children is a poorly studied area." (Speer 2017, p. 15), *Secondly,* although the importance of the child's socialisation context is emphasised and the lifeworld, milieu-specific or context-specific dimension of child health literacy in particular is repeatedly referred to, it is precisely these dimensions that no longer play any role at all when it comes to strengthening parental health literacy. Instead, there is a kind of health interventionist switch from the context of action within the family to a setting perspective, which is seen as promising here in terms of the good accessibility of vulnerable groups in their settings. A good example is the German National Action Plan on Health Literacy (NAG), whose progressive momentum of not fixing health literacy to health care settings is then redirected by a very strong focus on educational institutions.

The NAG distinguishes four fields of action, three of which are located in the clinical-medical-supply-technical area, the fourth area signals a lifeworld-milieu-specific approach under the keyword "*Promoting health literacy in all lifeworlds*". The following passages can be found under this heading by way of orientation and recommendation for action:

"What to Do?"

Firmly embed health literacy in the education and curricula of day-care centres, primary schools, secondary schools, higher education institutions, youth education and vocational training institutions, and adult education.

Conduct project weeks on health literacy in day-care centres, schools and other educational institutions and establish health as a school subject in the long term, if possible, but in any case integrate it into teaching as a cross-curricular, interdisciplinary aspect.

First aid combined with psychological, nursing and medical counselling in the form of school health care should be institutionally anchored in the educational and training institutions.

Enable staff of educational and training institutions through further training to contribute specifically to the promotion of health literacy" (Schaeffer et al. 2019, p. 31).

The lifeworld concept is first used to draw attention to the importance of the family context for action and then almost completely reformatted in the recommendations and strategies for action.[13] From *directly addressing family environments* to strengthen parental health literacy, which is supposed to be associated with a positive transfer to children's health literacy, it is switched to an *indirect influence in educational settings* through health literacy programmes in kindergartens, day care centres or schools. This somewhat strange and not openly discussed switch in the National Action Plan on Health Literacy is not an isolated case but exemplifies a specific system. For example, in the otherwise strong HBSC study by Matthias Richter et al. the word adolescent lifeworlds only appears in the title of the book (Richter et al. 2008). Similarly, Lena Paakkari and Shanti George's strong perspective on the ethical and moral dimensions of health literacy end up in the classroom (Paakkari and George 2018, pp. 3–4). And even a child-centred empowerment perspective on child health literacy addresses a health literate child primarily in the context of school-based health education, although the importance of parental framework settings is explicitly named (Rubene et al. 2015). Therefore, the following assessment by Dana Borzekowski, made over 10 years ago, is, in our view, still highly relevant today: "Although recommended initiatives to improve health literacy often include primary and secondary teachers, nurses, and librarians, the populations with whom these professionals work are hardly mentioned." (Borzekowski 2009, 284).

The picture that emerges with regard to children's and early childhood health literacy is that children are believed to have independent health literacy at a very early age, but that this remains largely dependent on the socialisation structure of parents and non-parents. Although the importance of parents, and especially the frequently emphasised importance of mothers for children's health literacy, is universally agreed upon, in order to strengthen parental health literacy, it is not families directly that are addressed, but rather educational settings as mediating instances (the situation is described similarly in a good current research overview in Austria; Maier and Felder-Puig 2017, p. 25). The mechanisms of the transition of health literacy within the families remain a black box. Studies on the individual availability of health skills of parents and children remain analytically separate. A concept like Family Health Literacy would be promising, which develops

[13] Raimund Geene points out that the family is not a setting in the sense of the WHO, although it is relatively often referred to as such, especially in public health; cf. Geene 2018 However, this depends very much on how precisely the concept of setting is defined. In our context, family is above all a pre-eminent locus of health socialisation and can be unproblematically linked to the setting concept insofar as the family directly represents the lifeworld of children and adolescents, is conceptualised in a supra-individual way, and can be considered a particularly promising area of public health and health literacy interventions.

intergenerational perspectives from the beginning,[14] but an elaborated theory and a developed concept of Family Health Literacy are not (yet) available (cf. for instance Levin-Zamir et al. 2017; Rosenbaum et al. 2007).[15] The massive tension between emphasising the *importance of family contexts* for the development of children's health literacy *and simultaneously ignoring those very contexts* is one of the central findings of our analysis of the state of research so far.

After presenting and discussing the literature on health inequalities and health literacy in childhood and adolescence, which is primarily based on quantitative studies, in the last section of this chapter we will discuss a topic that is specifically related to childhood and adolescence and that can be defined as digital health literacy, or a number of similar terms.

3.4 Child and Adolescent Health and Digital Health Literacy

The topic of digital health literacy is an integral part of health literacy research and debate and is becoming increasingly prominent. Particularly with regard to the health literacy of children and adolescents, so-called eHealth literacy plays a particularly central role because the younger generation has been described as "digital natives"since the early 2000s, i.e. as a generation that is socialised, as it were from birth, into the technical possibilities and achievements of the Internet and its digital advancements.[16] Digital media are already an everyday companion for

[14]This is in contrast to parental health literacy, which again refers to a one-sided directionality of simply transferring parental health literacy to the child and excludes the autonomous development of children.

[15]It should also be pointed out that in the existing work on Family Health Literacy primarily the parents and the child are considered, but the learning through and from the experiences of the sibling(s) has so far remained unnoticed. In this respect, the concept of Family Health Literacy lacks a realistic conception of family.

[16]Over the last 15 years, a larger number of proposed terms have proliferated: thus, one can find side by side the terms eHealth Literacy (classically: Norman and Skinner 2006), Media Health Literacy (e.g. Levin-Zamir et al. 2011), Electronic Health Literacy (e.g. Seçkin et al. 2016), Digital Health Literacy (e.g. Del Giudice 2017) or, even more specifically, Internet Health Literacy (e.g. Robinson and Graham 2010) and Mobile Health Literacy (e.g. Vaz 2017). For the purposes of this study, we will not pursue the fine ramifications of these terms, which are in any case due in large part to the attention economy of scientific production, but will use the common terms eHealth Literacy or, in a German translation, digitale Gesundheitskompetenzen.

children and young people. The reason why we are devoting a separate section to the concept of digital health literacy relates not only to the presence of the topic in public discourse but also to the fact that children's (and thus families'!) and adolescents' lifeworlds are more or less completely permeated by the Internet and the necessary connected devices for using it, such as smartphones, tablets, and so on. For Germany and Switzerland, it is true that the question of access to the Internet is no longer problematic for young people, but also increasingly for children: "Regardless of the distribution channel, all young people today have more or less unrestricted access to the Internet. And at the same time, the involvement in everyday life has increased again in 2018. 91% of 12- to 19-year-olds are online every day – a renewed increase on the previous year (2017: 89%, 2016: 87%). For the second time in a row, a slightly higher proportion of girls (93%) than boys (90%) are daily online, and the differences in age have weakened significantly." (mpfs – Medienpädagogischer Forschungsverbund Südwest 2018, p. 31). For Switzerland, the same findings apply. "'Access to the Internet has become less tangible for young people [. . .] and a matter of course." (Suter et al. 2018, p. 74).

Digital media allow access to the unlimited digital world, providing young people with opportunities for entertainment, interaction and information. Among them are numerous health-related offers. In contrast to earlier times, in the age of the Internet the basic problem for children and adolescents is not so much the scarcity of information and the provision of information, but rather the precise search for information and the appropriate evaluation of information, which, however, adds a further level of complexity to the already complex topic of individual health literacy. This is because studies indicate that children and adolescents must have a wide variety of skills in order to be able to deal adequately with digital health information. This does not only include skills that are based on the increasingly complex technical access that is associated with new media and the deliberate search for information. Going significantly beyond this, the question of the *content* and *reliability of the information* and the subjective ability to assess reliability is also discussed as a central eHealth literacy competence dimension. In this context, the "end of information scarcity" topic is particularly important.

> The ongoing health literacy crisis is not caused by lack of information. Information abounds in much of today's world – including for adolescents and children – as a consequence of globalization and the technology that supports rapid development of the internet and media. Children make use of the internet at increasingly younger ages, with a recent study from Finland revealing that 81% of the children aged seven to eight are allowed to use internet at home, and one third does so daily. Neither is the crisis about skills required to gain access to information, as was the case in the late twentieth century when information was limited, not easily available and took different forms.

> Now, in contrast, the internet's exponential development in a globalized world requires skills to use effectively an abundance of health information and to distinguish between information of varying quality through comparison, classification and assessment of credibility. (Paakkari and George 2018, p. 5).

In addition to the end of information scarcity, a second topic appears here that is significant for eHealth literacy in children and adolescents. In childhood and adolescence, individual health literacy and (critical) media literacy are obviously very much intertwined (as argued by Borzekowski 2009, p. 284; Bröder et al. 2017, p. 15).

3.4.1 Definitions of eHealth Literacy

The fact that media skills are seen as playing such a significant role in the maintenance of health, in health-promoting behaviour and in the establishment of a healthy lifestyle as early as childhood and adolescence is also illustrated by the pertaining attempts to define eHealth literacy (and its synonyms). The three most frequently used definitions come from Eng, Eysenbach, and Norman and Skinner. At the beginning of the health literacy debate, Eng introduced a brief definition that is very close to common general health literacy concepts, defining digital health literacy as "the use of emerging information and communication technology, especially the Internet, to improve or enable health and health care" (Eng 2001, p. 15). In contrast, Eysenbach defined eHealth literacy much more comprehensively, finding it to be an interdisciplinary field and taking it far beyond the utilisation of health-related information.

> ehealth is an emerging field in the intersection of medical informatics, public health and business, referring to health services and information delivered or enhanced through the Internet and related technologies. In a broader sense, the term characterizes not only a technical development, but also a state-of-mind, a way of thinking, an attitude, and a commitment for networked, global thinking, to improve health care locally, regionally, and worldwide by using information and communication technology. (Eysenbach 2001, e20)

The work and definition that still determines the discourse today comes from Norman and Skinner, who not only defined eHealth literacy in abstract terms, but also operationalized it in empirical terms. They describe digital health literacy "as the ability to seek, find, understand, and appraise health information from electronic sources and apply the knowledge gained to addressing or solving a health problem"

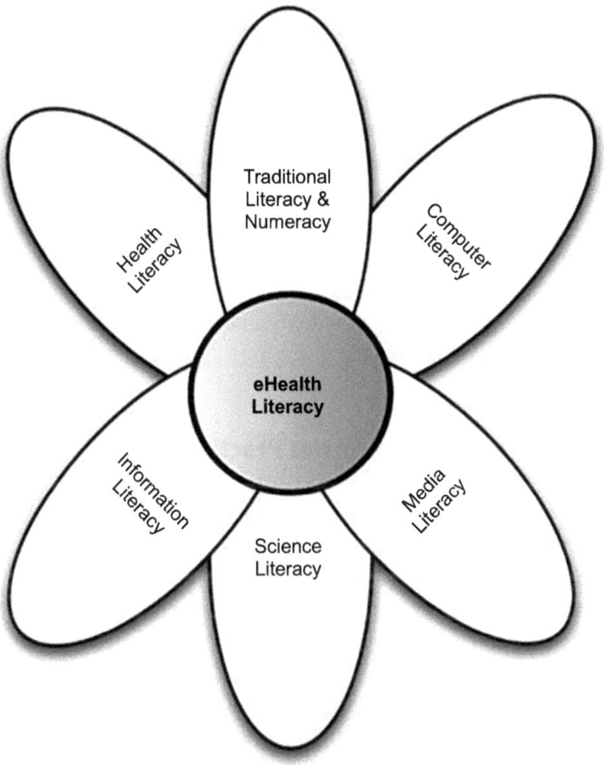

Fig. 3.8 ehealth literacy lily model. (Source: Norman and Skinner 2006, p. 3)

(Norman and Skinner 2006, p. 2). They further specified digital health literacy and created the Lily Model, which is still frequently used today as a standard for determining eHealth literacy (see Fig. 3.8).

In this model, six basic analytical and context-specific skills are arranged into an integrated competency model. As can be seen in Fig. 3.8, the analytical competencies include traditional literacy and numeracy, which relate to the formal level of education, reading and spelling and mathematical skills, and information and media literacy, which relate to the already application-oriented competencies that are aimed at dealing with information and new media. Beyond these dimensions, direct user competencies are also included as context-specific or context-sensitive competencies, which are understood as *computer literacy*. Strong is the inclusion of *scientific literacy*, which refers to a comprehensive understanding of science, including its sociological implications. This literacy concept is extremely ambitious: "For those who do not have the educational experience of exposure to scientific thought, understanding science-based online health information may present a formidable challenge. Science literacy places health research findings in appropriate context, allowing consumers to understand how science is done, the largely incremental process of discovery, and the limitations – and opportunities – that research can present." (Norman and Skinner 2006, p. 6). From our perspective, it is by no means clear that all those employed in the scientific field possess this dimension of competence as a matter of course. The last dimension is *health literacy*, which is quite orthodoxly understood as the execution of well-informed individual health decisions.

3.4.2 eHealth Literacy as Social Practice

In the meantime, the Lily model has also come under substantial criticism. For example, the action-theoretical foundation has been criticised as being too individual-centred. Gilstad in particular points out the subject-centred reduction. In this context, he proposes to include further competencies such as context-related and communicative competencies and extends the Lily model by the socio-cultural as well as situational context. According to Gilstad, it is precisely social factors such as social norms, belief horizons and shared ideas as well as socially shared values that significantly influence the use of digital health services (Gilstad 2014; Bautista 2015, p. 38, for example, argues similarly).

The emphasis on the social and cultural dimensions of technology use (Levin-Zamir et al. 2017) has advanced the discussion since Norman and Skinner and led to a more comprehensive definition of digital health literacy that focuses much more emphatically on the social embedding of individual technology use. John Robert Bautista provides the following most comprehensive definition of digital health literacy to date: "eHealth literacy involves the interplay of individual and social factors in the use of digital technologies to search, acquire, comprehend, appraise, communicate and apply health information in all contexts of healthcare with the goal of maintaining or improving the quality of life throughout the lifespan." (Bautista 2015, p. 43).

From our point of view, the emphasis on the social embedding of technology use is particularly significant for the health-related use of smartphones in childhood and adolescence, for example, because it draws attention to the fact that the popular idea of a lonely user is actually not true. First, the notion that the Internet outstrips the importance of peer socialisation must be rejected, precisely because under current socialisation conditions, the peer socialisation of children and adolescents itself has a digital dimension (Suter et al. 2018). Furthermore, the perspective of lonely user behaviour is a gross oversimplification because digital communication between children and adolescents is by no means a substitute, but rather a natural component of current communication – often enough simultaneous – alongside face-to-face communication.

In addition to the various contextual conditions within the peer group, the media behaviour of children and adolescents is also related to the sociocultural conditions within the family. Here, the migration background plays a significant role, at least for Swiss adolescents: Swiss adolescents without a migration background are significantly less likely to regularly do something with their family (25%) than adolescents with a migration background who live in Switzerland (36%) (Suter et al. 2018, p. 16). This significant difference should be taken with a grain of salt, however, because in both cases the clear majority of young people spend time with their families every day or several times a week. Nevertheless, this difference is important because it points to the importance of commonly shared values and norms in the familial, childhood, and adolescent socialisation process, along which distinction-relevant differentiators are anchored, in which individual technology use itself is embedded. And it points to something we will present in all three qualitative case studies, that at least for the (young) people we accompanied, family is the most significant resource for action not only in childhood but even in the context of adolescent health socialisation.

All in all, in the context of children's use of technology, it is very likely that in childhood the digital usage time allowed by parents is regarded within the peer group as a measure of autonomy and that owning a mobile phone at an early age represents a solid mark of distinction. The world of adolescents, on the other hand, is so permeated by the smartphone and being completely available around the clock that it requires justification to want to escape this as an adolescent and lead an analogue or at least limited digital life (it is not unlikely that at some point there will be such an analogue counter movement among privileged adolescents). Finally, the motif of social embeddedness leads directly to the relationship between digital health skills and social inequality.

3.4.3 eHealth Literacy and the Relationship to Social and Health Inequalities

As is often the case, the introduction of new technologies is associated with the hope of improving current ills, or with the suggestion that the latest technological developments tend to even deepen the rifts of social inequalities. In an extensive literature review, we found that the focus of the question about the relationship between social and digital inequalities in the context of health has shifted over the last 15 years, at least in highly industrialised countries. Until the mid-2000s, the question of *access* was still the focus of digital inequalities, health-related or not. Social inequality was operationalized as unequal access to the option spaces of the Internet (see, for example, Klein 2008; Cleppien and Kutscher 2004; Kutscher and Otto 2010).

Meanwhile, this focus has shifted significantly. As to the digital penetration of adolescent lifeworlds in Germany, the current JIM study shows that 97% of adolescents use the internet, 80% of adolescents aged 12–19 is online daily, 12% twice a week (mpfs – Medienpädagogischer Forschungsverbund Südwest 2018). Similar results come out in the James study for Switzerland. For example, 100% of households have a mobile phone, and 97% have internet access (Suter et al. 2018, p. 18), although overall device availability (e.g., ownership of tablet in the household) varies significantly by family socioeconomic status (Suter et al. 2018). Paakkari and George (2018, p. 5) also refer to the fact that the starting point of an at least partially autonomous use of the internet occurs at increasingly earlier stages of childhood. In the context of digital inequalities, there has therefore been a shift since the mid-2000s from the question of technical access to the question of content access and the question of concrete usage behaviour. Inequality is thus supposed to be generated by the use itself (cf. e.g., Klein 2016).

Following this direction, very different dimensions of social and, as a consequence, health inequality come to the fore. It should only be briefly pointed out at this point that in the central German-language reference studies for Internet use by young people – the JIM study and the JAMES study – the topic of health plays no role. In the current JIM study (mpfs – Medienpädagogischer Forschungsverbund Südwest 2018), the word health does not even appear, in the JAMES study it appears exactly once, in connection with an assumed but unexplained increase in adolescent health competencies in the context of an increase in the importance of Healthy Lifestyles (Suter et al. 2018, p. 74). The concept of *linking media education, health sciences, and health literacy research is, it seems to us at least, still very much in its infancy.*

In the context of children's and adolescents' now generally easy access to the Internet, the main issue with regard to health literacy is whether children or adolescents are also able to decode the information they find on Internet sites and to understand the meaning of the information. Henna Kim and Bo Xie show in a systematic literature review that (lacking) readability of content, and ease of use emerge as key barriers to accessing and using online health information (Kim and Xie 2017). With this focus, the conventional literacy of children and adolescents comes more clearly to the fore again in the middle of the field of application of digital health literacy and thus, for example in Germany, also the question of the school type-specific effects of digital health literacy which have, to our knowledge, not yet been researched. The findings presented above (Sect. 3.2) on the dependence of the individual health literacy level (on the Bielefeld scale, which has been shortened to 16 items and dichotomized) on the type of school to which young people aged eleven to fifteen belong are an indication in this direction.

Another inequality-relevant dimension paradoxically results from an increased usage time of digital media. In particular, this concerns the time that children and young people spend playing digital games, now usually online and worldwide. This can be done on specialised game consoles, which have long since been connected to the Internet, or on a normal PCs, laptop computers or internet-enabled television set. There are a number of studies that indicate that children and young people of low social status spend on average significantly more time in front of screens (screen time) than do children and young people from the middle and upper classes. The higher the screen time, the higher the level of physical inactivity. Particularly intensive use of the digital world in childhood and adolescence is then associated with pathological Internet addiction, which is certainly the extreme opposite of the eHealth literacy envisaged by optimists. The WHO has already included gaming and internet addiction (internet addiction, gaming disorder, pathological internet use or compulsive internet use are the frequently mentioned English-language terms) in the new ICD 11 disease catalogue (see e.g., WHO 2019). However, from our point of view, considerable caution is advised with regard to the readily conveyed image of excessive consumption of digital (or, classically, analogue media as well: daily soaps on television, etc.) media by the adolescent generation – preferably of the lower social classes, even if these are of course not the only ones affected – because they are associated with a host of implicit normative ideas about the good (health-oriented) life, which themselves need to be questioned (Bittlingmayer and Ziegler 2012; Schmidt 2017; Kühn 1993).

Finally, there is the classic distributional inequality dimension, which deals with the socially unequal distribution of digital health skills. Here, the state of research is not very well developed. One of the few elaborate studies comes from Israel and examines the availability of the so-called *media health literacy of* 11-, 13-, and 15-year-old adolescents. In particular, this study examined the correlates of media health literacy – a construct composed of Nutbeam's understanding of health literacy and the concept of media literacy – and dimensions of health behaviour (Levin-Zamir et al. 2011). The research team led by Diane Levin-Zamir first found that girls and children with an educated mother (more than 15 years of formal education) have high media health literacy. However, unlike many studies of adult health literacy, the research team found no associations between media health literacy and ethnicity, immigration status, socioeconomic status, or even health status (Levin-Zamir et al. 2011, p. 330). However, this could be due to the specificity of the media health literacy construct. Besides Levin-Zamir, only Wharf Higgins and Begoray (2012) deal more intensively with critical media health literacy and address the three areas of skill set, empowerment and competency of engaged citizenship. In general, the measurement of digital health literacy is not yet very advanced, partly because the available measurement tools are still comparatively underdeveloped when it comes to capturing the more complex social embeddedness of digital media use and linking it to a critical (media) health literacy perspective. The following presentation of the few available instruments reveals a large number of gaps.

3.4.4 The Measurement of eHealth Literacy

Only a few instruments are currently available to measure eHealth literacy, most notably the 8-item "eHEALS" (*eHealth* Literacy Scale), which Norman and Skinner used to operationalize their own eHealth literacy model.

> "The eHealth Literacy Scale (eHEALS) has been developed to address the need to assess eHealth literacy for a wide range of populations and contexts. The eHEALS is a self-report tool that can be administered by a health professional and is based on an individual's perception of her or his own skills and knowledge within each measured domain. The instrument is designed to provide a general estimate of consumer eHealth-related skills that can be used to inform clinical decision making and health promotion planning with individuals or specific populations." (Norman et al. 2006, e47)

The scale developed by Norman and Skinner is probably the most frequently used scale to measure eHealth literacy, at least in the international context: "Although there has been limited research, Norman and Skinner's model of eHealth Literacy (Lily model) and the eHealth Literacy Scale (eHEALS) are most frequently used in

Table 3.5 eHEALS scale reliability and factor analysis

Item	Factor loading	Mean item-total correlation
Q1: I know how to find helpful health resources on the Internet	0.77	0.68
Q2: I know how to use the Internet to answer my health questions	0.79	0.70
Q3: I know what health resources are available on the Internet	0.77	0.68
Q4: I know where to find helpful health resources on the Internet	0.84	0.76
Q5: I know how to use the health information I find on the Internet to help me	0.81	0.73
Q6: I have the skills I need to evaluate the health resources I find on the Internet	0.72	0.63
Q7: I can tell high quality from low quality health resources on the Internet	0.65	0.55
Q8: I feel confident in using information from the Internet to make health decisions	0.60	0.51
Variance accounted for = 56		
Coefficient alpha = 0.88		

Source: Norman et al. 2006

studies to evaluate eHealth literacy." (Chung and Nahm 2015, p. 152). The comparatively short scale for measuring eHealth literacy comprises the following specific questions (Table 3.5).

The response options of the eHEALS comprise a five-point Likert scale ranging from "strongly disagree" to "strongly agree". In our view, the frequent use of the eHEALS bears little plausible relationship to the complexity implied by the concept of digital health literacy. However, it is still considered an adequate instrument for measuring digital health literacy (e.g., Kim and Xie 2017, p. 1078).

A different approach to determining digital health literacy is through the measurement of a "Web Performance Test". To date, a wide variety of screening instruments have been used to determine individual eHealth literacy – but no instrument yet exists that can comprehensively map digital health literacy in the sense of the full range of competencies involved in digital health literacy (Kim and Xie 2017, p. 1078). In particular, to our knowledge, no quantitative instrument exists that captures digital health literacies as a *social practice,* either among adults or among children and adolescents. This is a serious shortcoming because, as suggested above, the notion of solitary technology use has very limited relevance to children's and adolescents' lifeworlds. This deficiency points to a more systematic problem within conceptual and empirical health literacy and eHealth literacy research, which has to do with the action-theoretical grounding of generally subject-oriented health decisions and the cognitivist grounding implicitly employed. Therefore, in the following chapter we will unfold somewhat more systematically the limitations of the approaches presented so far, as well as introduce an *alternative perspective on health literacy research in children and adolescents.*

Health Literacy of Adolescents and Families from a Health Ethnology Perspective: A Theoretical Framing

4

Abstract

Having presented the current state of health literacy research in the context of health inequalities in the previous two chapters, this chapter now aims to achieve a change of perspective, which seems appropriate in view of the vast majority of empirical studies presented. However, this change of perspective must first be prepared. Therefore, we will start with a critique of empirical health literacy research, in order to then develop theoretical starting points for health ethnological health literacy research (Sect. 4.1).

Having presented the current state of health literacy research in the context of health inequalities in the previous two chapters, this chapter now aims to achieve a change of perspective, which seems appropriate in view of the vast majority of empirical studies presented. However, this change of perspective must first be prepared. Therefore, we will begin with a critique of empirical health literacy research in order to develop theoretical starting points for health ethnological health literacy research (Sect. 4.1). In a second step, we will present approaches and arguments from the sociology of justice and inequality that seem relevant for this context (Sect. 4.2). Only in the third step will we trace a difference-theoretical variant of adolescent health literacy research and determine some of its central dimensions (Sect. 4.3). Only after these preparatory steps do we finally present our understanding of an appropriate theoretical framing of health literacy research and describe our position as a dialectic of difference and deficit (Sect. 4.4).

U. H. Bittlingmayer et al., *Health Literacy From A Health Ethnology Perspective*, https://doi.org/10.1007/978-3-658-42348-3_4

4.1 Critique of (Empirical) Health Literacy Research in Adolescents, Children and Families

Health literacy research, which is primarily quantitative and empirical, has its strengths in showing that there are socially unequally distributed health literacies on the basis of different questionnaire instruments and that it is precisely these very different vulnerable or marginalised social groups that frequently also have poorer scores on the scales used (Robards et al. 2018). Thus, the empirically visible deficits in the group-specific distributions of important health-related action resources resulting from current social conditions are very clearly pointed out and named (e.g., Pelikan et al. 2012b; Robert Koch Institute (RKI) 2015; RKI 2016; WHO Europe 2013). Moreover, quantitative health literacy research, very similar to research on so-called functional illiteracy in the adult population, has generated mass media attention mainly by identifying a relatively large number of the adult or, to some extent, adolescent population as having limited health literacy. In European countries such as Bulgaria, Austria or Spain, the majority of the population is affected by limited health literacy; in Germany, Poland or Estonia, the figure is over 40% (based on the HLS-EU-47 scale; Pelikan et al. 2012b). In Asian countries such as Afghanistan, even the vast majority of the population is affected (Harsch et al. in press).

The mass media attention thus generated has – and this is certainly positive – led to national programmes to strengthen health literacy in the population. The Scottish Government, for example, published a National Action Plan for Health Literacy in 2014, which established comprehensive health-related action programmes (The Scottish Government 2014). In Germany, a National Action Plan on Health Literacy has also recently been launched, albeit not as a government programme, but at the initiative of Doris Schaeffer and Ullrich Bauer from the University of Bielefeld, Klaus Hurrelmann from the Hertie School of Governance and the Federal Association of the General Local Health Insurance Funds (Schaeffer et al. 2019). These large-scale initiatives would not have come about without the representative surveys in eight European countries that were carried out in connection with the Health Literacy in Europe project funded by the European Union (Pelikan et al. 2012b; Sørensen et al. 2012b; WHO Europe 2013), and the topic of health literacy would not have been as significant a topic in the field of empirical health research as it is today.[1]

[1]The enormous increase in popularity of health literacy research also has to do with the persistent rumour that low health literacy causes enormous costs in the health care system. In

However, these studies also have downsides and weaknesses when it comes to their theoretical and empirical approaches to health literacy. The expansion of health literacy research from narrow clinical fields of application to health promotion and prevention behaviours, that is, to the non-clinical realm of everyday behaviour, was based on the insight that "the successful maintenance of health is the sum of many everyday judgments and activities outside of a hospital or outpatient doctor's office." (Chinn 2011, p. 61; own translation). However, the expansion of the scope of health literacy was, as it were, paid for methodologically, in that the testing procedures were switched from the simple language tests used in the clinical setting (primarily TOFHLA, REALM, NVS) to self-reports by the interviewees. Self-statements, from which measures of competence are then generated, are riddled with uncertainties, with exaggerations or understatements, or with estimations of action spaces far removed from experience (cf. also Speer 2017, p. 16).[2] This is illustrated *firstly* by the fact that young people attest to themselves a significantly higher level of health literacy than the adult population. And *secondly*, chronically ill people attribute to themselves a significantly lower level of health literacy than the average (Schaeffer et al. 2016), even though it can be assumed that people with a chronic illness have greater experience in the healthcare system and generally have to deal with their illness on a daily basis.

4.1.1 Critique of the Lone Informed Health Decision

In addition to the fundamental measurement problems of subjective competence attributions (and the test fairness in objective performance measurements), the choice of an action-theoretical foundation for the background models of health literacy is worthy of discussion. The concept of health literacy has not only been freed from the corset of correct pronunciation of medical vocabulary and clinical navigation and appropriate compliance but has come to include more and more

the policy paper Health Literacy – the solid facts, published by the European Directorate of WHO, for example, it is stated that limited health literacy is associated with costs of US$ 8 billion; WHO Europe (2013, p. 8) These health economic figures are gut-felt rather than seriously measured, but they form an important component in the promotion of health literacy worldwide. At least in highly industrialised countries, the costs of intensive care medicine in the last months of life are so significantly higher that the potential costs of low health literacy, compared, do not carry any serious weight.

[2] As discussed earlier, even so-called objective measures such as TOFHLA or REALM are not assumed to be bias-free instruments; see Nguyen et al. (2017).

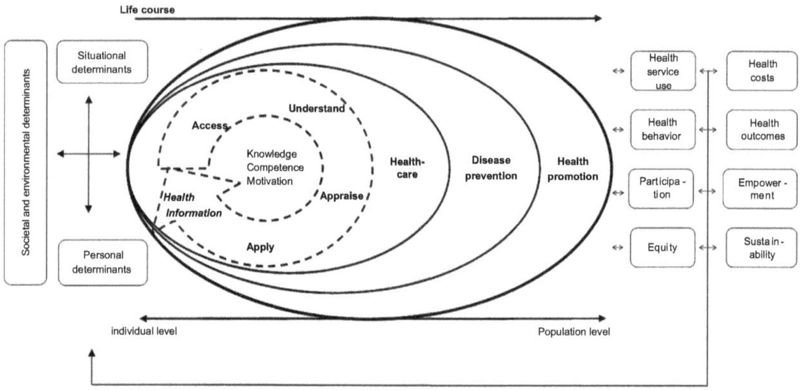

Fig. 4.1 Integrated model of health literacy. (Source: Sørensen et al. 2012a, p. 9)

domains and fields of action. In the process, the definitions have taken on an increasingly complex shape – a complexity in the determination of general health literacy that is best exemplified by the integrative and frequently cited model from the European Health Literacy Survey. The definition by Kristine Sørensen et al. already cited above reads:

"Health literacy is linked to literacy and entails people's knowledge, motivation and competences to access, understand, appraise, and apply health information in order to make judgments and take decisions in everyday life concerning healthcare, disease prevention and health promotion to maintain or improve quality of life during the life course." (Sørensen et al. 2012a, p. 3)

This comprehensive definition is linked to a complex theoretical model of health literacy, which is illustrated in Fig. 4.1 below. This model is currently regarded as a kind of international standard model (e.g., Duong et al. 2017), which is further applied, for example, to childhood and adolescence (Bollweg et al. 2020a, in press).

The formal framework model includes major dimensions and fields of action such as participation, empowerment, equality, sustainability or social and ecological determinants, but *first of all* it is not clearly explained how these dimensions and levels intertwine in actuality. This would require an anchoring in social theory, but this is completely lacking. *Secondly*, like the majority of health literacy conceptualisations, it remains embedded in a rationalist model of action.[3] Since

[3]It should only be mentioned in passing that in the widely discussed concept of health literacy, of all things, the concept of health itself remains very indeterminate to this day.

Nutbeam's famous definition of health literacy, health literacy has primarily meant 'correct' information processing from a public health perspective, which is then translated into appropriate health action more or less automatically. This understanding shapes not only the literacy and mathematics tests used as health literacy screening procedures, but also the integrated health literacy model of Kristine Sørensen et al. and a number of other proposed definitions and measurements, such as "The Calgary Charter on Health Literacy Scale" (Pleasant et al. 2018), which also takes its starting point from the *subjective* perception of health information in order to then move through the application of health information into a health-promoting action *normatively* described as appropriate. This basic understanding, which is characteristic of the majority of health literacy research, can be described as *cognitivist rationalism.*

What is problematic about this, from a sociological and action-theoretically informed perspective, is that people in their everyday lives do not spend most of their time thinking intensively about which options for action are available to them in a given situation, weighing up the pros and cons and then deciding on the most appropriate – for example, the most health-promoting – variant (Bittlingmayer and Bauer 2007b). The cognitivist-rationalist approach typical of health literacy research to date has to do with its early transfer of broad-based literacy studies (in adulthood) to the health context (Nutbeam 2000, 2009). Although this action model of rational choice, which underlies most health literacy models, can be readily transferred to quantitative empirical (large-scale) research – which is correspondingly considerably reduced in its theoretical complexity – it reflects everyday human actions only to a very limited extent (the recently published article Samerski 2019, p. 7, argues analogously).

If a broader understanding of health literacy is applied that is not limited to the context of health care activities, then none of the sixteen instruments examined for measuring children's health literacy in the period from 1980 to 2011 provides a comprehensive and overarching measurement of children's health literacy – according to the conclusion of a systematic review (Ormshaw et al. 2013, p. 450). For children and adolescents in particular, it is true that they find themselves in socialisation contexts that are difficult to grasp, and which structure their entire personality throughout, and have consequences for, among other things, "manners, preferences, lifestyle, manner of speaking, tastes, habits of thinking, feeling and acting." (Hehlmann et al. 2018, p. 86). Human agency can be described with Pierre

There are hardly any reasonable and clear theoretical anchors; cf. on this in more detail Saboga-Nunes et al. (2019).

Bourdieu's habit theory (Krais and Gebauer 2002) or with Mustafa Emirbayer and Ann Mische's agency theory (Emirbayer and Mische 1998) as *behaviours deeply embedded in social contexts* that follow certain *routines of action, regularities, and preferences* that are *not up for disposition every day,* and that do not falter merely because a person happens to notice a piece of health information, such as reading it himself, being told about it in person, or being presented with it on a screen in the tram. Without wanting to dive into Bourdieu's habitus theory or sociological action theory at this point (for more on this, see for example Lenger et al. 2013; Rieger-Ladich and Grabau 2017; Hehlmann et al. 2018, pp. 85–89; Sperlich 2016; Bauer 2012b), we believe we can state with regard to basic sociological theorems that the cognitivist-rationalist model of health literacy, often also referred to as health informed decision-making, and its quantitative-empirical implementation are fraught with some weighty problems, particularly when it comes to children and adolescents on the one hand and social disadvantage on the other (cf. on this also the strong contribution Bauer 2019b).

4.1.2 The (Underestimated) Importance of the Context of Action for Health Literacy

Within health literacy research as a whole, a strong tension can be discerned between the frequent emphasis on the importance of contexts of action (e.g. in Okan et al. 2017b, pp. 11, 14–15; Bröder et al. 2017, p. 20; Paakkari and George 2018, p. 4; Chinn 2011, p. 62) and the overwhelming number of measurement procedures that stop at the individual availability of competencies in the context of informed health-promoting decision-making. There is a common linking of the importance of context of action which often leads to a warning against relating health literacy only to individual skills and competencies, but there is no systematic consequence of integrating contexts of action into the study of health literacy itself. The tension between the availability of individual competencies and supra-individual contexts of action can be traced even in the case of literacy and mathematics competencies, which are considered to be absolutely basic. Janine Bröder et al. are of the opinion that "[m]ost articles recognize that health literacy requires being able to read, write, fill out a form or comprehend a text." (Bröder et al. 2017, p. 14).

But even the necessity of literacy skills for health literacy depends directly on the context of action. In a country like Afghanistan or Pakistan with very high illiteracy rates, it is by no means certain that literacy and numeracy are among the necessary prerequisites for high health literacy (Harsch et al. in press). The objection that health literacy models are primarily models aimed at highly industrialised societies, although they are considered generalised health literacy models, can be easily countered by the arguing that so-called (functional) illiterates live among us in large numbers through refugee and migration movements, but also through school refusal and (attributed) learning or mental disabilities (Feuser 2017; Mürner and Sierck 2013; Bittlingmayer and Sahrai 2019).[4]

The problem of the individual measurement of health literacy and the inherent model of the lonely but, preferably, well-informed health decision maker also becomes virulent with regard to contexts of action, for example when it comes to processes of deliberation and negotiation within families. "In some recent research undertaken in Pakistan, male heads of households are usually responsible for making any health related decisions that have financial implications. This complexity brings to light the question of 'whose health literacy' is the most important and relevant to actions? In the case of Pakistan, there might be a very health literate wife, but if her husband is the one making the decisions, it is his health literacy that ultimately influences how she engages with health actions and services." (Levin-Zamir et al. 2017, p. 135). It would not only be foolish to assume that this situation described by Diane Levin-Zamir et al. does not occur in Germany because we have overcome patriarchy. This situation, which is about asymmetrical agency with regard to health-related behaviour, can also be transferred to everyday situations of children and adolescents living together with adult heads of households who, in addition to informal socialisation processes, also impose direct restrictions on children's and adolescents' actions – usually, it must be admitted, in order to avert harm from them – within the framework of specific educational ideas.

A somewhat different example, but no less significant for individual health action, is action in peer groups. Sociological research on adolescence has frequently described the adolescent phase as a more or less rigorous process of detachment from parents with the aim of increasing individual autonomy and liberation from parental restrictions (we will see later in the case studies that this picture is problematic; see Chaps. 6 and 7). However, it is undisputed that the adolescent phase is initially about securing friendship and mutual acceptance (Richter 2005, pp. 55–57; Hurrelmann and Quenzel 2012, pp. 143–171). The associated processes of recognition and the fear of experiencing disregard led to a situationally considerable pressure from the peer group, which has to be reconciled with one's own

[4]For years, a repeatedly quoted figure was 7.5 million functionally illiterate people; cf. Grotlüschen and Riekmann (2012); in the meantime, the number of functionally illiterate people is said to be declining and, according to a press release, "only" amounts to 6.2 million.

preferences and predilections, should they deviate from the group opinion. If, for example, the afternoon activity is shisha smoking, which is certainly not conducive to good health, then the insight of a young person who realises that this is a possibly unhealthy leisure activity will probably not be listened to and the person – despite their better knowledge – will not want to risk attracting the ridicule of the group.

These few examples, which are intended to make plausible the importance of contexts of action and the embedding of individual action in social units such as families, educational institutions or peer groups, indicate that the hitherto customary measurements of individual health literacy cannot capture the contextual conditions of everyday decision-making processes.

4.1.3 Health Literacy and the One-Dimensionality of Inequality Determination

A second, systematic problem of inequality-oriented health literacy research in particular lies in the one-dimensional conceptualization of social or health inequalities. The health literacy measurement instruments used determine a more or less adequate or limited measure of individual health literacy with the progressive health policy intention of adequately empowering those with low health literacy. Hidden in this basic model is the intrinsic difficulty of the so-called deficit construction of specific, statistically produced groups. Somewhat crudely formulated, the mechanism follows a specific pattern: first, a methodological asocialisation of people is carried out to measure individual competence, which, as shown, abstracts from the highly relevant contexts of action. In a second step, effects and correlations of individual variables or summarised scales are determined on the basis of advanced statistical procedures – and then associated with health literacy, for example – and compared with social determinants (cf. Fig. 4.2 for one arbitrary example of a very large number of possible illustrations).

This then leads to statements such as: Academics have a higher level of health literacy, (optionally male or female) children and adolescents with a Turkish migration background have an increased risk of being overweight or obese, or it is stated that (autochthonous) male adolescents attribute a higher level of health literacy to themselves than do female adolescents. In a final, usually implicit step, the statistical correlations of increased risk or lower competencies are then used to generate group constructions with specific group characteristics, which then describe Turkish children and adolescents as overweight, groups with little schooling or socio-economic underprivilege as having little health competence, or girls as reticent in their assessment of their own competencies. This *double construction*

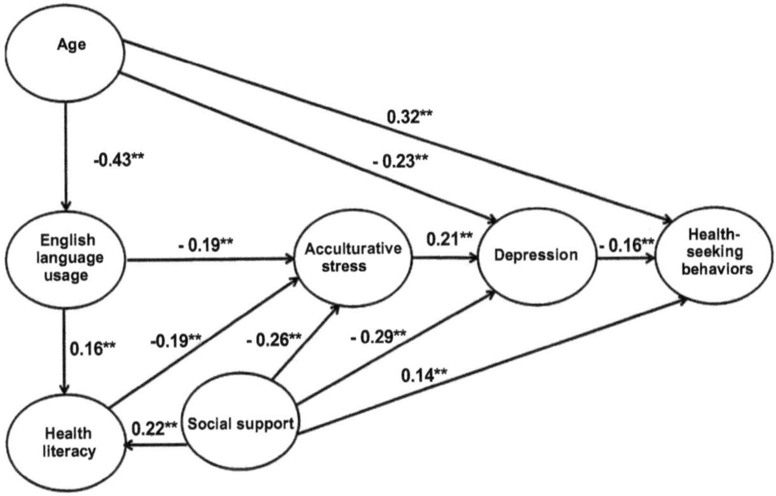

Fig. 4.2 The relationship between health literacy, social support and acculturation stress. (Maneze et al. 2016; cited in Levin-Zamir et al. 2017, p. 140)

process of methodical individualisation and subsequent group construction has all the characteristics of radical constructivism, which is, however, rarely associated with quantitative-statistical social research.

But even without a process of essentialization of group characteristics, the conceptualization of a one-dimensional health literacy scale, which in the end is able to distinguish between groups of people with excellent, sufficient, problematic and inadequate health literacy, is too simplistic, because it takes insufficient or no notice of the *different* horizons of meaning and meaning-making processes of "real social groups" in connection with health, as they are common in the various large social groups, nor can it adequately address the multidimensionality of inequality structures and processes. In the following section, we want to be a little more specific about what this multidimensionality consists of and what we want to use it to focus on.

4.2 Remarks on the Multidimensionality of Inequality from a Sociological and Philosophical Perspective

The multidimensionality of inequality relations was initially discussed more broadly in the sociology of social inequality (I) and more or less in parallel and independently in justice theory or political theory (II). The following remarks are only exemplary in character – it is not possible here to provide a detailed tracing of the broad discourses and diverse positions in the sociology of justice or inequality and their respective ramifications or further developments. For our purposes, it is particularly important to justify the necessity of a "theory of difference" approach and to unfold it more precisely with respect to public health and health literacy. Furthermore, it should be made clear that the study of social inequalities is theoretically enormously demanding, even if one believes that pure fact-gathering could help here (such a comparatively brutally positivistic idea in public health can be found, for example, in Prüss-Üstün et al. 2006, p. 41; on the normative complexity of inequality research, see Zinn 2008). Looking at the exploration of inequality relations and measures of justice is intended to help sound out a perspective focussing on difference that is complementary to the one focussing on deficit.

(I) As early as the 1970s, Pierre Bourdieu differentiated a vertical from a horizontal axis of domination with regard to differently functioning forms of domination, and precisely described forms of symbolic domination (Bourdieu 1982; Bourdieu and Passeron 1973; cf. on this also the contributions in Schmidt and Woltersdorff 2008), which is characterised in particular by its proximity to official educational institutions. In the 1980s and 1990s, German sociology of inequality and social structural analysis discussed the existence and continuity of social inequalities very broadly. The initial observation was that vertical social inequality relations can no longer be described empirically along the lines of classical major social groups such as strata and classes, going as far as stating that social origin no longer has a particularly strong impact on individual biographies (relevant to this is Beck 1986; critical of this is e.g., Vester et al. 2001). This idea has been strongly questioned not only within the sociology of inequality discourse,[5] but also by health science and social epidemiology (Elkeles and Mielck 1997).

Another line of discourse pursued the distinction between horizontal and vertical inequality structures (Kreckel 1993). Horizontal inequalities were supposed to be primarily based on so-called “askriptive”, i.e., ascribed, characteristics such as gender or ethnic origin, which, unlike disposable monthly income, cannot easily be placed in a clear linear hierarchy. Inequality researchers who looked at society less from the perspective of social structure analysis and its inherent theories of stratification and class, but rather from a feminist perspective or from the

[5] It also seems important to point out that the problematisation of the social structure analytical categories of class and stratum is a specific feature of the German inequality discourse of the 1980s and 1990s. In the Anglo-American and Francophone parts of the world, as well as in Spain or Portugal, the existence and significance of these major social groups was not questioned.

perspective of postcolonialism or migration research, argued in this direction. Here, too, massive social inequalities were identified without these inequalities necessarily being related to available economic capital. From the 1990s and 2000s onwards, the *theoretical and empirical relationship between the different dimensions of inequality* was discussed in particular (Rademacher and Wiechens 2001; Krönert-Othman and Lenz 2002; Souza 2008). A central consideration of all these approaches has been the embedding of empirical inequality relations along their different dimensions in more general theories of domination and power (Young 1996; Bourdieu and Passeron 1973). Currently, relatively often reference is made to the intersectionality approach of as a background theory or framework guiding empirical research, which is also concerned with how the different dimensions of domination are interwoven in their respective concrete empirical relationships (fundamental for the German-speaking area Winker and Degele 2010).

It should have become clear from these remarks that health inequalities can hardly be arranged along a single dimension and that such attempts are obvious reductions of real social conditions. It is no exaggeration to state that the term social inequality is frequently used, but not deeply understood in public health research and that the term often remains empiricist and superficial. The motif of social inequalities becomes even more complex when the reference to equity is made.

(II) In political theory, with the study by John Rawls "Theory of Justice", which is still fundamental and worth reading today, basic questions of moral philosophy were also brought close to the question, pertaining to the theory of inequality, of the just distribution of goods and services (in Rawls' terminology: basic goods) in the 1970s (Rawls 1979). John Rawls' theory of justice has been discussed very broadly and controversially in the 1980s and 1990s, culminating in the so-called communitarianism debate, in which – in short – one of the central questions was to what extent the theoretical construction of a Rawlsian individual, characterised by Charles Taylor for instance as atomism (cf. Taylor 1995), is at all compatible with empirical individuals, and to what extent the justificatory theoretical connections to justice (especially in the figure of the "original position") are at all relevant to actual people in the constraints and opportunity structures of their life worlds (cf. for example the critiques in Bellah et al. 1985; Taylor 1996).

For our considerations on the *multidimensionality of unequal health competence*, some arguments from the debate on communitarianism (Honneth 1994), which is still extremely instructive today, and a further development of the Rawlsian approach (although the extent to which this is a further development at all is disputed among genuine Rawls fans) are significant.

Firstly, with his comprehensive theory of justice, which he wants to see anchored in the context of liberalist, and thus libertarian, theoretical approaches,

John Rawls made a point of paramount importance with regard to a multidimensional concept of unequal health literacy, which is particularly virulent in the context of possible empowerment-oriented interventions. In a sense, Rawls radicalises the notion that each individual has a fundamental right to pursue his or her own conception of the good life and that the state or state institutions have no right of intervention here, regardless of whether such an intervention would be health-promoting or not (a direct transfer of Rawlsian theory of justice to the health field is provided by Daniels 2008; see also Bittlingmayer and Ziegler 2012 for more detail). The state must therefore behave neutrally in view of individuals' conceptions of the good life and provide resources, goods and services that enable individuals to pursue their conception of the good life in a sustainable manner (always assuming, in line with Kant's reasoning, that it does not harm any other individual conception of the good life in its realisation).

Secondly, the so-called Capabilities Approach by Amartya Sen and Martha Nussbaum follows up on these considerations, both of whom see their respective variants as further developments of the Rawlsian approach and are anchored in the same tradition of political liberalism. In this context, it is first of all exciting to note the remark by socialisation and youth researcher Heiner Keupp that the capability approach shows great analogies and compatibilities to Aaron Antonovski's salutogenic approach (Keupp 2012, pp. 24–30). Moreover, it is worth mentioning that Amartya Sen very explicitly developed a theory of justice built on the concept of *complex equality*. The simple, as well as convincing, starting point is that the individually available resources for action do not provide the central measure for justice, but that resources for action such as income, wealth or educational titles are only *means to* the *end of* being able to pursue and implement the self-imposed goals of a good life (formulated for instance in Sen 2010, p. 282). If such a change of perspective on distributive justice is carried out, i.e., from available resources for action to the realisation chances of real freedoms of action, the heterogeneity of people and their needs comes more into view. Sens' and Nussbaum's basic idea is that people need different amounts of action resources in order to enjoy the same freedom of action. Sen's standard example refers to the area of individual mobility: in order for a person who is in a wheelchair to be able to realise the same degree of mobility (understood as realised freedom of action), the person needs significantly more resources for action in order to be able to realise this freedom, namely to get from A to B, than a person who is not in a wheelchair. An equal distribution of resources – or in Rawlsian terminology: basic goods – would therefore, despite good intentions, be accompanied by socially unequal consequences for the freedom of action of individuals with different needs (cf. on this Pauer-Studer 1999, p. 18).[6]

However, while Sen deliberately leaves open the determination of what is to constitute freedom of action for people more specifically, Martha Nussbaum provides a list of capabilities that is intended to apply to all people and to be a comprehensive account of "what seems to constitute a life that we regard as a human life" (Nussbaum 1999, p. 49). The box below shows the list of Capabilities that Nussbaum uses to try to determine a general theory of the good life (Table 4.1). In the meantime, the list has been supplemented several times, widely discussed and applied to health as a subject area (cf. among others Bittlingmayer and Ziegler 2012, pp. 52–64). However, we are less concerned here with a discussion of Nussbaum's theory of the good life than with the heterogeneity dimensions that can be found in the list itself.

Table 4.1 List of basic human abilities according to Martha Nussbaum (1999, S. 235)

1. ***Life***. *Being able to live to the end of a human life of normal length; not dying prematurely, or before one's life is so diminished as to be not worth living.*
2. ***Bodily health***. *Being able to have good health, including reproductive health;* to be adequately nourished; to have adequate shelter.*
3. ***Bodily integrity***. *Being able to move freely from place to place; to be secure against violent assault, including sexual assault and domestic violence; having opportunities for sexual satisfaction and for choice in matters of reproduction.*
4. ***Senses, imagination and thought.*** *Being able to use the senses, to imagine, think and reason – and to do these things in a „truly human" way, a way informed and cultivated by an adequate education, including, but by no means limited to, literacy and basic mathematical and scientific training. Being able to use imagination and thought in connection with experiencing and producing works and events of one's own choice, religious, literary, musical, and so forth. Being able to use one's mind in ways protected by guarantees of freedom of expression with respect to both political*

(continued)

[6]The idea of equal opportunities, which originates in the neoliberal and neoconservative cosmos and plays a very important role today with regard to labour market and social policy, but also with regard to health policy, is similarly situated. As Thomas Nagel, one of the most important contemporary philosophers, unsuspected of left-wing radicalism soberly notes, "[equality of opportunity] entails unequal outcomes.[...] The main question about inequalities is: what kinds of *causes of inequality* are unjust? [...] What *methods of* intervening in inequality are legitimate." Nagel (1990, pp. 66, 68).

and artistic speech, and freedom of religious exercise. Being able to have pleasurable experiences, and to avoid non-necessary pain.
5. ***Emotions***. *Being able to have attachments to things and people outside ourselves; to love those who love and care for us, to grieve at their absence; in general, to love, to grieve, to experience longing, gratitude, and justified anger. Not having one's emotional development blighted by fear and anxiety. (Supporting this capability means supporting forms of human association that can be shown to be crucial in people's development.)*
6. ***Practical reason***. *Being able to form a conception of the good and to engage in critical reflection about the planning of one's life (which entails protection for the liberty of conscience).*
7. ***Affiliation.***
A. *Being able to live with and toward others, to recognize and show concern for other human beings, to engage in various forms of social interaction; to be able to imagine the situation of another and to have compassion for that situation; to have the capability for both justice and friendship. (Protecting this capability means protecting institutions that constitute and nourish such forms of affiliation, and also protecting the freedom of assembly and political speech.)*
B. *Having the social bases of self-respect and non-humiliation; being able to be treated as a dignified being whose worth is equal to that of others. This entails protections against discrimination on the basis of race, sex, sexual orientation, religion, caste, ethnicity, or national origin.*
8. ***Other species***. *Being able to live with concern for and in relation to animals, plants and the world of nature.*
9. ***Play***. *Being able to laugh, to play, to enjoy recreational activities.*
10. ***Control over one's environment.***
A. ***Political.*** *Being able to participate effectively in political choices that govern one's life; having the right of political participation, protections of free speech and association.*
B. ***Material.*** *Being able to hold property (both land and movable goods); having the right to seek employment on an equal basis with others; having freedom from unwarranted search and seizure. In work, being able to work as a human being, exercising practical reason and entering into meaningful relationships of mutual recognition with other workers.*

To be sure, Nussbaum's own transfer of the socio-institutional and health policy consequences arising from her own list remains peculiarly pale:

> Required are a comprehensive health care system, wholesome air and water, security for life and property, and protection of citizens' freedom of choice regarding important aspects of their medical treatment. What is required is adequate food and housing, and these things are to be arranged so that citizens can arrange their food and housing

> according to their own practical reason. (This would mean, for example, emphasizing health education, drug education, etc.). What is needed is protection of the ability of citizens to regulate their sexual activities according to their own practical reason and free choice. (Here, too, the promotion of sex education programs would probably play a crucial role.) (Nussbaum 1999, pp. 60–61)

Nussbaum obviously has little sense of the fact that, at least with regard to health and health inequalities, educational programmes hardly benefit underprivileged social groups in particular. But Nussbaum, on the other hand, has a clear idea that people concretize their list of capabilities in very different ways in the practice of action and develop very different ideas of the good life. Here she can take up Rawls and make him clearly more precise by outlining, at least in the abstract, the field of possible lifestyle-relevant differentiations.

The discussion about the idea of the good life, set against the abstract individualism in the tradition of political liberalism (especially John Rawls, Michael Sandel; Ronald Dworkin; Amartya Sen; Martha Nussbaum), is considerably more specific. Heterogeneity, already present in the approaches from the spectrum of political liberalism and emphatically justified in its normative dimension, is once again given a more prominent place by the critics and connected with a critique of the imaginary worlds of (too) abstract social institutions. Against the idea that social institutions should support and safeguard all individual conceptions of the good life in an equally neutral way, the communitarian critique of liberalist theories of justice formulates a critique similar to the one we have formulated here against the rationalist cognitivism which in our view underlies most theoretical models of health literacy (see above under Sect. 4.1). The criticism relates to the fact that the conceptualization of human beings as rational, conscious, context-free and, in this sense, personal ahistorical decision-making machines, which is built into the Rawlsian theory of justice, is quite possibly a more suitable foundation for a contradiction-free justification of norms of justice, but largely misses the conceptualization of empirical subjects. This is, of course, extremely significant when it comes to a proper understanding of health action. Without wishing to elaborate on communitarianism here, the spectrum of communitarian positions is essentially concerned with *perceiving and thus taking seriously existing cultural heterogeneities that result from membership in various large social groups.*

Somewhat pointedly, it can therefore be said that the deficits in the distributive justice of contemporary societies can be specified and pinpointed through the approaches of political liberalism, but at the same time they remain too abstract in relation to the real actions of social actors. The strength of communitarian positions lies in directing the view to the individuals situated in specific social contexts and to correct the idea that designs of the good life are individual (atomistic) projects.

For the transfer to the health sciences in general and to health literacy research in particular, all arguments developed so far signify above all that the prevailing (competence) deficit perspectives, focussing on unequal resource endowment, must be supplemented by a perspective that *firstly* includes other, more symbolically negotiated inequalities, *secondly takes into* account the social frameworks of individual life plans, and *thirdly* perceives and takes seriously cultural heterogeneities. Catching up with these dimensions theoretically/conceptually therefore requires, in our view, the adoption, complementary to the deficit perspective, of a perspective of difference, which is already present in the health sciences, but is itself linked to quite different positions. In the next section, we will develop the possible linking points and specifications of the difference perspective in public health.

4.3 The Difference Perspective as Overcoming the Deficit Perspective?

In contrast to, positions that are located in the context of the paradigm of the health sciences (Schnabel 2007a) take a very different approach from the one which proceed the strong socio-epidemiological deficit perspectives. For the *positive* paradigm, health *instead of* disease, which goes beyond the critique of a medical or medical-police view of the world, as carried out, for example, in the studies of Michel Foucault, there can be based on two theoretical foundations.

Firstly, in several policy papers, the WHO has presented a positive description of health that focuses not only on comprehensive individual well-being, but also on societal structures as a whole and links health, for example, to the individual's ability to shape his or her own living environment (Saboga-Nunes et al. 2019). The concept of health advocated by the WHO is, if taken seriously in terms of theory, quite radical. If social structures are present that considerably limit the potentials of social actors, then it is no longer possible to speak of a healthy society, quite independently of average life expectancy (as Marcuse already argued in 1968, pp. 7–11). This has consequences for the theoretical evaluation of individual risk behaviour or health literacy deficits, which are much less important than they are in the medical-oriented or social epidemiological studies in relation to burdensome social structures.

Secondly, the work of Aaron Antonovsky, to whom the paradigm shift from the analysis of disease to the analysis of health can be traced, is highly relevant (Antonovsky 1987; BZgA 2001). His concept of salutogenesis examines conditions under which people are able to maintain their health, whether they are ill in the medical sense or not or have a high or low level of health literacy (cf. on the relationship between health literacy and salutogenesis Saboga-Nunes et al. 2019). Within the framework of the WHO documents and Antonovsky's salutogenesis, it is crucial for the constitution of a difference perspective in the health sciences to turn consistently to the individual resources for action that maintain or promote health.

It is the explicit claim of a health science or salutogenic perspective to overcome the usual focus on deficit, as it is also welded into the mainstream of health literacy research. Commanding low health literacy can also be understood and traced from a classic risk factor logic. The salutogenic approach, however, takes a different path: from a salutogenic perspective, social actors are to be conceptualised *primarily as bearers of individual resources for action,* to which salutogenic approaches can be applied. More important than the analysis of risky or uninformed behaviour is the investigation of subjective action competences, the existence of which is in principle attributed to all social actors.

What is significant about this seemingly small difference for an applied or practice-oriented science such as public health is that the basic orientation of health literacy programs and public health interventions differs considerably depending on whether the aim is to eliminate risky behaviours, which remains in the context of a paradigm of medicine-oriented risk factor research, or whether it is a matter of concentrating on the expansion of already existing strengths and resources for action and then hoping for *indirect, non-determinable effects* towards improved individual health (specified, for example, in the so-called life skills approach) (authoritative on this: Schnabel 2007a). According to the WHO and Antonovsky, salutogenesis is programmed to aim at the strengthening of individual action resources, which are labelled as generalised resistance resources and which overlap strongly with classic social-psychological action resources such as self-confidence, self-esteem or the strengthening of internal control beliefs (Antonovsky 1997; BZgA 2001). In public health, the turn to individual competencies and action resources that are always already positively available is the direct consequence of attempts to overcome the medical profession's inscribed deficit orientation. However, within public health, different variants can be distinguished with which a deficit perspective can be countered. These will now be presented in more detail.

4.3.1 Three Variants of a Difference Theory Perspective in Public Health

On the basis of the negation of deficit orientation, a rough distinction can be made between three variants. The first variant, which to a certain extent can be regarded as a direct negation of the deficit perspective, can be described as a consistent resource orientation. It refers to the strict turn towards a resource-oriented view of social actors. As indicated above, in the context of resource orientation, the focus is not on deviant or irrational lifestyles, but on the resource base available to each social actor. *Social actors* are constructed *as having* very different competencies, which are brought to *bear* in different areas of their lifeworld, education, occupation, work or family. Health-preserving competences are subject-related competences such as a high self-esteem, a lot of self-confidence or internal control beliefs, i.e., the ideas of being able to affect something in the world in the desired direction through one's own actions, or the sense of coherence developed by Antonovsky, which should have the highest possible level.

A more positive interpretation takes the place of a direct deficit orientation, because every person, one could say slightly too pointedly, is regarded as a bearer of action competences, only in one case the action competences have already been fully developed, in the other case they still need health-promoting interventions in order for the social actors themselves to become adequately aware of them and to develop them further.

The direct resource orientation must be described overall as a rather weak variant of the difference perspective, because it ultimately remains bound to the same logic as the deficit perspective, even if the social actors are now depicted more positively according to their resources for action. But the sorting of those who have a lot of health-preserving or health-promoting action resources and competences against those who have few action resources and competences is homologous to the sorting from a deficit perspective. For as soon as health inequalities or an unequal endowment with health competencies come into play, a distinction must be made between more competent and less competent social actors, even within the competency orientation. Even if the focus is consistently on individual potential for action, members of certain social milieus, ethnic groups or older people are obviously less likely to succeed in maintaining a positive state of health than others, for example because they make less use of preventive services or behave more frequently in ways that are detrimental to health (Bauer 2005: Chap. 1). From the perspective of resource orientation, too, deficient lifestyles can thus be defined by simple analogy, just as those inscribed in the deficit perspective, insofar as the life practice of the individuals is not carried out in a health-oriented manner. In Hagen Kühn's still impressive study, for example, the accurate criticism of the comprehensive risk factor model and the identified healthism in the United States ultimately becomes a comprehensive deficit description of resource-weak social actors:

> To sum up, social classes and strata are consistently distinguished by the degree of restrictiveness of living conditions in a quite comprehensive sense, including subjectivity, habitus and conditions [. . .]: Thus, the lifestyle of a university professor has far more degrees of freedom than that of the automobile worker. The latter has more restrictive work arrangements, his income allows him only a small apartment, less travel, his lower education (e.g. foreign languages) hinders perceptions of opportunity, etc. That is why the habitus acquired in the upper classes is not only 'different', but also more flexible [. . .]. Behaviour is far less fixed. There is a greater potential of behavioural reserves. (Kühn 1993, pp. 111–112).

What is significant about this quotation is that even from a health-oriented perspective, critical of medicine and risk factors, a deficit view can follow as a consequence, which weakens the turn towards a consistent resource orientation. The blanket attribution that the habitus of a university professor is more flexible than a lower-class habitus must be countered with regard to behaviour-oriented health literacy, for example, by the significantly higher alcohol consumption of higher social classes. This notion not only appears to be substantially too crude, but from a scarcity of resources for action to infer a limited complexity of individual behaviour is a jump to conclusions that is quite problematic especially in the context of available health competences.

The *second variant of the difference perspective* goes a bit further and postulates that there is clearly more than one single understanding of health and illness. It can be described as a cultural anthropological variant of the difference perspective (Stollberg 2001, pp. 19–24). Social actors not only have *different* competencies and resources in terms of maintaining their well-being and health. They *also* have *different ideas about what they understand by health and illness in the first place.*

In a cross-cultural and cross-national comparison, this point is immediately apparent. If, for example, illness is understood as insulting the gods or angering the ancestors, who must be appeased by professional shamans, this perspective has little in common with either the medical-biopsychological or the salutogenic view. From the ethnological perspective, the western-modern industrial and medical-professional meaning system concerning illness or health is only one of many and thus not an unproblematic starting point from which deficits in lifestyles or in resource endowments could be established with universal validity (Evans-Pritchard 1988).

The cultural anthropological variant, however, goes beyond the abstract comparative cultural approach when it is aimed at one's own society (cf. Reichmayr 2003: Chap. 3). The "ethnology of one's own society" as expressed in the tradition of the US-American ethnomethodologists (cf. on this classically Garfinkel 1967; Goffman 1980, 1996, 2008; cf. as a good introduction also Mullins 1981) and in the writings of Pierre Bourdieu (Bourdieu 1979, 1982, 1987) is decisive here. If one follows this perspective, then it becomes clear that *quite different concepts of illness and health prevail* even *within modern societies.* The difference in the conceptions of health and illness of social actors within a society most likely follows the common structuring principles of contemporary Western societies – gender, class, ethnicity (cf. as a good theoretical overview Rademacher and Wiechens 2001) – even if a considerable need for research can be stated here. Comparatively better theoretically conceptualised, but still little empirically researched in the health sciences are gender-specific differences, for example, with regard to gender-mediated body concepts or health-related competence profiles that go beyond a deficit perspective (for example, in the life expectancy of men and women) (cf. on this, for example, Butler 2001; Bourdieu 2005; Gugutzer 2004, pp. 124–130; with direct reference to public health Kolip 1997, 2000; Kuhlmann and Kolip 2008; Kolip et al. 2013; Babitsch 2009).

Less known and researched are differences (not deficits!) with regard to *class- or milieu-specific health (competence), disease or body concepts.* The best-known example of such a difference is certainly the study by Paul Willis (1979), which arose in the context of cultural studies and points out that a certain lifestyle in adolescence, which certainly does not gain widespread approval from a health promotion and prevention perspective (heavy alcohol and tobacco consumption, risky behaviour), can claim functionality and thus legitimacy in the context of preparation for physically very stressful working conditions in later life. The emphasis here is thus on the fact that, depending on the class-cultural position in the social space, there are different connectable health competence concepts which actors can relate to and which are reflected in different somatic cultures (cf. on this Boltanski 1976; Kolip 1997; see also the section below). From this difference perspective, the practices that tend to cause concern from a health promotion perspective are first of all framed more neutrally as individually and socially meaningful behaviours. The study by Willis, which will not be discussed specifically here (cf. on this the strong anthology by Dolby and Dimitriadis 2004), can be understood as a particularly good example of how, depending on the class-cultural position of the social actors, differentiated concepts of body and health can be "suitable for everyday life" and, precisely for this reason, meaningful (cf. as a general theoretical frame of reference Schütz and Luckmann 2003; cf. on the connection between knowledge, meaning and socialisation Grundmann et al. 2003; Grundmann et al. 2006; cf. the descriptions of body concepts, postures, diets etc. in Bourdieu 1982b).

Finally, the *ethnicity-specific difference perspective* points to the fact that, not least in the course of mass migration in the twentieth century, a large number of social actors with different cultural backgrounds immigrated to the core countries of Western capitalist societies (see, among others, Treibel 2003; Han 2016; Lange and Polat 2010). According to more recent findings from the micro-census, it can now be assumed that more than 20%, rather than the previous standard figure of 10% of households in Germany have a migration background, which means that research on migration- or ethnicity-specific differences from a health science perspective is aimed at a significant proportion of the citizens living in Germany. As for Germany, the majority of migrants immigrated as a result of European and Eurasian labour and internal migration. This leads to the co-existence of etiological understandings. Thus, in a German-Greek or German-Turkish comparison, considerable differences in the understanding of health and illness can be postulated. For example, the "evil eye" is a normal component of everyday etiological explanations of headaches and other general complaints among Greek or Turkish migrants in Germany, in contrast to the autochthonous population. A consistent difference perspective would take this etiological model seriously and understand it as a component of the cultural processing of specific physical conditions. Research on such differences, however, is in its infancy. Overall, little is known about ethnicity-specific differences in health and illness perceptions or about the existence of ethnicity-differentiated health literacy within industrial contemporary societies – in contrast, for example, to the increasingly collected social epidemiological ethnicity-specific probabilities of illness (Razum 2006).

The *third variant of the difference orientation* argues from a normativity-critical perspective and opposes the strong standardising effects associated with a deficit perspective on health and health literacy. On the one hand, from a principled medical-critical perspective, the standardising view is criticised, which evaluates every behaviour and every lifestyle of social actors according to the risk of disease. The medical gaze is postmodernly deconstructed and decoded as a gaze that exercises domination (Foucault 1988, p. 55). This perspective is truly radical, and it certainly contains potential that has been very little exploited so far, especially for applied health science. For deconstructivist work not only deals with the archaeology of the medical gaze but can also be related to the standardising (and certainly well-intentioned) empowerment programs that are launched in the context of public health. Just as – according to Foucault – "sick people" or "crazy people" are discursively constructed on the basis of arbitrary symptoms in order to let bourgeois reason shine in bright light, so too people in need of empowerment are first produced or at least co-produced by the preventive or health-promoting programs themselves. This argument is not settled by reference to an evidence base, for it is precisely the practice of basing on evidence itself that is likely to appear from this perspective to be part of the generating act of construction (for a critique of basing on evidence from an action research perspective, see Wright 2016).

The third variant is thus directed against standardizations in general and standardising constructions of deficits in particular and asserts that, for example, the very notions of "behavior detrimental to health" or "the systematic ignorance of certain social actors with regard to preventive offers" cement a view of domination that do not even take note of *different* rational (counter)notions (I go to the doctor when I am sick, not before, etc.) or devalue them as deviant, irrational, etc. It is precisely this analogy between illness or lack of health literacy (deficit) and deviance (understood and defined as normatively questionable or legally punishable practices) that is at the heart of the third variant.

The strength of this variant consists in particular in drawing attention to the discursive acts, interwoven with mechanisms of domination, of constituting and constructing, for example of the "sick person", the "person in need of empowerment" or, in our context, the "individual equipped with only little health competence". In some respects, therefore, this perspective is also connectable to the justice theory ideas from the spectrum of political liberalism briefly alluded to above, even if the theoretical underpinnings are quite contrary. This also points to an aspect that is rarely discussed in the application-oriented health sciences: the offers of health-promoting or preventive courses that are supposed to lead to an increase in (population-wide) health literacy create their own demand, at least in part, especially among groups that are close to or accustomed to education, and divide the social world into social actors who are willing and unwilling to participate in voluntary prevention courses. Inherent in this division is always the idea that those social groups that have not yet been reached or addressed will in future come into view as particularly important target groups of any measures. In the process, however, underprivileged groups are usually labelled as difficult to reach, while other groups that are even more difficult to reach, such as the super-rich, Bundeswehr soldiers on foreign war missions, or parliamentarians, are not mentioned, even though their participation rates are likely to be significantly lower than those of underprivileged groups. A consistent difference perspective would be considerably more cautious here, because it does not want the spectrum of what is considered an individual conception of the good life to be restricted by pre-standardizations.

But strong as the (also epistemologically) sceptical arguments of such a discourse-theoretical or deconstructivist perspective might be, for example in the analysis of the construction of social groups, the standardised idea of health-promoting behaviour or the deficit constructions within the common health competence models, they always find a kind of objective limit in the unequal mortality rates of different large social groups such as social classes, men in contrast to women or ethnic or minority groups. A radical constructivist variant, which, for example, out of an impulse critical of domination, does not regard alcoholism as a problem but simply as an alternative way of life within the framework of a different conception of the good, must include the very material consequences of a shortened lifespan and the strain on social relations in order not to become itself ideological. And it is precisely *between these poles, symbolic domination through healthism* (Kühn 1993; Bittlingmayer and Bauer 2007b; Schmidt 2017) *and material health inequalities, between different conceptions of life and deficient resource endowments, that we believe health literacy research must also operate if an adequate understanding of health inequalities is to be achieved in the context or shape of unequal health literacy as well.* In the following section, which concludes the chapter, we will define our perspective on health literacy research in more detail.

4.4 The Dialectic of Deficit and Difference as a Theoretical Framework for Health Literacy Research

So far in this chapter, we have provided an intrinsic critique of the deficit-oriented health literacy research perspective along the most common measurements and models, and shown that sorting people or children, young people and families along a single linear dimension of competence is problematic (Sect. 4.1). We then briefly introduced the theories and perspectives of the sociology of inequality and justice theory, which point to the complexity and multidimensionality of social inequality relations. Furthermore, we pointed out that, especially against the background of the plurality of conceptions of the good life, we can expect more than one variant of a successful life plan, but rather an enormous heterogeneity of differently weighted capabilities as components of the good life (Sect. 4.2). The consideration of a difference perspective within health literacy research can, we further argued, be associated with different strands of theory that *substitute,* more or less radically, differences for deficit and empirical inequalities. The multidimensionality of social inequality relations must be given just as much attention in health literacy research as the heterogeneity and differences in the conceptions of a good life, according to our core argument developed so far.

The consideration of cultural heterogeneity in the broadest sense, and symbolic dimensions of domination is, in our opinion, for reasons both conceptual and theoretical, unfeasible within the written-language performance tests (REALM, TOHFLA, etc.) dominant in the context of health care action, as well as within the psychometric health literacy scales based on self-reports and self-assessments (HLS-EU-47 scale, HELMA, The Calgary Charter on Health Literacy scale, etc.), which are meanwhile widely used. Especially if a broad understanding of health literacy is taken as a basis, such as is common in current comprehensive health literacy models, quantitative empirical measures are not able to catch up with the implicitly addressed dimensions of action. We can refer here once again to the conclusion of the systematic literature review on the precise measurement of health literacy in children and adolescents by Michael Ormshaw and others, who sum up in their study: "When this broader view of health literacy is considered, it is clear that none of the 16 selected studies provided a comprehensive assessment of health literacy" (Ormshaw et al. 2013, p. 450).

This aspect is reflected in an increasing number of publications that emphasise the importance of the social context in which health literacy-relevant attitudes (rarely actions) are embedded and in the emphasis on the difference between attitudes and actions (e.g. E.g. Chinn 2011, p. 65; Okan et al. 2017b, pp. 11–16; Paakkari and George 2018 passim; Wharf Higgins et al. 2009; Bröder et al. 2017, pp. 20–21; Levin-Zamir et al. 2017). It is no coincidence, however, that calls for increased attention to context come primarily from the spectrum of conceptual and theoretical contributions and are comparatively rarely directly reflected and implemented in empirical studies. A rare example is the empirical research of Uta Papen, who has focused her research interest on the importance of the context of action and meaning within the scope of health literacy. According to Papen, health literacy cannot be reasonably understood as an isolated competence (skill), but rather as a practice directly embedded in social contexts: 'health literacy is always situated' (Papen 2009, p. 28). In a study that included both a large number of interviews ($N = 45$) and ethnographic fieldwork of selected interviewees ($N = 6$), Papen was able to show that people with low literacy skills (usually due to recent migration) are not adequately described and understood in the field of care provision if, because of their low literacy, they are firmly defined as having a deficit in their health literacy. She argues for a view of health literacy that more closely follows a strictly resource-oriented perspective, because "it is important to see that patients, including those commonly represented as having limited basic skills, are not without resources when it comes to dealing with the literacy and language demands of health care settings." (Papen 2009, p. 26). The observation of specific actions within contexts of action almost necessarily provides a view of social actors as persons who are usually able to act, in a resisting or affirming manner , but in any case actively in contexts of action.[7] Such research shifts the focus of analysis from the measurement of specific skills to the overarching forms of meaning-making of subjects within contexts of action and requirements for action (cf. also Okan et al. 2017b, p. 17).

The second aspect in Uta Papen's analysis that is crucial to our own study, and which was further confirmed in a recently published study of a similar nature (Samerski 2019), is also mentioned at first glance in a variety of other publications in different directions. There is frequent critique of the individualistic bias in health literacy concepts and orthodox measurement methods (Chinn 2011; Bröder et al. 2017). Critically oriented work on health literacy, especially on the health literacy of children and young people, points out that organisational embeddedness is more relevant than individual skills and abilities. Especially when it comes to the idea of empowerment through health literacy promotion, supra-individual and formal structures and fields of action such as schools, kindergartens/day-care centres or organisations such as sports clubs come into view, which should provide reasonable protective structures for individual (and family) health literacy development (Paakkari 2015; St Leger 2001; Chinn 2011; Paakkari and George 2018; Wharf Higgins et al. 2009). The main point made in this variant is that organisations massively shape individual agency and therefore, by analogy with the classic setting perspective in health sciences, organisational structures should be changed with a

[7]To be distinguished from the direct observation of actions are attempts to identify social contexts as a background variable for explaining individual health literacy levels or to integrate them into the operationalization of quantitative health literacy measures. Tetine Sentell and others recently presented a review of the quantitative evidence of social context for determining health literacy, examining 34 studies: "We found three distinct perspectives on the intersection between health literacy and social context. Most common ($n = 23$) were studies measuring an *association* between individual health literacy and individual social capital, social support, or social engagement, particularly whether social support varied by health literacy and/or if this relationship mediated health outcomes. Another group of studies ($n = 6$) took the perspective that being health literate by *definition* included social context, including access to and/or use of social support as a domain in individual health literacy assessment. Five studies considered the social context of health literacy as an independent *property* measured beyond the individual level." Sentell et al. (2017, p. e41). However, although the social context was central to the 34 studies evaluated, the real-world context of action was not addressed in any of the studies; instead, the operationalizations and measurements of health literacy are made along standard measurement lines.

view to maximising health literacy development. In a similar direction, recent indications and considerations aim to interlink health literacy development in practice more closely with community- or district-based interventions and to assign significantly more importance to the community level (e.g., Levin-Zamir et al. 2017; Okan et al. 2017b).

However, the perspectives provided by Uta Papen (2009) and Silja Samerski (2019), which are directly applicable to our own study, in specific ways go beyond reminding us of the importance of formal or supra-individual contexts of action. Papen criticises not so much the overly individualistic perspective of analysis, but rather the whole notion of a singular – in Taylor's terminology: atomistic – individual, each possessing individual skills and abilities. According to Papen, health literacy is not an individual but a "shared resource frequently achieved collectively by groups of people, for example families. [. . .] One of the most common strategies [. . .]; of people with limited literacy; the author] was to draw on others who could help them with the literacy tasks involved in dealing with ill health. They drew on family members, friends and neighbours as literacy mediators." (Papen 2009, pp. 19, 27). This means that measurement at the level of an individually completed self-report or written language performance test does not represent a realistic assessment of the action repertoire of individual persons, be they adults, children or adolescents. This systematic curtailment has already been elaborated on for agency in the care sector by Papen and Walters (Walters and Papen 2008). All the more justification for a perspective that is not focussed on isolated individual action, but on its necessary social, institutional and situational embedding, and takes the concept of health literacy beyond health care action to the realm of everyday life.

The two reference studies presented here clearly identify the problematic theoretical and conceptual foundations of the mainstream in health literacy research. Methodologically, they have therefore taken a different path and primarily conducted qualitative, semi-standardised interviews, from which both studies infer everyday practices. Papen additionally conducted ethnographic research and followed six individuals primarily in the care setting. If the argumentation we have unfolded up to this point is at least to some extent correct, then there is a worrying lack of studies that analyse the contexts of action *in* which health competencies are transformed *in actu* into everyday practical action. This requires ethnographically based monitoring, which should take place as far as possible in the lifeworld environments – in the living environment, in extra-institutional everyday life, in group-specific gatherings or in family interactions – in order to sound out the interplay of individual action, opportunity structures and action restrictions, social embedding and social framing more precisely than would be possible with standardised instruments.

With the ELMi and ELiS projects, we have attempted to catch up with these perspectives. In doing so, we did not fall into the fallacy of believing we were developing and conducting health literacy research that is now correct and better than questionnaire research. As we have already seen above, we ourselves work with standardised surveys in order to make tangible the measure of the unequal distribution of individual action resources. Rather, we wanted to find out more precisely, in the context of basic research, *what exactly we see when we look in* a *(methodologically) different way.* An ethnographically based reconstruction of the spaces of action – in our studies: of young refugees from Afghanistan, of young people with a Turkish migration background in Germany, and of Latin American migrant families with young children in Switzerland – is a major challenge even for a theoretically well-informed praxeological or practice-theoretical perspective.

In this context, the theoretical-conceptual spectrum of difference and deficit, which we understand in our studies as a dialectical one in the sense of Theodor W. Adorno's negative dialectic, is once again of great importance.[8] This means, *first,* a concentration on the analysis of mediating processes between widely divergent and partly contradictory initial motifs and, *second,* the maintenance of a relationship of tension decisively initiated by two contrary concepts, without a rash resolution in favour of either of the two poles (cf. on this also Müller 2011), with full awareness that both poles in their conceptual purity represent ideologies as soon as they are extracted and detached from the relationship of tension. In more specific terms, this means for the interplay of deficit and difference that, with regard to health literacy, it is to be expected that deficits can indeed be detected in the most diverse areas and fields of action – with varying degrees of probability among different groups of actors – the ignoring of which would suggest a misconceived idea of solidarity with persons and groups who are weaker and underprivileged in terms of action resources. Deficits, as they are expressed in the spectrum of individual or family resources for action – along the lines of income, educational resources or even literacy and health skills – must be made visible as such. This is the independent and irreplaceable justification of a perspective that analyses the unequal distribution of resources for action.

It becomes problematic, however, when individuals or groups of people are defined exclusively in terms of a deficient resource endowment. In this case, all the

[8] We will not attempt a detailed consideration of the concept of dialectic here, but refer to the recent relevant literature, in which the concept of dialectic is reasonably elaborated. In our view, the studies Ritsert (1997); Müller (2011); Ritsert (2017) are authoritative; cf. also the instructive contribution Holzer (2019); as well as, of course, the initial work by Adorno 1966.

available individual and group-related resources for action and competences that were not part of a usually specific measurement are faded out and the spontaneity and creativity of human action are suppressed as a matter of principle (Joas 1996). Adopting a difference perspective is also necessary because health literacy research cannot blindly adopt the scientific constructions of high and low competencies in people without running the risk of simply reproducing inherent symbolic relations of domination and thus counteracting the critical visualisation of specific differences in competence within the framework of the deficit approach. These symbolic relations of domination consist, for example, in the fact that people with low literacy and/or low health literacy are denied the ability to think and act in the same complex way as "high scorers". Furthermore, an unreflective deficit perspective always encourages a meritocratic distribution logic, which at the end of the chain of reasoning explains the differences in salaries and the resulting differences in resources for action with the different individual competences and thus at the same time legitimises them – a simple circular argument. Finally, a closely related problem, which now also appears more frequently in the health literacy literature (for example, in Okan et al. 2017b; Paakkari and George 2018; Bittlingmayer and Sahrai 2019), is that structural problems and overall societal injustices are reformatted as individual differences in competence (Bittlingmayer 2016). This almost necessarily installs a "blaming the victim" process that simply flips the responsibilities for structural disadvantages.

For all the reasons that have only been cursorily explained here, a deficit perspective must, *in* our opinion, be combined with a difference perspective that attaches importance to the identification of existing resources and competences and that is in the tradition of a salutogenic or critical-pedagogical perspective. The adoption of a difference perspective stands first of all for the perception and acceptance of cultural differences in the broadest sense (cf. on this also the strong anthology by Schmidt 2014). With such a perspective, it is no longer possible to whole-heartedly propagate one-dimensional behaviours, nor to maintain the construction of a single reasonable health-oriented lifestyle. In this context, the lifestyles pursued in the lifeworlds are to be valued as equal in *principle,* and the conceptions of the good life of individuals, families or social groups are to be respected and honoured. Thus, an understanding and a more reconstructive strategy with regard to existing health competencies that become relevant in everyday practice becomes more central.

However, the strengthening of a difference perspective itself has its limits. First of all, it must be kept in mind that the relationship between deficits in resources for action and differences in life plans and strategies for action is not symmetrical. Here it is still true that social structures exert a preponderance, a clear predominance, over the overwhelming number of members of society. The tracing of available resources for action of underprivileged groups should not make the complementary mistake of constructing an autonomous, formerly underprivileged subject. Furthermore, it would be foolish to try to undermine the symbolic hierarchies and power relations inherent in everyday practices and lifestyles (Bourdieu 1982 still authoritative on this) by using health literacy research to sustainably raise the acceptance and recognition of the life practices of disadvantaged social groups. This ignores the sharpness of existing symbolic class struggles, which cannot be silenced with references to the, in principle, equal worth of different lifestyles.

From what has been said so far, crucial central orientation markers can be formulated for the research we are pursuing on the everyday frameworks of health literacy among young people with a migration or refugee background and migrant families with young children:

1. We are entering new territory (at least) in (German) health literacy research with our ethnographic approach to the health literacy of migrant youth and migrant families as embedded social practices outside of the classic institutional settings of observation such as health care delivery or educational institutions.
2. In doing so, we pursue a dialectical perspective between difference and deficit which, primarily in the tradition of salutogenesis, attempts to identify the existing resources and competences for action without, however, overlooking the structural and situational barriers to which the people we ethnographically accompany are exposed.
3. Our aim is not to establish the best health literacy research of all time, but above all to explore what actually comes into view when one accompanies people for several months and attempts to determine the existing competencies, contexts of action, opportunity structures and barriers to action more precisely.

In the following chapter, we present our methodological approach before focusing on the individual case studies.

The Ethnographic Study of Health Literacy: Methodological Notes

5

Abstract

The previous chapters have, from a theoretical perspective and on a broad literature basis, presented in detail how health literacy can be understood, which operationalisations (with their respective strengths and weaknesses) are available, which inequalities (can) occur, what relevance is attributed to parents, family and peer socialisation. In doing so, we listed the theoretical considerations of a meaningful health literacy research up to Adorno's negative dialectic. Such a theoretical pre-construction, which in our view is always necessary, inevitably creates the danger of a massive anti-climax when it comes to empirically catching up with all these perspectives.

The previous chapters have, from a theoretical perspective and on a broad literature basis, presented in detail how health literacy can be understood, which operationalisations (with their respective strengths and weaknesses) are available, which inequalities (can) occur, what relevance is attributed to parents, family and peer socialization. In doing so, we listed the theoretical considerations of a meaningful health literacy research up to Adorno's negative dialectic. Such a theoretical pre-construction, which in our view is always necessary, inevitably creates the danger of a massive anti-climax when it comes to empirically catching up with all these perspectives. We can openly admit that we will hardly succeed in doing so in the following chapters, but that we believe our case studies will contribute to bringing theoretical considerations and empirical research on health literacy among adolescents and families with young children closer together.

With regard to the connection between health literacy and everyday health actions of adolescents and parents with young children, we have noted that there

U. H. Bittlingmayer et al., *Health Literacy From A Health Ethnology Perspective*, https://doi.org/10.1007/978-3-658-42348-3_5

is a widespread lack of knowledge about the development of health literacy and its use in everyday life. The visualisation of social influences, of individual processes of meaning-making and attribution of meaning always exist only in their social and contextual frames of reference. The aim of our research was to observe these more closely and reveal them. Therefore, the choice of an ethnographic research agenda suggested itself as a method that can accommodate this theoretical overload. In this chapter, we will first briefly discuss the importance of ethnography in public health research and health literacy research (Sect. 5.1) and then present the methodological framework of this research approach (Sect. 5.2). We will then briefly introduce the three research projects (Sect. 5.3), before outlining the specific research procedures and the research process, including the difficulties and constructive modifications (Sect. 5.4).

5.1 Ethnographic Research in Public Health and Health Literacy Research

If health literacy is understood as a social practice within the family as its (major) social context and frame of reference (as explicated in more detail in the writings of Street, Papen, Santos), then it quickly becomes apparent – as in the studies presented previously – that the quantitative approach has its limitations. If we assume, from a difference-theoretical perspective, that complex resources for action are present in all subjects, then statistical relations are important in order to make broader trends visible, especially in the context of health and health literacy-related inequalities. But neither does this say anything about the interplay of dispositions, ideas and actions of a single individual (or smaller minority groups), nor is it possible to make the context of action visible in its structural and situational complexity.

Therefore, methodological procedures that take the subjectivity of individuals, their self-interpretations and explanatory patterns seriously are more appropriate for our approach and theoretical considerations. To meet the complexity of our purpose, the entire arsenal of qualitative research methods is to be used. Through the use of qualitative interview techniques such as the narrative (cf. e.g., Rosenthal and Loch 2002) or guided interview (cf. e.g., Helfferich 2019), the perspective and interpretations of the target group (or the experts) can be made visible and brought to bear.

On the other hand, there is a structural limit to interviews, and it lies in the fact that interviews can only tap explicitly accessible knowledge and the subjective interpretation of one's own attitudes, preferences or actions. This does take into account the subjectivity of people, which is considered part of the object of research. However, subject status should not be exaggerated in the context of social science research, because as reflective as – regardless of formal education! – people are, no one is completely transparent to himself or herself. This is shown not only by the psychoanalytically oriented research tradition, which, to express this opaqueness, coined the concept of the (deep-seated) character structure, but also by the phenomenological tradition, which shows, for example, that subjective relevance is mostly not decided on consciously, but is predisposed by socialisation and prior experience. Thus, in their introduction to the studies on authoritarian character, Theodor W. Adorno, Else Frenkel-Brunswik, Daniel J. Levinson and R. Nevitt Sanford keep the subjective parts of an action and the structural framings in a relationship of tension and conceptualise the – partly unconscious – character of an individual as an organising principle of his or her own opinions, values and preferences and, with regard to subjective actions, as a potentiality (cf. on this Adorno 1973, pp. 1–10). More or less analogously, though not on a psychoanalytical basis, Alfred Schütz argues that the consciousness of individuals follows some constitutive limitations and that the reflection on one's own behaviours may possibly lead to the elucidation of the specific genesis of this or that opinion or behaviour but does not reach the constitutional conditions of the genesis itself (Schütz 1971).

These limitations in the self-transparency of subjects are usually countered by reconstructive procedures. The most convincing procedure from our point of view is the objective hermeneutics developed by Ulrich Oevermann, which he himself classifies as a reconstruction-logical procedure. According to Oevermann, the basis of objective hermeneutics "consists in the authenticity of an expressive figure that is integral in itself, whose reconstructible latent structure of meaning validly embodies the case structure of a life practice, which in turn can be explicated in such a way as to bring to light the law of the case structure that determines the process of formation of this individual case, which generates the case structure of this individual case both as a general type and as a variant of a case structure that characterises the lifeworld or milieu to which this individual case belongs." (Oevermann 2010, p. 9). In other words, a specific procedural technique makes visible the structural framings of which the subjects themselves are not necessarily aware, and which turn subjective individual cases into *examples of something* in the sense of representations of certain structural logics. Oevermann provides a method based on the theoretical foundation of Adornite social research and aims to make visible the structures that structure every subject in all his actions and utterances. Oevermann himself describes his methodological approach succinctly in an essay that has received little attention to date:

> We begin the reconstruction of the objective structure of meaning of a specific utterance within the framework of objective hermeneutics by first telling stories about as diverse and contrasting situations as possible that are consistently in line with an utterance, that pragmatically fulfill its conditions of validity. In the next step, these told stories, which represent implicit thought-experimental constructions, are explicitly generalised in terms of the common structural properties they express, and in the third step, these general structural properties are compared with the specific contextual conditions in which the analysed utterance was made. (Oevermann 1983, pp. 236–237)

What is so convincing about this specific reconstructive procedure is without doubt the way in which structural framings of individual action are carefully unfolded. For our purposes, however, a procedure that limits structural reconstruction to the analysis of interview material is not quite ideal, although, in our view, Oevermann's objective hermeneutics deals with the tension between individual degrees of freedom, subjective competencies and objective (domination) structures in the best possible way in.

5.1.1 Health Literacy as Social Practice: Methodological Approaches

With regard to researching the health literacy of children and adolescents *as a social practice*, a method of direct observation of actions seemed particularly promising to us, not least because the communication patterns of young children and adolescents are somewhat specific. For conceptualising health literacy as a social practice, it is therefore, in our view, indispensable to accompany the children and adolescents in their lifeworld and to trace the processes of meaning and sense-making relevant for the role of health and health literacy. In terms of methodology, this is usually done in the form of an ethnographic study.

In order to be able to record, describe and understand conscious and unconscious interactions and meanings over a long period of time, approaches other than questionnaire research and statistical modelling are needed – as explained in Chap. 4. Proper research for this purpose must therefore take place in the "natural", lifeworld or milieu-specific environment, cognitive interest in must be pursued through an exploration of the processes, and it must be characterised by open-mindedly exploring the actual phenomenon and not by testing a preconceived hypothesis (Hammersley and Atkinson 2007). And research must not confine itself to the collection and analysis of interviews, as important as interviews (and conversations) are in the research process itself. This approach can be drawn straight from ethnographic research. Relevant ethnographic studies have explored the possibilities of illuminating lifestyles and lifeworlds in a more differentiated way and of analysing and reconstructing the processes of meaning-making and forms of action from the perspective of the participants themselves.[1]

However, ethnography cannot only serve to describe people and phenomena in detail but can also be helpful in the planning of interventions. For example, in the medical and health fields, international ethnographic studies, including medical ethnology, have made valuable contributions to improving treatment and healing outcomes by showing how decisions and behaviours are influenced by multiple conditions and how they can be adequately addressed. In recent years, ethnographic research has also been (re)discovered in the health sciences (see, among others, Papen 2009; Dilger and Dohrn 2016; Samerski 2019).

Although health ethnology and the use of ethnographic approaches is quite a common research practice internationally, it is still quite undeveloped in Germany; in the context of health literacy research, this approach has been largely ignored. Especially when it comes to groups of people who are considered high-risk and "hard to reach", ethnographic research designs can be described as complex and insightful approaches that capture the life situation, decision-making processes, the search for and the use of health-related information and its transformation into action, as well as the role of the social environment, as the present ethnographic studies on people with a migration background and/or refugee experience will show (cf. Chaps. 6, 7, and 8). In the following, we will briefly explain possible approaches and lines of tradition of health-related ethnographic research.

5.2 Approaches to Health-Related Ethnographic Research

Ethnographic approaches to researching health literacy among families with young children and adolescents can make reference to different traditions in medical and health anthropology. Points of reference would include Franz Boas' historical particularism, which emphasises the emic perspective in interpreting cultural practices, that is, the primacy of subjective sense-making over the objectifications by the researcher. The second point of reference is functionalism, represented by the work of Bronislaw Malinowski, one of the founding fathers of modern ethnographic research, a theory that has migrated deeply into standard sociological argumentation

[1] Still worth reading are reference studies such as Paul Willis' "Learning to Labor" or Annette Lareau's "Unequal Childhood"; Willis 1979; Lareau 2003.

(via Talcott Parsons, for example). The basic idea is that all cultural practices serve an overarching function, i.e., to reproduce the culture as a whole, without this having to be apparent to the researcher nor to the subject him/herself. In the context of social science research, Paul Willis argues analogously in the aforementioned study that the working-class children and adolescents' rebellion against educational institutions and their countercultural emphasis on (masculine) physical strength takes on the socialisation function of preparing young men for their, in all likelihood physically demanding occupational biography as dockworkers (Willis 1979; see also Dolby and Dimitriadis 2004; Willis 2004). More generally, as strange as it may seem from a public health perspective, unhealthy behaviour can be functional, for example in order to gain recognition in the adolescent peer group (see also Grundmann et al. 2006).

Finally, Clifford Geertz's interpretive anthropology, with its methodology of dense description, provides a particularly sharp focus on the social framings of even the simplest individual actions, arguing that a great deal of knowledge of the research field is necessary to place actions and utterances in the right context. All three traditions provide valuable inspiration for our perspective. In terms of the empirical research itself, we are guided by a catalogue that summarises the following features of ethnographic research (following Hammersley and Atkinson 2007):

- People are researched in their everyday living environment ("naturalism");
- "everything is data" – everything is considered and included as data material; data includes self-collected data (such as field notes, interviews), already existing data (documents, artefacts, diaries), as well as "unsystematically" collected data and information, which can also consist in WhatsApp groups, chat histories, etc. as additional, and increasingly important data from the digital universe;
- the data collection is 'unstructured' compared to other research methods both in the process and in the interpretive categories that adapt to the group being researched;
- (only) a small number of cases are explored, but in great detail and depth;
- the analysis of data includes both the interpretation of meanings, functions, consequences of human behaviour and institutional practices in a broader given context.

Consequently, the importance of the open-ended approach to exploring the social and contextual conditions of family and adolescent health literacies, and the interactions relevant to them, is strongly emphasised, for gaining a complex and theoretically based understanding – which includes subjective understandings and health actions, and how these relate to contextual conditions. Instrumental to our epistemological interest is Clifford Geertz's dense description methodology, which suggests a comprehensive description and analysis of contextual conditions (Geertz 2015). We try to do justice to this in our case studies by introducing the social (discursive) framings, such as the situation of the population with Turkish roots in Germany or typical conditions of Latin American immigration to Switzerland. In the following, we present the actual approach in the research projects in a little more detail.

5.3 Research Projects and the Identification of Target Groups

The aim of the research projects presented here was, on the one hand, to observe health-related action processes through direct participation in the lifeworld of adolescents or families, to generate knowledge and to obtain a deeper understanding of the connections between ethnic origin, health behaviour and competences, new social media/social media and health inequalities in adolescence or childhood socialisation (ELMi project).[2] A preliminary methodological decision in the ELMi project was that we wanted to recruit adolescents who were friends with each other, because typical extra-institutional everyday situations of adolescents take place in (small) groups and friendship should also be associated with a reasonable degree of security vis-à-vis university research; to accompany a single adolescent ethnographically, on the other hand, would, in our view, require justification and would take the misguided idea of social individualization at face value.

On the other hand, we wanted to examine more closely the socialisation-theoretical question of parental health competences and their relevance for the health competence development of young children in order to determine the intergenerational forms of transmitting competence. The target group was families with young children from Latin America residing in Switzerland (EliS project).[3] It should already be mentioned here that this research objective could only be

[2] The full name of the ELMi project is: eHealth Literacy and Minority Health: An Ethnographic Study of Health-Related Benefits of New Media among Disadvantaged Youth with Turkish and Afghan Immigrant Backgrounds.

[3] The full name of the EliS project is: Ethnography of Health Literacy as Social Practice. Health Disparities, Health Promotion, and Health Literacy among Latino Families in Switzerland: A Health Exploratory Ethnographic Study.

achieved to a limited extent because the study had to be terminated prematurely due to staff leaving.

In the ELMi project, we determined the target groups from an inequality theory perspective along the inequality dimensions of social origin, ethnicity and gender affiliation (without fixing these categories too much in advance) in the sense of an intersectional approach (Winker and Degele 2010). We defined these intertwined dimensions of inequality as design variables and focused on socially disadvantaged, female and male youth of non-German ethnicity. In the EliS project, the target group was theoretically predefined in analogy and confined to families with young children who immigrated to Switzerland from Latin America. On the basis of our initial findings, the criterion of economic social disadvantage was not used as a strong criterion for this group, but rather related to the people's respective residence status, because this played a relevant and somewhat decisive role for the target group.

Since we referred to ethnicity in defining the target group, we would like to make a few remarks beforehand in order to prevent misunderstandings. In principle, we represent a social constructivist (but not a radical constructivist!) approach with regard to the structural category of ethnicity (cf. e.g., Rademacher and Wiechens 2001). Although we did select people on the basis of their ethnicity (as well as other criteria), we do not understand ethnicity in the sense of a cultural essence, but as a socialisation framework (this is how we understand the milieu approach by Michael Vester and colleagues; cf. on this Vester et al. 2001; Bauer and Vester 2015). This socialisation framework *can be* situationally significant, *can* play a central role in the development of a child's or adolescent's identity, as a rule always depending on the social environment, and can lead to a clear positioning within a minority, but it does not have to. Trying to fix young people of the third or fourth generation to the cultural or ethnic origin of their (great)grandparents would be a grave mistake indeed. At the same time, it would also be strange to ignore existing cultural differences of large social groups, such as different beliefs, eating habits and group-specific taboos. Because migrant populations or ethnic minorities are frequently attested lower health literacy in socio-epidemiological studies, we explicitly considered this inequality dimension. The language skills of the researchers were the decisive criterion in the selection of ethnic origin. According to the available language competences Turkish, Spanish and Dari (Dari-Persian), young people with a Turkish migration background, families from Latin America and young people from Afghanistan were chosen as target groups. The researchers assigned to each group of adolescents from Afghanistan and Turkey were themselves from the respective ethnic groups. The researcher for the ethnography in Latin American families in Switzerland was Swiss, but with very good language skills, a personal connection to Latin America and well connected within the Latin American community in Switzerland.

Furthermore, we chose a gender-specific approach in selecting the target group, on the one hand due to socio-epidemiological findings, as many studies show that female and male adolescents differ significantly from each other (cf. e.g., Kolip et al. 2013). We assigned to each of the target groups a researcher of the same respective gender. Because it was to be expected that parents would have considerable reservations about a young male researcher exploring the everyday practices of girls, we designed the ethnography to be same sex. This means that a female researcher accompanied girls or mothers with (small) children and that a male researcher accompanied boys in their everyday lives.

Finally, in the context of the relevance of social practices, which in our study was more of a focus than skills-based individual endowment, the ethnography was concerned with getting a "feel" for the social environment of families and adolescents. Adolescents, as previously mentioned, are always part of a larger network consisting of social relationships and loose contacts, which includes family, friends, school, as well as other spare-time contacts. Although the main focus was on young people and families with young children, the target persons as representatives of the target groups cannot be described separately from their social relations in their real-life world, and their opinion-forming, meaning-making processes and behaviours can only be understood in the light of their embedding in their social context. We pursued a strategy of "de-individualization" here by framing our research as milieu studies. The *overarching goal was to make the contexts of action visible, to gain insights into the otherwise closed black boxes of family or peer group, and to trace the intergenerational dimension of health literacy*.

To this end, we focused on three groups accessible to the research team but had to make some adaptations in the course of the project phase due to the usual field-specific restrictions and difficulties in recruitment. In the two projects, ELMi and the Swiss sister project ELiS, we accompanied the above-mentioned target groups over a period of up to nine months in 2016 and 2017.

In the first sub-project of ELMi, Zeynep Islertas accompanied two female adolescents with a Turkish migration background for nine months in their free time and in different settings. The group of people with a Turkish migration background represents the largest of the migrant populations living in Germany and amounts to 14.4% of the total of 19.3 million people with a migration background. A large number of young people with a Turkish migration background are part of the third (or even, depending on the census, the fourth) generation living in Germany and are still significantly more likely to belong to a rather low and precarious class socio-economically than do Germans with no migration background. Contrary to what was theoretically projected in advance, it was not possible to recruit female adolescents with a Turkish migration background from secondary schools or special schools. The cultural distance and symbolic barriers to participating in a university research project were too great, so that only a female Realschule student and a female Gymnasium student were accompanied in the study.

In the second ELMi sub-project, Elias Sahrai accompanied young people from Afghanistan. Allowing for minor simplification, the population of Afghan origin residing in Germany can be divided into three groups. The first group consists of people who fled the Soviet invasion, the second group consists of people who had to flee the Taliban, and the third group consists of Afghans who recently immigrated to Germany after 2014 in the course of the so-called refugee crisis. The Afghan minority that immigrated to Germany in the 1980s to 2000s was (and still is) considered an example of a socially well integrated group that also does well when it comes to educational success. In the course of the project, we wanted to recruit male youths from the first two groups. We did not succeed, although we used all conceivable recruitment strategies (mosque visits, incentives, etc.). Instead, we were able – rather surprisingly for us – to recruit male Afghan adolescents from the third group for the study. They have their own immigration history and a recent successful escape behind them, so that their available health competencies can be significantly impaired by flight experiences or a problematic residence status (more on this in the case study in Chap. 7).

The group of Afghan asylum seekers has been repeatedly in the focus of mass media attention, because Afghanistan is not classified as a civil war country in the interpretation of political decision-makers, unlike other civil war countries such as Syria, Iraq or Somalia, whose asylum seekers currently have a high probability of remaining. People from Afghanistan usually only receive a toleration issued for a few months, and recently there have been repeated deportations to Afghanistan "staged" with an eye on media attention. This problematic residence status of current Afghan asylum seekers is probably also an important factor influencing adolescent health literacy. On the other hand, almost nothing is known about the health literacy of refugee adolescents (see as one of the very rare studies Wångdahl et al. 2015, 2018). Therefore, in the end, we accompanied male adolescent asylum seekers, fully aware that the research would take on a more exploratory character.

Finally, in the Swiss EliS project, families with young children from Colombia were originally intended to be the target group, as comparatively good field access to the Colombian community was available and people with a Colombian migration background represent the third-largest Latin American group of immigrants to

Switzerland (Bundesamt für Statistik 2019). Again, however, despite an intensive recruitment phase lasting several months, it proved particularly difficult to convince only Colombian families to participate in the EliS project. Therefore, the target group was expanded to include people from all over Latin America. This approach, which had not been planned in this way, was inspired by field experiences themselves, because people from different South and Central American countries describe themselves in a homogenic manner as a "Latino community" due to their small numbers in Switzerland. The constituting criterion – apart from Catholicism – is Spanish, their common first language, against the background of which the national differences, present within South and Central America *initially* recede in Switzerland. In the concluding section of the methodological part, we describe the technical research procedure before presenting the case studies in detail in the next chapters.

5.4 Recruitment

Before the ELMi study was conducted, we submitted a detailed outline of the research project to the ethics committee of a major university in Baden-Württemberg for review. The vote of the ethics committee was positive (the decision was made in April 2016), no legal or ethical concerns were raised. In order to explore the research fields, the ELMi project, for example, not only did the usual extensive literature research, but also conducted interviews with experts from child and youth welfare as well as interviews and focus groups with young people.

In order to gain an insight into the extra-institutional life-worlds of young people, experts in open youth work, especially social workers from youth centres, were asked about current youth cultures, the role of youth centres, characterisation of young visitors, recurring leisure activities with young people, health behaviour, understanding and influencing factors, health-related offers and the use of new media. Furthermore, individual interviews and focus group discussions with young people with and without a migration background were conducted with regard to their understandings of health, everyday coping strategies, approaches to health issues, the role of school lessons, use of the Internet and social media, among other things.

A wide range of measures and recruitment strategies were used to explore the field of investigation within the ELMi project, to gain access to the field and to recruit young people. These included inviting experienced ethnological field researchers or creating an urban youth map to visualise places where young people spend time. Of course, the usual repertoire was also used and multilingual (German-Turkish; German-Dari) information flyers and posters were produced. The flyers for the recruitment of male Afghan youth were distributed, for example, in Asian supermarkets and restaurants as well as (in a later recruitment phase) in asylum seeker shelters to Afghan families. Furthermore, access was sought through gatekeepers from the social work, education and religious communities. For example, social educators from youth centres, contact persons from various social institutions, school social workers, school administrators, coordinators of teachers for Turkish language instruction, contact persons from German-Turkish parents' associations, and imams from various mosques were specifically approached as part of the recruitment process. Finally, the existing networks of the researchers were used to inform about the project as well as to recruit potential participants.

The recruitment of the Turkish girls was successful through the mediation of people who are active in mosque communities. In the end, the successful recruitment of and contact with the Afghan refugees was brought about in each case thanks to the help of a refugee aid volunteer.

Different strategies were also used in the ELiS project to recruit participants for the interviews. Different settings were identified in which Latin American migrants were present and contact was made with them. Flyers and information letters were distributed in different places where it was assumed that migrants from Latin America were present.

In order to avoid redundancies between an outsourced methodology chapter and the three case studies, further methodological details will be explained and taken up in the case studies. In the following three chapters, then, the question of what exactly we saw after a conversion of the methodological gaze will be answered in detail.

Part II

Case Studies

6 Health Understanding and Health Competences of Two Girls with a Turkish Migration Background

Abstract

The fact that Germany is an immigration country can be exemplified by various historical events in the Federal Republic. First and foremost, the promotion of labour migration after the Second World War should be mentioned. The Federal Republic signed various recruitment agreements with Turkey and seven other countries between 1955 and 1968 in order to meet the economic challenges in the country. As early as 1964, the millionth guest worker was admitted to Germany (Seifert, 2012).

Germany is the most popular immigration country in Europe. (OECD 2018)

6.1 Introduction

The fact that Germany is an immigration country can be exemplified by various historical events in the Federal Republic.

First and foremost, the promotion of labour migration after the Second World War should be mentioned. The Federal Republic of Germany signed various recruitment agreements with Turkey and seven other countries between 1955 and 1968 in order to meet the economic challenges in the country. As early as 1964, the millionth guest worker was admitted to Germany (Seifert 2012). Due to demographic change, Germany has again been dependent on workers from abroad for several years. For example, as early as 2000, during the international computer trade fair CeBIT, the then German Chancellor Gerhard Schröder announced the introduction of a German green card in order to be able to bring foreign experts in the field of

U. H. Bittlingmayer et al., *Health Literacy From A Health Ethnology Perspective*, https://doi.org/10.1007/978-3-658-42348-3_6

information technologies into the country with as little red tape as possible (Brodmerkel 2017). Eighteen years later – in 2018 – Germany is described by the Organisation for Economic Cooperation and Development as the most popular immigration country in Europe. It is emphasised that the majority of immigrants are labour migrants from Europe (OECD 2018).

The economically stable Federal Republic of Germany has a population of about 82 million people in 2017. If the population composition is examined more closely, it can be stated that 23.6% of the population have a migration background. People with a Turkish migration background represent the largest group of the population with a migration background in Germany, ahead of people from Poland and Russia (Bundeszentrale für politische Bildung 2018).

Despite the economic stability and the well-developed social and welfare systems in the country, the various population groups in the Federal Republic do not have the same living conditions at their disposal. For example, around 14% of the population is at risk of poverty. Among children and young people, this proportion is as high as 17% (Lampert and Koch-Gromus 2016). People with a migration background in Germany are more often affected by a low socio-economic status than the native population in Germany (Lokhande 2016; Nold 2010).

Social epidemiological studies outline the relationship between the "social inequalities" (Hradil 2012) just outlined and the health of the population (see in detail Chap. 2). The majority of available studies show that low socioeconomic status is associated with poorer health, a higher risk of physical and mental illnesses, as well as functional restrictions in everyday life and an impaired health-related quality of life (Lampert and Koch-Gromus 2016; Lampert and Kroll 2010).

In addition to economic and social conditions as well as educational status, which are related to health, the dependence of health on a person's gender has been discussed. For example, gender-differentiated studies in the field of health very clearly point to differences between men and women with regard to health and disease behaviour, disease profiles and living conditions (Ministerium für Arbeit, Soziales, Gesundheit, Frauen und Familie Brandenburg 2018; Regitz-Zagrosek 2018; Babitsch et al. 2017).

6.1.1 Health of the Turkish Migrant Population

When looking at the studies that illustrate the connection between health and the health-relevant framework conditions of people or population groups in Germany, it must be noted that a comparison is made between the health of autochthons and people or population groups with a migration background, as well as a comparison within the "group with a migration background". Here, people with a Turkish migration background are described as particularly vulnerable (Lampert and Koch-Gromus 2016; Knipper and Bilgin 2009). They are said to have a lower economic and educational status and more often deficient social conditions compared to the autochthonous population in Germany as well as compared to people from Italy, Spain and Portugal living in Germany (Bundeszentrale für politische Bildung und Statistisches Bundesamt 2016). In addition, they are declared to be a "difficult group to reach" for health promotion programmes. Borde and Blümel (2015) report that health promotion programmes reach people with a migration background less frequently than they do the autochthonous population in Germany.

The described health-related vulnerability of people with a Turkish migration background is also confirmed by the most recent quantitative health literacy studies. These studies illustrate that people with a migration background have a low level of health literacy and consequently face difficulties in searching for, finding and evaluating health information and in implementing or transferring newly acquired health-related knowledge into their everyday lives (Horn et al. 2015; Messer et al. 2015; Quenzel et al. 2016a).

Qualitative research on health literacy and studies on the health literacy level of migrant children and adolescents, on the other hand, can hardly be found. Thus, the health literacy level of children and adolescents within the existing studies is usually derived from the parents, and the connections of a person's health literacy level with health behaviour, health outcomes and health status are presented. According to Faltermaier et al. (1998b), however, qualitative studies are a relevant and necessary addition to quantitative approaches in the empirical health field, since a large part of health-relevant everyday behaviour is shaped by the unconscious or barely conscious interaction of different socialising influences. Thus, (health) behaviours are social practices rather than conscious behaviours. In addition, Johnson et al. (2011) report that the complex relationships between health literacy and health behaviour or health outcomes can be better illustrated and understood through qualitative study designs.

Within the qualitative youth health study "ELMi" (eHealth Literacy and minority health), funded by the Federal Ministry of Education and Research, we followed this recommendation. Two female adolescents with a Turkish migration background and their social environment were ethnographically accompanied over a period of nine months in order to be able to understand and describe how health is implemented in their everyday lives, what meaning-making processes they pursue in this context and what role new media (Holly 2000) play in their health-relevant everyday actions. Essential results are presented and discussed in this chapter.

In order to be able to place the target group and the health-relevant framework conditions they encounter within German society as a whole, the first step (Sect. 6.2) – without claiming completeness – provides a historical outline of how the guest workers from Turkey and their health were reported in the 1970s. In the following, Sect. 6.3 presents current data and health-related findings on this population group in Germany. After outlining the state of socio-epidemiological research, the next Sect. 6.4, deals with the results of the ethnographic-salutogenic youth health study on female adolescents with a Turkish migration background in Germany. Here, the connection of their health with their lifeworld (Thiersch 2012) will be described by going into the political situation, the socio-economic framework conditions, the social networks and the lifeworld settings (World Health Organization 1986; Altgeld 2004a), as well as outlining the role of new media in their health-related everyday actions. In Sect. 6.5, the results will finally be related to the studies already available, as well as discussed.

6.2 The "Guest Worker" ... and His/Her Health

> Manpower has been called, and human beings are coming. (Frisch 1965).

Germany promoted labour migration in the past and now has a long history as an immigration country. The reason for this is, among other things, the number of citizens killed in the war and the resulting loss of workers who were needed for the reconstruction of the Federal Republic. In addition, the shortage of workers came to a head as a result of the "economic boom" that followed the Second World War and which is still proverbial today. In order to prevent the positive economic developments after the Second World War from flattening out and to ensure that strong economic growth was sustained, additional workers were recruited abroad. Thus, the government of the time under Konrad Adenauer concluded the first recruitment agreement with Italy on December 20, 1955. This was followed by agreements with Greece and Spain (1960), Turkey (1961), Morocco and South Korea (1963), Portugal (1964), Tunisia (1965) and the former Yugoslavia (1968). The initiatives for this came from the recruiting country as well as the applicant country: Germany needed people to support the economy with their labour during the boom, and the countries with which a recruitment agreement was concluded were affected by social and economic upheaval, high population growth, and severe underemployment, which led to high "emigration pressure" at home (Brodmerkel 2017; Luft 2014; Seifert 2012). The Turkish government expected the agreement with the Federal Republic of Germany to provide urgently needed foreign currency earnings in addition to relieving the pressure on its own labour market, as well as a boost to modernisation from returning guest workers who would have acquired the relevant qualifications. Thus, from the perspective of the country of origin, as well as the Federal Republic, employment was to remain temporary (Brodmerkel 2017; Gieler 2017; Hunn 2005; Luft 2014; Seifert 2012). Between 1961 and 1973, more than two and a half million applications for emigration to the Federal Republic were received from Turkey. One in four of them, about 625,000 people were admitted. The foreign workers were mostly employed in the mining, metal and textile industries, i.e., industries with low qualification requirements (Gieler 2017; Luft 2014; Seifert 2012).

At the end of the 1960s, the economic situation in the Federal Republic changed – a recession set in. When the economic crisis reached its first peak in 1973, Germany stopped recruiting guest workers. At the same time, many companies had a strong interest in not laying off the workers they had recruited and trained, so many foreign workers brought their families and settled in for a permanent stay. Also, contrary to the original plans of the Federal Republic of Germany and Turkey regarding the repatriation of Turkish migrant workers, the majority of people with a Turkish migration background living in Germany decided against returning to their country of origin (Brodmerkel 2017; Gieler 2017; Hunn 2005; Luft 2014; Seifert 2012).

When the arrivals were referred to as guest workers, this was also associated with expectations that were or are related to the health of these people. For example, the health examinations already carried out in the home countries were intended to ensure that only young, healthy workers came to Germany (Razum et al. 2011). Acute physical illness and impaired ability to work were to be ruled out by certain diagnostic procedures. Thus, the German healthcare system was mainly concerned with the physical health or disease status of the guest workers. Mental illnesses were neglected due to a lack of time resources, and the challenging nature of diagnoses and therapies (Knipper and Bilgin 2010).

Guest workers in the Federal Republic of Germany often suffered from so-called psychosomatic illnesses, which manifested themselves in physical symptoms such as back, joint and muscle pain and/or gastrointestinal illnesses, without any organic causes to be found. In one of the first systematic studies on the mental illnesses of guest workers, Häfner et al. (1977) recorded that a quarter of the guest workers examined became mentally ill three months after their immigration and a third after 18 months. The initially predominant depressive syndromes almost exclusively turned into psychosomatic complaints.

In addition, in the 1970s, a so-called "guest worker ulcer" was discussed. In this context, an attempt was made to establish a connection between the occurrence of ulcers in the stomach and the duodenum, and the migration background of the respective patients, since guest workers suffered disproportionately often from this disease, for which psychosomatic disease theories in particular suggested themselves as explanatory models (Hartl and Pürgyi 1975; Horn and Herfarth 1978). Among the explanations discussed at the time were psychosocial stresses resulting on the one hand from sociocultural "uprootedness" as a consequence of separation from the "homeland" and the social environment left behind, and on the other hand from social isolation in the "host country" and difficulties in "acculturation" in a society with a foreign language and a foreign system of communication and values (Bilgin et al. 1988; Böker 1977; Häfner et al. 1977). However, with the discovery of a bacterial cause and the development of corresponding therapeutic approaches in the 1980s, the migration-related psychosomatic pattern of interpretation largely faded into the background, although the link between psychological stress and gastrointestinal disorders has not been refuted (Leiß 2001).

Looking back at the debates in the 1970s, it becomes clear that the guest workers were not expected to "integrate" into German society, but at best to "partially adapt" for the duration of their stay. This also seemed necessary from a medical point of view in order to avoid the pathogenic consequences of being "uprooted", especially since the linguistic and cultural barrier between the population and the guest workers was considered "relatively high". In addition, it was pointed out at the time that due to such a situation, considerable social and above all psychological problems were to be expected for the guest workers in the long term, from which their children born in Germany in particular would have to suffer (Häfner et al. 1977; Riedesser 1973; Knipper and Bilgin 2009).

6.3 People with a Turkish Migration Background in Germany: Facts and Figures

In 2016, 18.6 million of the 82.4 million inhabitants in Germany had a migration background. 69.6% of these people represented the first generation and 31.4% the second or third generation. Compared to the first generation, they have no migration or immigration experience of their own (Bundeszentrale für politische Bildung 2018).

Followed by people from Poland, Russia and Italy, people with a Turkish migration background represented the largest group with a migration background in the Federal Republic, accounting for 15.1% of the 18.6 million overall, yet they can by no means be considered a homogeneous group (Bundeszentrale für politische Bildung 2018).

If the age structure of Germany's overall population is examined more closely, it can be seen that demographic change caused by the decline in births and rising life expectancy represents one of the greatest socio-political and health policy challenges in Germany. Thus, in 2016, 17.5 million people in the Federal Republic were 65 years old and older. At the same time, the number of people under the age of 18 was 13.3 million (Statistisches Bundesamt 2019, 2018b).

Consequently, the question of the future of the healthcare system in Germany is being discussed against the backdrop of demographic change and the rising number of cases of illness (Peters et al. 2010). According to Peters and colleagues, age-related changes in the overall population will increase the so-called widespread diseases and the prevalence of particularly cost-intensive diseases such as osteoarthritis, dementia, cancer or renal insufficiency by 2050. The gender aspect is not to be neglected either when considering health policies. For example, according to Babitsch et al. (2017), a difference can be observed between men and women in terms of health behaviour, health outcomes and health status. Females represent a slightly larger proportion of the total population in Germany than males. In 2016, 41.8 million women and 40.7 men lived in the Federal Republic (Federal Statistical Office 2018a). If only the population group with a migration background in Germany is considered, it can be stated that they represent a younger group compared to the autochthonous population and show a slight (two percent) surplus of men (Woellert and Klingholz 2014).

In addition to gender and age, people's educational status, economic and social conditions, as well as their use of new media are related to the health of people or population groups in Germany (Lampert and Kroll 2010; Lampert and Koch-Gromus 2016; Horn et al. 2015). In the following section, the (formal) level of education of the overall population and of people with a Turkish migration background in Germany is discussed, before other health-relevant aspects such as socio-economic status and the role of new media in (health-related) everyday life are addressed.

6.3.1 Education and Vocational Training

International comparative studies such as PISA (Programme for International Student Assessment) and IGLU (International Primary School Reading Survey) show that educational success and educational opportunities in Germany are strongly dependent on social origin or migration background. Thus, an important indicator for the socio-economic status of children seems to be the educational attainment of their parents (Bundeszentrale für politische Bildung and Statistisches Bundesamt 2016; Statistisches Bundesamt 2016; Schulze and Preisendörfer 2013).

On average, foreign youths have a significantly worse school education than native Germans (Bundesministerium für Arbeit und Soziales 2005; Organisation for Economic Co-operation and Development 2018; Britz 2007; Schulze and Preisendörfer 2013). However, there are also differences between the various migrant groups and their educational status. A comparatively high level of education is found in people with a Polish or Russian migrant background. The educational indicators for people with a Turkish migration background have improved slightly since 2005, but they do not reach the average of all migrants or natives. Current statistics show that 35.5% of people with a Turkish migration background have a lower secondary school leaving certificate. Only 11.8% have a specialised baccalaureate or the general university entrance qualification (Statistisches Bundesamt 2018c). By contrast, only 27.7% of the autochthonous population acquire a lower secondary school leaving certificate and 32.1% an advanced technical college or university degree (Statistisches Bundesamt 2018d).

If the educational parameters of adults with a migration background in Germany today are examined in more detail, it can be seen that 68% of working age people with a Turkish migration background who moved to Germany during the period of the recruitment agreement still have no vocational qualification and 33% have no school-leaving qualifications. A similar picture can be seen among people from Turkey who came to Germany after the recruitment stop, mostly by way of family reunification (Bundeszentrale für politische Bildung und Statistisches Bundesamt 2016). One possible explanation for this "low" level of education may be the history of the Turkish migrant group: the population group that decided to migrate to Germany from Turkey was composed of people who lived under economically and culturally poor conditions in their country of origin (Herburger 2010). In addition, there was no systematic schooling in Germany for the guest workers who were integrated into their fields of work and workplaces, so that they could not acquire the language skills that are unanimously considered necessary today for the chance of further education and for successful social integration (Maier 2012; Sauer 2007). Furthermore, after the arrival of family members and after the second generation had been born in Germany, migrants as well as most Germans believed that the language problems would get solved simply by integrating the children into the German school system (Goldberg and Sauer 2003). The reason for this was that parents attached particular importance to language classes for migrant children in the German education system, and Turkish parents therefore placed a high degree of trust in the German school and expected it to make a significant contribution to their own social integration (Sahrai 2010a; Deutsches Institut für Internationale Pädagogische Forschung 2016; Bittlingmayer and Bauer 2007a).

6.3.2 Household Structure and Household Income

According to the results of the 2009 Microcensus, 28.4% of all families in Germany have a migration background. Families in which at least one family member has a Turkish migration background make up the highest proportion of families with a migration background at 21% (Statistisches Bundesamt 2010). Compared to native families, families with a migration background show "more traditional family ties", in which marriage with children is the dominant form of family cohabitation. Alternative forms of living, such as unmarried heterosexual or even same-sex couples with children and one to two person households are rare (Bundesministerium für Familie, Senioren, Frauen und Jugend 2009; Uygun-Altunbaş 2017).

According to estimates, about two thirds of families with a migration background live in a household with one or two children, in which regard they do not differ from German families. However, the number of families with three or four children is 20%, while this proportion is 12% among families without a migration background. If a distinction is made according to the origin of the families with a migration background, it can be seen that the rate for Turkish married couples with three or four children is above average compared to other migrant groups (Bundesministerium für Familie, Senioren, Frauen und Jugend 2009).

A clear difference can be observed with regard to the per capita income of people with and without a migration background. 26% of people with a migration background have a monthly net income of less than €500. Among the autochthonous population in Germany, the number is 17%. Among the native population without a migration background, 32 per cent have a monthly net income of between €1300 and €2600, as opposed to 26% among migrants. Only 3% of people with a migrant background earn between €2600 and €4500 per month. In this income group the difference between the autochthonous population and people with a migration background amounts to four percentage points (see Fig. 6.1) (Statistisches Bundesamt 2018e).

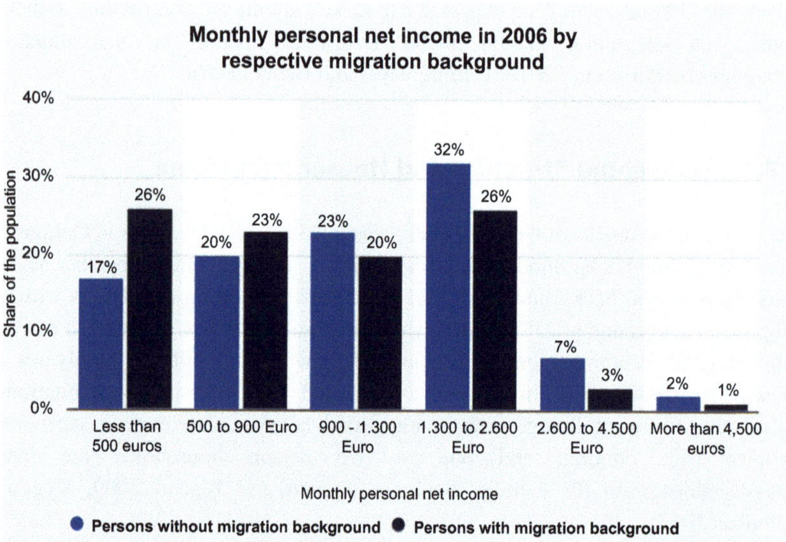

Fig. 6.1 Federal Statistical Office: Monthly net income per capita per year

6.3.3 Religion/Beliefs

The assumption that a person's religion and/or faith can be related to their health is supported by numerous studies. It has been repeatedly described that a person's religion/faith can be regarded as a health-promoting aspect (Klein and Albani 2007; Hefti 2010; Reich 2003). Some studies discuss the connection between individual aspects of health and a person's religiosity and it has been pointed out that a holistic exploration of the connection can be useful for the treatment of illnesses (Klein and Albani 2007).

There are no precise figures on how many Muslims actually live in Germany. This is because exact figures on people's Islamic denomination cannot be found via the Federal Statistical Office (Uygun-Altunbaş 2017). According to the Federal Office for Migration and Refugees, the number varies between 4.4 and 4.7 million (Stichs 2016). If an attempt is made to describe the religious affiliation as well as degrees of devoutness among the people with a Turkish migration background in Germany, the numbers, with a few exceptions, are the same as in Turkey (Sauer 2007). Thus 95% of people with a Turkish migration background living in Germany belong to the Muslim faith. About 1.5% of this group of people identify as Christian or of other faiths. 2.5% identify as non-religious (Sauer 2007).

If we take a closer look at the group of people who describe themselves as belonging to Islam, Sunnis (74%) and Alevis (13%) represent the two largest subgroups among Muslims (Haug et al. 2009). In this context, 50–60% of the population group with a Turkish migration background describe themselves as religious. Furthermore, 62% of people with a Turkish migration background state that religion is important to very important for them in their daily lives. The majority also define themselves not only as formally belonging to Islam, but also emotionally. If the gender aspect is considered more closely, women are more likely than men to declare their close religious affiliation (Sauer 2007).

These rough figures show that, *on average,* religion has a different status in the Muslim population in general and in the Turkish population in particular than Christianity in its two main denominations has for the majority of the German population. As will be shown below, Islam is also extremely relevant for the two female adolescents participating in the study, both in their everyday lives and for their actual health behaviour, and it serves as an orientation framework for their everyday actions that does not require legitimation in their Turkish-Muslim lifeworld.

6.3.4 The Internet as an Information Platform

Health information is accessible to a large part of the world's population via a wide variety of media. There are television channels, various radio stations and also websites exclusively devoted to health-related topics (Kryspin-Exner and Stetina 2009). Health-related websites were among the most used sites on the Internet early on (Wilson 2002). About three quarters of adults in the USA use the Internet to obtain health information and the majority of them consider the use of the Internet to be a helpful tool for making health-related decisions. In Germany, too, the hardware available in households is used to obtain health-related information. For example, Zschorlich et al. (2015) report that middle-aged women with above-average levels of education and income are most likely to search for health information on the Internet. However, electronic health information plays a very important role in the daily lives not only of adults, but of young people, too. Wartella et al. (2016) report that this population group uses the internet-enabled devices available to them to obtain information on topics such as wellness/lifestyle, sexuality, pregnancy, fitness, nutrition, piercing/tattoos and skin care. In addition to the health apps used here, there are various favourite websites. Here, it is not exclusively the written information provided online that is of interest to the young people. The internet is also seen as a platform for direct communication with health experts as well as other affected people (Zschorlich et al. 2015). If the results of studies on the internet use of young people with a Turkish migration background in Germany are examined in more detail, it can be seen that there are major overlaps with the behaviour patterns of autochthonous young people. For example, the quantitative study by Trebbe and colleagues describes young people with a Turkish migration background as using the Internet as a communication and entertainment platform as well as a source of information (Trebbe et al. 2010). However, empirical findings on whether the target group also uses the Internet to obtain health information are hard to come by.

6.3.5 Health of People with a Turkish Migration Background in Germany

People with a migration background are a heterogeneous group in terms of their countries of origin, migration motives, ethnic and cultural backgrounds, socioeconomic status and health behaviour (Razum et al. 2008; Knipper and Bilgin 2010). Furthermore, heterogeneity can also be observed within the different ethnic groups. Thus, it is difficult or impossible to speak of "the Italians", "the Turks" or "the Russians".

For scientific or technical reasons, many health studies use quantitative approaches. Within this approach, the health of people with and without a migration background has been compared, or various migrant groups have been compared that way (see also Chap. 3). The all but universal finding in all of these studies seems to be that people with a migration background exhibit increased health risks, more frequently "inadequate" or "risky" health behaviour and poorer health outcomes compared to the native majority population. Migration alone is not used as an explanation for this, but also the circumstances of migration and the living and working conditions of people with a migration background in Germany (Razum et al. 2008). In addition to the above-mentioned relation-oriented/external explanations, behaviour-oriented explanations such as lower physical activity or a low health literacy level are cited and the connection with health status is discussed (Razum et al. 2008; Horn et al. 2015; Messer et al. 2015; Quenzel et al. 2016a). In the following, some target group-specific findings will be briefly outlined.

"Turkish families are too fat" (Daniel 2009) read the headline of an article in the media. But it is not only the public discourse that draws attention to the prevalence and consequences of overweight and obesity in the population as a whole and describes people with a Turkish migration background as particularly vulnerable. Existing studies have repeatedly shown that the body mass index values of middle-aged and older women with a migration background are higher than those of native women in Germany (Razum et al. 2008; Statistisches Bundesamt 2007, 2010). Particularly women with a Turkish migration background are described here as a vulnerable group who frequently exhibit obesity and a low value of "good cholesterol", the so-called HDL value, and are thus exposed to a high risk of suffering from coronary heart disease (Razum et al. 2008). However, it is not only adult women with a Turkish migration background who are frequently overweight or obese. Even children and adolescents with a Turkish migration background are described as significantly more often affected by overweight or obesity (Zwick et al. 2011).

In addition to the description of physical health, there are currently also numerous studies that deal with the mental health of people with a Turkish migration background. Socioeconomic status and nationality are used to explain the prevalence of mental illness. For example, Schouler and colleagues (2015) report that socioeconomic status and perceived discrimination may be associated with mental health. In their study, people of Polish, Vietnamese and Turkish nationality are mentioned as being particularly at risk.

In another report, a low socioeconomic status of women with a Turkish migration background in the first and second generation is associated with a large emotional stress burden (Bromand et al. 2012). In addition to socioeconomic status, the influence of nationality on mental health has been discussed. Merbach et al. (2008) describe citizenship as a possible predictor of depression and anxiety. Social problems and anxiety also lead to mental distress among the same population group in Germany, according to Bermejo et al. (2010). According to a federal health survey, for instance, women with a Turkish migration background seem to show an increased prevalence of mental disorders.

In addition to health status, the health-related studies also address health behaviour. For example, it is shown that increased psychological stress and less favourable living conditions can lead to a higher degree of risky behaviour, such as alcohol and cigarette consumption as well as drug and medication abuse, especially among young people from families with a migration background (Walter et al. 2007). Migrants from Turkey and Russia seem to be most affected by drug problems (Walter et al. 2007). With regard to alcohol consumption, it should be mentioned that newly immigrated young people drink less alcohol than young people with a Turkish migration background who were born and grew up in Germany (Schouler-Ocak et al. 2015). However, the alcohol consumption of young people with a migration background equals that of autochthonous young people in the long run (provided they continue living in Germany). If female and male adolescents are compared, it can be noted that female adolescents with a migration background drink less alcohol, than both male adolescents with the same migration background and female autochthonous adolescents (Schouler-Ocak et al. 2015). Religious affiliation is cited as an explanation for the lower consumption of alcohol by female adolescents with a Turkish migration background (Brettschneider et al. 2015; Boos-Nünning and Siefen 2005).

In addition to alcohol and cigarette consumption, a prevalence of suicidal behaviour and psychological morbidity is reported. In this context, an increased risk of attempted suicide among young women with a Turkish migration background in Germany compared to their autochthonous peers has been reported (Schouler-Ocak et al. 2015; Razum et al. 2008; Montesinos et al. 2010).

6.3.6 A Summary of the State of Research

Numerous quantitative studies show that socioeconomic conditions and gender are associated with an individual's health behaviour, health outcome and health status. For instance, studies describe people with a "high" socioeconomic status as showing a "better" health than people who find "worse" economic and social conditions and have a low educational status. Reports on health within the total population of Germany compare "population groups" with each other. Here it is shown that people with a migration background are exposed to worse overall conditions and consequently show poorer health more frequently than the autochthonous population. People with a Turkish migration background are described as particularly vulnerable in this respect. This deficit-oriented representation of health in quantitative studies raises the question of whether people with a migration background, and especially people with a Turkish migration background, have no or significantly fewer health-relevant resources or whether their resources cannot be grasped with quantitative methods. In the following, selected results from an ethnographic and salutogenic milieu study on the health literacy of female adolescents with a Turkish migration background will be presented.

6.4 Ethnographic Milieu Study on Health Literacy: Using the Example of Female Adolescents with a Turkish Migration Background in Germany

Within ethnography, the analytical approach refers to the area of practical and publicly practised sociality, situated between the micro-phenomena of interaction analysis and the macro-phenomena of social structure analysis of complex societies (Breidenstein et al. 2015). Accordingly, the immediate units of ethnography are not limited to individuals, but extend to situations, scenes and milieus in which the everyday life of individuals takes place – following an order and logic of its own. The basic methodology of this kind of ethnography requires the seeking out in person of lifeworlds in order to be able to obtain adequate data about the authentic behaviour of individuals in their lifeworlds (cf. Breidenstein et al. 2015). This is achieved through the observation of and interaction *with* the "objects of observation" in their "natural environment". In order to understand and describe these idiosyncrasies in the context of the health of female adolescents with a Turkish migration background in Germany, two female adolescents – Leyla and Meryem – were ethnographically accompanied in their life worlds.

The ethnographic monitoring, which lasted nine months and involved a total of 220 h, took place at the times and places that the young people preferred. In this way, an attempt was made to explore the lifeworld of the young people and to keep the distortion of social practices (Reckwitz 2003) in everyday life, which can already be caused by the very presence of the ethnographer (Breidenstein et al. 2015), at a minimum. Also, in order to keep the distortions during the ethnographic monitoring as minimal as possible, the form of communication according to Socrates (Stavemann 2008) was chosen in the interactions with the young people and their social environment. Thus, the researcher held back her own opinions and tried to understand and describe the observable health-relevant social practices of the adolescents, as well as and the underlying meaning-making processes.

Analysing the settings that were visited by the young people with the ethnographer within these nine months, three categories emerge. The largest proportion of time can be attributed to the setting "private household". This category summarises the homes in which the adolescents and their family members resided. In addition, during the ethnographic monitoring, there was a desire on the part of the adolescents to see how the ethnographer lived. Thus, the category "private apartment" subsumes not only the time spent in the apartments where the adolescents resided with their families, but also the units of time spent in the ethnographer's apartment. 70 h were spent in the "mosque" setting and 50 h "outside", meaning in

Fig. 6.2 Percentage distribution of total hours among the settings in which the ethnographic research took place; N = 220 observation hours

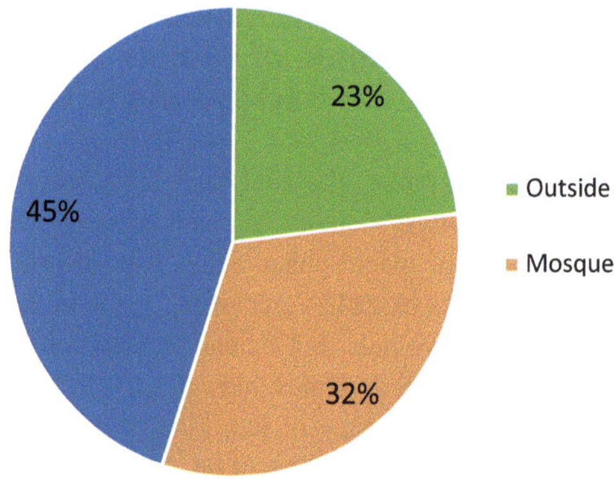

semi-public or public spaces such as cafés, parks and shopping centres (see Fig. 6.2).

In order to be able to adequately locate the lifeworlds of the female adolescents and to describe the relationship-oriented aspects, the "transnational diaspora" (Halm 2009) will be discussed, which developed through the immigration of people from Turkey to Germany and within which social, cultural and political elements from Turkey mixed with the elements to be found in Germany, causing the two societies and political systems to influence each other. Based on this description, which outlines the cross-national relationship between Turkey and Germany, thus primarily describing the *political situation* within the young people's lifeworlds, *the settings and social networks* that individually represent proportions of the young people's perceived lifeworlds will be mapped. In illustrating these health-relevant conditions, the significance of these aspects within Leyla and Meryem's health-relevant everyday actions will be outlined at the same time. Finally, the role of the media in relation to the adolescents' health decisions and actions will be presented.

This approach aims to provide a holistic understanding of the health-relevant interrelationships between micro-level and macro-level phenomena in the everyday life of female adolescents with a Turkish migration background and to make the meaning-making processes within their health actions comprehensible.

6.4.1 The Political Discourse About Turkey in the Lifeworld of Leyla and Meryem

Before an account of German-Turkish relations is given, they need to be defined. They can be contacts between the "Germans" and the "Turks" or contacts between

Germany and Turkey (Lüdke 2017). This distinction attempts to reduce the complexity of the "German-Turkish" relationship by focusing on either "public" or "political", as the case might require. Despite this attempt at simplification, there can be no doubt that both "types" of contacts are in fact interrelated and do influence each other.

Within this section, the "relationship" between the two states will be briefly outlined without aiming to achieve a holistic account. Following the American philosopher and writer Santyana (1863–1952) who claimed that *"if one does not know the past, one cannot understand the present and consequently cannot shape the future"*, the "relationship" between Turkey and Germany in the past will be outlined at the beginning before the current discourse is discussed.

6.4.2 The German-Turkish Relationship Yesterday ...

As soon as an attempt is made to locate the first contact between the two states, definitional difficulties arise: For what is to be understood by Germany and Turkey? Is "Germany" the "Holy Roman Empire of the German Nation" or only the empire existing from 1871 and its successor states? For the "Turkish side", there is still the question of whether the Ottoman Empire, which legally ceased to exist in 1923, should be referred to as "Turkey" or as "Old Turkey", or whether "Turkey" refers in the narrower sense to the Turkish Republic proclaimed in October 1923 (Lüdke 2017).

It has often been documented that the "bilateral relationship" up to the seventeenth century can essentially be described in terms of warlike conflicts. The first contact between "Turkey" and "Germany" can be dated to the eleventh century. Back then, the Rum Seljuk Sultanate came into contact with the Holy Roman Empire of German Nations during the First Crusade (Jaspert 2013). Among the other "encounters" taking place up until the seventeenth century, the warlike confrontation during the conquest of Constantinople in 1453 and the siege of Vienna in 1529 and 1683 (Neubauer 2011) are perhaps the most prominent.

At that time, war was launched against "Turks" not just because they were regarded as people of another nation (Neubauer 2011). Religion, and thus Islam, played a special role here: *"In addition to a military threat, it is above all the cultural-religious "other" and the alienness of Islam that frightens and unites the West, although, or precisely because, Western knowledge about Islam, at this time, is low and primarily reflects its (the West's) own prejudices and fears"* (Walter 2008, p. 43). Thus, in the perception of the public, there was a widespread "equation of the Turks with Islam" which, according to Andrea Polaschegg, is not surprising, *"the Turks [being] the first and for a long time the only Muslim nation [...] with whom one came into contact in the German lands, while the countless polemics and pamphlets of the churches against the pagan Turks contributed their part to the connection of the two concepts"* (Polaschegg 2005, p. 127). This equation remained constant over many centuries, which can be seen, for example, in the naming of David Friedrich Megerlin's Koran translations from 1772 as "The Turkish Bible" (Megerlin 1772).

Despite the perception of various "differences" between the "Germans" and the "Turks", political, military and economic cooperation was established between the two states in the nineteenth century. For example, Prussia maintained relations with the Ottoman Empire since the Congress of Vienna in 1815 (Neubauer 2011). Furthermore, during a state visit, Wilhelm II "declared Germany's friendship with the Islamic world in a solemn speech" (Schneiderheinze 2004; Neubauer 2011).

Moreover, during the First World War, which was fought between 1914 and 1918 in Europe, the Middle East, Africa, and East Asia, and in which Germany, Austria-Hungary, the Ottoman Empire, and Bulgaria, among others, were considered important participants, Germany and the Ottoman Empire entered into a brotherhood in arms (Bayaz 2002).

Another important role in German-Turkish relations was played by the Turkish state's acceptance of German exiles between 1933 and 1945. During the National Socialist regime, Turkey, which remained neutral for a long time during the Second World War, was a place of refuge for many German scientists and artists (Neubauer 2011). After the war, the Federal Republic of Germany resumed its relationship with Turkey in the 1950s, and "the mutual certainty of a reliable partnership emerged on the basis of political, economic and military cooperation" (Hesse and Steinbach 2002). Consequently, in 1961, the Recruitment Agreement was concluded as a significant expression of this reliable partnership.

6.4.3 The German-Turkish Relationship Today ...

Today, both states continue to have a close relationship. For example, they are joint members of the Council of Europe, the Organization for Security and Cooperation in Europe, the Organization for Economic Cooperation and Development, and the North Atlantic Treaty Organization. Thus, they continue to have political, economic, and military cooperation, as well as a certain "mutual dependence".

Germany appears to be of crucial importance for Turkey in the context of the country's negotiations for accession to the European Union. Turkey's possible accession to the European Union has been under discussion since the foundation of the European Economic Community. As early as 1999, it was granted the status of an official candidate country. Even today, from the point of view of the other contracting states, Turkey has not achieved the "adaptation of political, economic and legal standards to EU regulations" described by the European Council as prerequisites.[1] The Turkish mass media are dominated by allegations of Germany in particular repeatedly blocking these accession efforts (Kazim 2014). This perception is also reinforced by the fact that the Federal Republic of Germany is seen as the "representative of Europe", which must be specifically addressed as a point of reference in the accession negotiations (Incesu 2014).

In turn, the importance of Turkey for Germany can be illustrated by the refugee agreement between the European Union and Turkey: Since the Syria crisis, the European Union and especially Germany have been dealing with the resulting refugee issue. Especially since 2015, the ongoing refugee movement from war and crisis zones has become one of the dominant topics in summit meetings and crisis areas. In Germany, this issue has repeatedly and controversially been discussed and reported on. Turkey is considered to play a key role in controlling or mitigating the refugee migration. To this end, numerous summits have been organised between representatives of the European Union and Turkey, but also specifically between Germany and Turkey. As a result, an agreement on the repatriation of refugees was signed between the European Union and Turkey in Brussels in 2016. According to this agreement, Turkey is obliged to take back all refugees who reach Greece and the European Union via Turkey. In return, the European Union is to take in Syrian refugees from Turkey in a "one-to-one" ratio and distribute them among the European member states. In addition, it was agreed that the European Union would provide Turkey with a total of six billion euros in subsequent years to cover the housing and caring expenses for refugees. Explicitly for the Turkish population, this meant that after an examination of the conditions, they would be eligible for visa-free travel to the European Union from June 2016 (Keskin 2017). Thus, this agreement marked the opening of another chapter in the hitherto faltering negotiations on Turkey's membership in the European Union.

Among other things, it was hoped that this agreement would significantly reduce the illegal and uncontrolled influx of refugees, put an end to the business of so-called smuggling gangs and prevent human trafficking (Keskin 2017). However, this agreement also met with some criticism. For example, the UN Special

---

[1]This is a very sensitive issue because, in the course of the eastward expansion, states have been granted EU membership that are autocratic and certainly no more democratic than Turkey.

Rapporteur Peter Sutherland said: *"collective deportations without having regard to the individual rights of those who claim to be refugees are illegal"* (Gayle 2016). An opinion shared by Spiegel-Online commentator Maximilian Popp (2016), who added: *"[It] has shifted the problem of refugees from the centre of Europe to the periphery."* Moreover, it seems that the strong refugee movement, in which around one million people were taken in by Germany in 2015, has led to the radical right-wing populist or neo-fascist parties in Germany and other EU member states gaining a strong following. In the state elections of 13 March 2016 in Baden-Württemberg, the right-wing populist party "Alternative for Germany" (AFD) achieved considerable success. However, not only in Germany, but also in France, the Netherlands, Austria and Sweden, parties that take strong stances against Islam and refugees have been successful and thus have a visible influence on the discourses about the successful integration of ethnic minorities (Keskin 2017). These framework conditions can have direct consequences for the self-descriptions, forms of action or patterns of interaction of, for example, headscarf-wearing young people who, according to these discourses, are not compatible with the normative ideas of the majority society and can thus come under pressure to legitimise themselves.

In addition to the negotiations on how to deal with refugees, other events in the recent past have shaped the relationship between the two countries. For example, the "Böhmermann affair" in March 2016, the criticism surrounding the attempted coup in the same year, the events at the central commemoration of the arson attack in Solingen 29 years ago, and the numerous prevented appearances by Turkish politicians in Germany before the elections in Turkey, which were at least partially banned by the German government.[2] Particularly against the backdrop of the freedom of opinion enshrined in Article five of the German Constitution, these events provide occasion for controversial discussion.

Furthermore, the way in which the "political" and "public" debates interlock can be seen from the diverse descriptions of the Turkish population on a political level. Referring to the recent elections in Turkey, Cem Özdemir, the former federal chairman of the party "Die Grünen" (The Greens), said that people with a Turkish migration background in Germany who vote for Recep Tayyip Erdoğan expressed their rejection of liberal democracy. He said he saw some overlap with the behaviour of members of the right-wing populist party "Alternative for Germany" (Tagesschau.de 2018). In contrast, Federal Justice Minister Heiko Maas described

[2] Of the 1,445 million people with a Turkish migrant background who are eligible to cast their own vote in Turkish elections, 717,992 did so (Diemand 2017; Önder 2018).

"the Turks" at the central commemoration ceremony in Solingen as "part of our country" (TRT Deutsch 2018). The question of what exactly motivates politicians at different times to use these mutually exclusive descriptions will not be explored further here.

It can hardly be denied, however, that within this "national" debate religion plays a fundamental role in the political discussions staged by the mass media even today. In a variety of ways, some of them massively contradictory, Islam occupies a prominent position in the political arena. In Baden-Württemberg, for example, "Islamic religious instruction" was introduced as a model project in 2006; in Lower Saxony, Islamic religious instruction was made a regular subject in 2013 after almost 10 years of pilot projects; Hesse introduced Islamic religious instruction in the same way in 2013; and the first generation of Islamic teachers is being trained for primary schools in Giessen and for secondary schools in Frankfurt. In Baden-Württemberg, one of the first institutes for Islamic theology was established in 2006 at the university of education in Freiburg (Mediendienst Integration 2018). In addition to these rather "inclusive" measures, more "exclusionary" voices are also being heard, for example when parties such as the Christian Social Union of Bavaria and the "Alternative for Germany" postulate that Islam does not belong to Germany (Alternative für Deutschland 2018; CSU 2018).

From this sketch of the bilateral relationship, it becomes clear that German-Turkish relations are currently not free of tension and that the motives within the interaction processes are not easy to understand. Within these debates, so-called "differences" and "deficits" are primarily emphasised, which are attributed to the "nation" or the "religion" – without it being clear what is to be understood by this. These debates, which are primarily conducted on the political level, can influence the way citizens live their lives within Germany. If the lifeworlds of Leyla and Meryem are examined more closely in this regard, it can be seen that within the urban population with a Turkish migration background – especially when the German media report critically on the government in Turkey – the risk of public-political polarisation increases. Although no direct correlations or even health-relevant consequences could be established in the two female adolescents' everyday life, the political situation in Turkey and Germany as well as social integration or exclusion in the country of immigration nevertheless became a topic of conversation in the adolescents' everyday lives from time to time.

6.4.4 The Socio-economic Framework Within the Lifeworld Environment of Leyla and Meryem

The *large city*,[3] where the female youths with Turkish migration background and their families reside, is said to be of increasing importance for the growing together of Europe, due to its being the seat of consulates and honorary consulates of various European states. The city, which is governed by the Green Party, is an economic centre and one of the cities in Germany with "high chances for the future".

Between 2005 and 2016, the proportion of people in employment, which includes all people who work as employees or self-employed people or as family members assisting in an economic activity, increased by around 20% and the proportion of employees subject to social insurance contributions increased by 20% to 30%. The unemployment rate increased slightly between 2011 and 2016, averaging around six per cent in 2016.

If the "group of people not in employment" is looked at more closely, there has been stability within the gender ratio since 2005 in the city, whose population is made up of 50% women. In 2016, the proportion of male unemployed was just under 60% and the proportion of female unemployed was just under 40%. In this context, in the city, where the proportion of people with a migrant background is 30% and people with a Turkish migrant background represent the third largest group after people from Italy and Romania, the proportion of the native population without an employment relationship has been steadily decreasing since 2012. In turn, the proportion of unemployed foreigners has risen in the same period.

If we take a closer look at the age of the "non-employed", we can see that the proportion of people aged 55 and over has risen by around eight per cent in the last 11 years. In contrast, the group of those aged 25 or younger who are unemployed has fallen by around two per cent over the same period. Thus, in 2016, about 5% of those 25 and younger were unemployed.

In the big city, whose inhabitants have an average age of 40 years and the under 18-year-olds represent a share of about 20%, it can also be noted that the majority of households are "one-person households". Households with five or more people are comparatively rare. Children live in about a quarter of the households.

As to the religious affiliation of the city's population, it should be noted that approximately 60% of the population identify as Christian, of which approximately 35% identify as Catholic and 20% as Protestant. Approximately 40% of the city's population is either non-denominational or a member of other denominations or

[3]For privacy reasons, this section is not referenced with sources.

religions. There are several Islamic organisations of different origin and religious orientation as well as several synagogues and Buddhist centres in the city.

The families of Leyla and Meryem reside in this city. Leyla, 16 years old, lives with her parents and a younger (13) and an older brother (19). She is aiming to graduate from high school and then study to become a teacher. The father, who immigrated to Germany 31 years ago with his own parents, is 43 years old. He works in a company as an employee. The company where he works is described by Leyla as a company "where various devices are assembled". The mother has lived in Germany for 23 years. She is now 41 years old and works as a cleaner. Leyla's younger brother is aiming for the secondary school leaving certificate. The older brother has attended offers of the transition system (Schultheis 2014) after graduating from secondary school and is looking for an apprenticeship. Leyla lives with her nuclear family (Fuchs-Heinritz 2013) in a four-room apartment. In addition to the nuclear family, uncles and aunts as well as paternal cousins live in Germany. The paternal and maternal grandparents, as well as aunts, uncles, cousins and maternal cousins live in Turkey.

Meryem, who is also 16 years old, lives with her mother (43), her brother (18) and with her maternal grandmother in a three-room apartment. The father (44), who was born and raised in Germany and works as a construction worker, moved back in with his mother, who resides in another city in Germany, after a divorce 10 years ago. Meryem's mother, who was born in Turkey, immigrated to Germany with her own parents and married Meryem's father in Germany at the age of 20. Today she works as a cleaner. Meryem, who is aiming for the Abitur, would like to study medicine or education. Her brother is also aiming for the Abitur. Apart from her mother, father, brother and maternal and paternal grandmothers, Meryem also has uncles, aunts, cousins living in Germany. But she also has relatives living in Turkey.

Meryem and Leyla's families came known to each other through the mosque congregation that both families attend. Their mothers are good friends according to the young people. When describing their relationship network according to Beushausen (2012), Leyla and Meryem told the ethnographer that the important parts of their lives take place in the settings of private home, mosque and school and named people they meet in these settings who are significant to them. At the same time, the networks differ markedly between the two friends, both in their structure and in their interpretation of the network map itself. Thus, for Leyla, family members, people from school, people from the mosque and friends represent her subjectively perceived social network presented to the researcher, with her mother, class teacher and friends with the same migrant background described by Leyla as the most important people. It is true that for Meryem, the social network is also

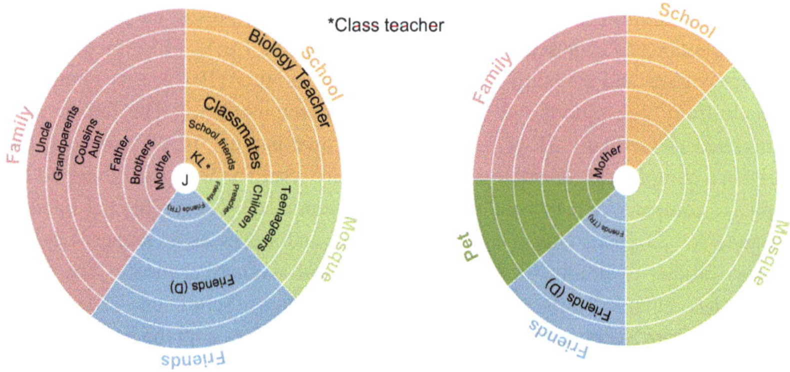

Fig. 6.3 Leyla's relationship network Meryem's relationship network

composed of family members, people from school, people from the mosque and friends. But Meryem's entries are much sparser. Meryem named her mother and friends with the same migration background as the most important people. (see Fig. 6.3).

The correlations between socio-economic conditions and the health of female adolescents with a Turkish migration background refer to social conditions as well as religious/cultural norms and values that are related to the health of the adolescents. In this context, the people described by the adolescents as "important" as well as the settings in which they shape their everyday life take on a significant role.

In the following, excerpts from the qualitative findings are presented in order to show the connection between the social conditions and the health of Leyla and Meryem.

6.4.5 Health-Relevant Significance of the Social Network and Religious/Cultural Norms and Values in the Everyday Life of the Young People

The young people attribute an overriding importance to the family, and in particular to the parents. Leyla answers the question: "What do you think, what people are important to you?

> So of course, first of all family, my mother, my father and my brothers and sisters, that kind of thing. So of course, they are in the foreground (. . .). So, my mother, first of all my parents, they raised me, they taught me a lot. And I don't know, the role of mother and father, they are different again. But both are just as important to me (. . .). So mum is important when I have questions about health and household and dad for school questions and general questions. (Islertas 28.06.2016, lines: 189–207)

For Meryem, only her mother plays a special role within her family. The health-related significance of the mothers for Leyla and Meryem can be further differentiated. Thus, in addition to being (1) an adviser on health issues, she is (2) the person who controls and regulates the health-related behaviour of her own children based on her own knowledge, as well as evaluates their health status. An interview excerpt with Leyla's mother clearly outlines this role: "I currently have to watch out for my sons not to eat too much. I stop them sometimes and mean, 'you've already eaten quite a bit, I think that's enough'. The two boys are both developing paunches right now. Leyla is chubby but she eats the least" (Islertas 27.08.2016, lines 31–34). Moreover, she is (3) the person who guides and instructs the young people. During a conversation with Meryem, the ethnographer learns that she cooked according to her mother's recipe: 'I ask Meryem what she has been doing since her mother, grandma and brother left, if she was bored. She said: "No, not really, I tidied up the flat a bit, went shopping and cooked for us. We are having spaetzle with mushrooms. Meryem cooked the dish according to her mother's recipe. Before the mother left, she explained to Meryem how she should proceed with the cooking (Islertas 08.10.2016, lines 48–52).

Finally, the mother is also (4) the person who provides health-related care for her own child. The ethnographer learns that Meryem was suffering from pain due to menstruation before a common day and the mother took care of her: *"When asked if she took painkillers, Meryem replied no, she did not take painkillers. The mother had given Meryem a hot water bottle and covered her well" (Islertas 10.07.2016, lines 65–70).*

For Leyla, friends with the same migration background, who were also assigned to the category of "most important people", are advisers on health-related questions (in addition to her mother). More exactly, they are preferred advisers on "youth-specific" health-related questions: *"Yes, yes for example so now especially in puberty or so, some questions are perhaps more embarrassing and there you rather ask friends who perhaps also already had experience with it" (Islertas 28.06.2016, lines 288–290).* In contrast to Leyla, Meryem does not mention female friends as advisers on health issues.

However, the friends with the same migration background are available to Leyla not only as advisers on health issues. Female friends with the same migration background are also the people with whom Leyla and Meryem spend a large part of their time away from school. The girls meet to hang out, barbecue, cook, bake, dance, shop, but also to swim. The places where they meet are mostly the flats where the young people live or a garden attached to one of the flats. These premises or places used for recreation represent the spaces where the young people can move freely. This means dancing, laughing and behaving as boisterously as they like without a male person being able to observe them doing so. Using such a space for recreational activities is particularly important to adolescent girls. Therefore, if a meeting is planned in an apartment and there is a male family member in that apartment, they are asked to leave the house for that time: *"The younger brother is at the open-air swimming pool, the older brother Leyla sent out of the apartment because she has a visitor, he is to go shopping and stay outside." (Islertas 23.08.2016b, lines 24–25).*

Cooking and baking are done from recipes found on the Internet or according to the instructions of the mother. In addition, the young people can grill on their own. They have learned how to use the grill from their parents. When buying food, it is important for them to buy only products that are "halal". In conversations with Leyla, the ethnographer learns: "Leyla and Eda, a friend of Leyla's, make sure that they buy halal meat. For this purpose, they always go to the same shop" (Islertas 05.08.2016, lines 36–37). Apart from meat, they also make sure when buying drinks, pastry and sweets, among other things, that they do not take any products that are counted among the forbidden foods from a religious perspective.

Grocery Shopping in the City Centre

On a sunny Wednesday in August, Leyla and the ethnographer meet in the city centre. Via WhatsApp Leyla suggested a pharmacy in the middle of the city centre as a meeting place. At 3 pm, the two meet in front of this pharmacy. After saying hello, the ethnographer asks Leyla what they should do in the city and where she would like to go first. Leyla decides to take a stroll first, so the two of them walk down the shopping street, which is linked to the left and right with a wide variety of shops and is easily accessible by tram, as there are tram stops in the immediate vicinity. They pass a large department store, a jeweller, an optician, a shoe shop and various fashion stores and talk. Leyla talks about how school is going and what she has been

(continued)

doing the last few days. After strolling, Leyla wants to look around a drugstore and a fashion store. The ethnographer follows her. Leyla looks at clothes, DVDs and cosmetics, but doesn't buy anything. After three hours downtown, Leyla wants to buy a little something for her father and younger brother. She decides on Haribo for the brother and Marshmallows for the father. To get these, Leyla and the ethnographer visit a discount grocery store that is also in the shopping street. The two find what they are looking for here. Before Leyla purchases the goods, however, she looks at the ingredients and discovers that there is gelatine in both of the products she chooses. She leaves both products behind and decides to shop at a Turkish store located just outside of the city centre. Leyla and the ethnographer, in order to get to this supermarket, take the tram. After about 15 min they reach the store and look for Haribo and Marshmallows. Leyla finds both products. As they do not contain gelatine this time, she buys them.

Not only is it important for the young people to eat "halal" goods themselves, but also to offer "halal" goods or give them to others. Leyla, for example, drew the ethnographer's attention to the characteristic of gummy bears when she was at her home: *"Haribo [do] not contain gelatine, you can eat them without hesitation if you want to" (Islertas 16.07.2016, lines 19–20).*

For swimming, the girls use the indoor and outdoor swimming pools, on days when only female customers are allowed in. Despite this restriction, however male lifeguards may still enter the swimming area on these days. These situations can pose challenges to the girls.

Going Swimming with friends

On a warm September day, Leyla goes to the open-air swimming pool with two friends of Turkish origin. The swimming facility, which is easily accessible by public transport, is about a 30-min tram ride from the city centre. The facility is well attended on this day. There are a few bathers on the large lawn surrounding the 25 m pool, which is equipped with occasional deck chairs. They are either dressed in a bathing suit or in a bikini. Some women, however, sunbathe only in bikini bottoms, so that their torsos can get a

(continued)

complete tan. Leyla and her friends spread out their towels on a free spot on the sunbathing lawn and undress, so that they only have their bathing suits on, which they have already been wearing underneath their clothes. After an "in-the-sun warm-up", Leyla wants to go swimming. Before she does so, she discusses with her friends what they should do if a male lifeguard – gets in the pool at the same time as one of the girls. They agree to let each other know so that the one who is in the water can take a deep dive.

The circle of friends, described as especially important, the values and norms to which nutrition, exercise and interaction are subjected, make the importance of cultural/religious norms/values within health-relevant everyday activities clear. However, not only in individual health-relevant activities, but also in the structuring of everyday life, religion takes on a special significance for Meryem, as she prays five times a day. It is particularly important for her to pray at the appropriate times – as soon as there are not really more important things that cannot be postponed.

In addition to their female friends with the same migration background, their mothers and the cultural/religious values and norms to which they refer for orientation, new media and the Internet take on a special significance in the (health-related) everyday life of Leyla and Meryem. New media are used for entertainment, communication and information purposes. In addition to her mother and friends, Leyla also refers to the Internet as an information platform for health-related questions: *"(. . .) Or when I have a question like that, I type it into Google and the answer comes up immediately (. . .) For example, I have a headache. Then I type in, I've had a headache for an hour, what can it be and then I click on search" (Islertas 28.06.2016, lines 92–101)*. After "Google", her preferred search platform, Leyla uses the homepage "gutefrage.net" as a source of information: *"Well, I look, well, usually the best always comes first, but then I just keep looking on my favourite site, gutefrage.net. And those are just, so also, like, normal people who just give answers to your questions (. . .) And if I did not get a good answer there, then always on the first thing that comes up" (Islertas 28.06.2016, lines 108–112).* Leyla thinks she can tell if a page is good by the language used to present the content: *"I think it always depends on how the person wrote it, if they wrote, like, matter-of-factly, so well, then I just think it helps me more than when someone wrote using, I don't know, juvenile words" (Islertas 28.06.2016, lines 125–127).*

This is a crucial statement, because addressing young people in a target group-specific way is a natural part of trying to reach young people. However, Leyla sees a lack of soundness when youth language is used and then does not use the site. Of course, it must be taken into account here that Leyla's level of education is high and her educational aspirations are pronounced, so that she hardly belongs to a particularly vulnerable group in this respect. However, the fact that youth language is regarded as a flaw with regard to the search for health information is still very remarkable. When describing Leyla's health-relevant use of new media, it should be noted that she uses those media to search for medical information and health-promoting aspects.

Meryem also uses online platforms quite naturally to view health-related information. Meryem, who prefers Turkish-language books to German-language books, as she feels that her "own cultural and religious norms", to which she feels she belongs, are more clearly represented in these books (Islertas 22.08.2016, lines 35–39), also uses German-language electronic platforms to obtain health-related information. In doing so, she does not look for information that is important for explaining and understanding pathogenic conditions such as pain or other ailments but moves within what might be called the health information and health literacy domain that is intended to promote health. For example, Meryem reports that she prefers the Internet to books when looking for cooking recipes because the search is easy and because the Internet offers a larger selection: *"In the case of Turkish cookbooks, she mentions that she likes the books very much because they are colourful and look nice and she likes the books. Only she doesn't look in there so often after all, because it is easier to pick out recipes online and she does have a large selection there" (Islertas 23.08.2016a, lines 53–55).* Apart from nutrition, Meryem also seeks out online information related to exercise and sport. During the ethnographic monitoring, she reports: (...) she has gained weight, and you can see it on her belly, that's why since yesterday she has been doing a workout she found on YouTube: *"15 min is good, not too long and the exercises are not hard" (Islertas 23.08.2016a, lines 83–87). It is* clear from these examples that health is an integral part of both young people's everyday lifestyles, which is not identified and discussed by way of an independent issue.

6.5 Health, Health Literacy and Health Behaviour of Female Adolescents with a Turkish Migration Background: Summary and Overarching Motives

In the 1970s, when describing the health of people with a Turkish migration background in Germany, primarily psychosomatic illnesses of guest workers were discussed in connection with economic conditions, or with their being "uprooted from the homeland" and from the "social environment", or with the linguistic and cultural barriers in the host country. In their 1977 study, Häfner and colleagues drew attention to the fact that the children of parents with a Turkish migration background, who were born and socialised in Germany, suffered from social and psychological problems (Häfner et al. 1977).

Recent findings on the health of people with a Turkish migration background show that a high prevalence of diabetes mellitus and coronary heart disease can be found in this population group. These are associated with elevated LDL levels and are consequently at least in part related to the diet of these individuals. Primarily women with a Turkish migration background seem to be affected by this (Razum et al. 2008). However, not only in nutrition, but also with regard to the acquisition of health information, people with a migration background appear to have difficulties, which may also be related to their health-related everyday actions (Horn et al. 2015; Messer et al. 2015; Quenzel et al. 2016a). However, compared to the autochthonous and also people with other migration backgrounds, this population group is not consistently described as vulnerable. For example, according to Schouler and colleagues (2015), female adolescents with a Turkish migration background consume less alcohol than their autochthonous peers. This health-related behaviour is explained by their religious faith and the importance young people attach to it (Boos-Nünning and Siefen 2005). If the studies describing the health literacy level of people with a migration background are collated with those dealing with alcohol consumption, the question can be asked as to why health-relevant behaviour and quantitatively surveyed health literacy level do not correlate positively, as is actually assumed in health literacy research.

In addition to their health-relevant everyday actions and their physical state of health, recent studies report on mental illnesses among people with a Turkish migration background. For instance, women are primarily affected by depression and anxiety. The reasons given for this are (emotional) stress, perceived discrimination, nationality and economic conditions (Schouler-Ocak et al. 2015; Merbach et al. 2008; Bermejo et al. 2010). In addition, the suicidality rate among young women with a Turkish migration background seems to be higher compared to autochthonous adolescents and adolescents with other migration backgrounds in Germany (Schouler-Ocak et al. 2015; Razum et al. 2008; Montesinos et al. 2010).

Whether the more recent findings support the hypothesis put forward at the beginning by Häfner and colleagues cannot be answered, as a comparison between socio-epidemiological studies of people from Turkey would be necessary for this. From the older and more recent findings, which for the most part show a quantitative approach and offer a deficient description of the health of people with a Turkish migration background in Germany, it can be concluded, however, that health is related to the life worlds of the people, the settings in which they shape their everyday life and the norm and value system to which they refer for orientation in their health-relevant everyday actions.

6.5.1 What You See When You Look Differently: The Example of Young Women with a Turkish Migration Background

An ethnographic-salutogenic approach was used to understand and describe the role of health in the everyday life of female adolescents with a Turkish migration background. The focus of the findings presented in this chapter is on exploring the relation between health and the lifeworld (Thiersch 2012) of female adolescents.

If we take a closer look at the settings within which the ethnographic monitoring took place, it can be stated that these are settings that were described by the young people as "significant" and included in the relationship networks according to Beushausen (2012). The respective living environment is assigned a special significance here, but the mosque is also assigned crucial significance, which is why the cultural-religious norms and values that differ from those of the majority society are also of particular relevance within the girls' health-relevant everyday actions. The accompanied young people spend a significant amount of time each week in settings in which they have the opportunity to communicate in both Turkish and German and also practise both languages in the interaction processes. Both cultural "worlds" are synthesised unproblematically, depending on the action at hand, and the girls' easy natural navigation in two cultural reference systems was perceived, at least by the ELMi researcher, as a health-relevant everyday resource, rather than an acculturation burden.

However, the importance of cultural/religious norms and values in shaping the health-relevant everyday actions of female adolescents with a Turkish migration background is not only made clear by the description of the settings in which they shape their everyday lives. The relevance of cultural/religious norms and values to the ethnic minority is felt in all health-relevant everyday routines such as nutrition, food shopping, inter-gender interactions, the selection and forms of sporting activities or in the direct acquisition of health information, whereby the findings acquired in our qualitative ethnographic study appear to support the studies by Boos-Nünning and colleagues (2005). In the acquisition of health information, the mother and friends with the same migration background, with whom Turkish and/or German can be spoken, who were either socialised in Turkey and migrated to Germany and/or, like the participating adolescents themselves, were born and grew up in the Federal Republic and have a Turkish migration background, take on a special significance. Thus, when acquiring health-related information, the participating female adolescents prefer advisers who, like themselves, move between two cultural/religious norms and value systems. The mothers and female friends, who are preferred here, take on different roles and functions within the process of acquiring health information, as shown.

Cultural/religious norms and values can also be crucial in selecting an online information platform on health-related topics. With regard to written electronic health platforms, German-language sites are preferred by adolescents. Content preference, however, differed significantly between the girls when it comes to electronic information sources, at least at the time of the survey. Meryem primarily searches the web for topics related to health promotion, while Leyla acquires medical knowledge online. Thus, based on the qualitative findings on the health literacy of female adolescents with a Turkish migration background, it can be concluded that the adolescents can search for, find and evaluate health information online and decide on practical measures on their own.

6.5.2 Some Final Overarching Themes

The intensive and long monitoring of the two female adolescents with a Turkish migration background reveals that – in line with theory – the idea of health literacy as an isolable discreet entity is problematic. It is too difficult to separate health-related aspects from everyday life for health literacy to be meaningfully linked to distinct domain-specific knowledge and action competencies. In this respect, quantitative instruments ultimately provide a rather arbitrary extract from the conceivable spectrum of health-relevant actions, at least if the concept is not only related to health care actions.

From a socio-epidemiological perspective, the female adolescents participating in the study can at least partially be defined as vulnerable in advance – they belong to a statistically constructed at-risk group with an increased likelihood of suicide and overweight and lower levels of physical activity. In one case, the family structure also deviates from the clearly established nuclear family norm in the Turkish community due to a divorce. However, the picture presented by both female adolescents over three quarters of a year had little to do with official members of a risk group. Rather, both were very well able to use their own resources for action, such as bilingualism, as well as health-promoting facilities such as swimming pools, even if there was the possibility of a male lifeguard entering the bathing area, which would violate their own and the group-specific gender norms.

At the same time, the young people showed that health is also, and perhaps especially so, welded to motivational factors and meaning-making processes in the area of everyday actions. Intending to bring something back for the brother and father from the city can perhaps still be categorised as social skills, but then to forego the obvious offer from a large supermarket and instead get gelatine-free food that is compatible with their religious dietary rules, and to put in an entire extra hour's worth of effort doing so, presupposes quite a strong intent. This simple example shows vividly how much general health behaviour is also permeated by cultural norms and values and that it can only be restricted to information processing to a very limited extent. In summary, it can be concluded from the present study that, in addition to formal education, informal educational pathways as well as the aspect of bi-culturality and the associated systems of norms and values, which provide the organisational framework for everyday actions, play a significant role in how health is understood and practised.

7 The Health Literacy of Male Adolescent Refugees from Afghanistan and the Exploration of Existing Scope for Action

Abstract

As mentioned in the state of the research, when it comes to refugees in general and refugee children and adolescents in particular, very little is known about the health literacy they might have available regardless of how it is measured. In the two ELMi subprojects, we originally wanted to study and relate adolescents from two cultures with different Muslim backgrounds, primarily to examine what exactly are the differences between adolescent groups with Muslim backgrounds. Because we did not succeed in convincing young people and parents from the established Afghan diaspora community to participate in our study, we had to fall back on the group of recent refugees in the end, happy that we were able to maintain the original plan of accompanying young people from different Muslim traditions at all.

... if my family is doing well, I'm doing well ... good. (Bari, Afghan refugee, 17 years old)

7.1 Introduction

As mentioned in the state of the research, when it comes to refugees in general and refugee children and adolescents in particular, very little is known about the health literacy they might have available regardless of how it is measured. In the two ELMi subprojects, we originally wanted to study and relate adolescents from two cultures with different Muslim backgrounds, primarily to examine what exactly are the differences between adolescent groups with Muslim backgrounds. Because we did not succeed in convincing young people and parents from the established

U. H. Bittlingmayer et al., *Health Literacy From A Health Ethnology Perspective*, https://doi.org/10.1007/978-3-658-42348-3_7

Afghan diaspora community to participate in our study, we had to fall back on the group of recent refugees in the end, happy that we were able to maintain the original plan of accompanying young people from different Muslim traditions at all.

However, the inclusion of young refugees with ongoing asylum application procedures ultimately led to a number of shifts in the original research interest and made the question of available health literacy and digital health literacy considerably more complicated once again. *Firstly,* because refugees, unlike young people who are continuously socialised in one country, cannot develop a stable preference structure. Rather, their preferences, behaviours and values get fairly shaken up by flight and arrival in a foreign country. The findings on available health competences are therefore strongly influenced by general orientation in the host country and the need for language acquisition. Both are dimensions for which it is not entirely clear to what extent they are related to health literacy, and whether health literacy facilitates reorientation (and perhaps also language acquisition) or whether, conversely, successful social integration leads to well-developed health literacy (see also the following case study in Chap. 8).

Secondly, it can be assumed that young people who have fled are confronted with extraordinary, above all mental health burdens. Direct experience of flight, a residence status that frequently remains unresolved for a long period of time, the necessity of restructuring one's social capital and fragmented family, in which relevant third parties (e.g. aunts, uncles, cousins, grandparents, friends) usually remain in the home country, combined with concern for the well-being of those still in the home country, and finally the readjustment of existing skills, many of which are no longer equally useful in the destination country, all lead to a great potential for stress. We say *potential,* because the idea that *all* asylum seekers are severely traumatised is not realistic and would also contradict the salutogenic approach pursued here, according to which a person's ability to cope with the escape experience and to readjust to the destination country is dependent on the degree of individually available generalised resistance resources (Antonovsky 1987; cf. on the correlation between health literacy and Salutogenesis Saboga-Nunes et al. 2019).

For all these reasons, research on health literacy among the group of refugee adolescents obviously poses great challenges. We are very aware that we are only providing a first, modest start with this case study, but because there is nothing available on health literacy among refugee youth in the German-speaking world so far, we believe that we are contributing to health literacy research among youth with this study, despite all limitations. The entire fieldwork and the interviews with the adolescents and their families and relatives was done in Dari. The focus group interview with the adolescents was conducted in German, only some passages were translated into Dari by me during the interview.

The case study is structured as follows: We start with a brief description of the global situation with regard to flight and displacement (Sect. 7.2). We then relate the context of flight more closely to our health focus (Sect. 7.3). Only then do we introduce the accompanied adolescents in more detail (Sect. 7.4), before presenting selected results from the ethnographic field research (Sect. 7.5) in relation to family social (Sect. 7.5.1) and health perceptions (Sect. 7.5.2). Because the smartphone obviously plays a central role in young people's everyday lives, we re-focused our results once again with a view to digital health skills (Sect. 7.5.3). In the following section, we try to identify health-related competencies (Sect. 7.5.4). Because one of the young people kept in touch with us even after the official end of the field phase, we provide a brief update on developments after the end of the field phase (Sect. 7.5.5). Finally, we discuss the results as a whole and look at limitations, challenges and future questions (Sect. 7.6).

7.2 The Significance of Afghanistan in the Context of Global Forced Migration

Globally, never before have so many people been on the run as in the last decade. At the end of 2016 – during the period covered by our ethnographic survey – a total of 65.6 million people worldwide was displaced or forced from their homes (UNHCR 2017a, b), more than had ever been recorded before. According to daily updated data from October 2019, the number has continued to rise massively, with 70.8 million people now so-called forcibly displaced persons, according to the UN Refugee Agency (UNHCR – The UN Refugee Agency 2019). According to the UN, 25.9 millions of these were fleeing to another country or were residing in foreign countries as refugees for an extended period of time, while the vast majority is described as internally displaced persons. The flow of refugees over the past 4–5 years has been so high in part because of severe unrest in Syria, Afghanistan and South Sudan in particular. According to UNHCR statistics, more than half of the refugees come from these three countries. Globally, refugees from Afghanistan (2.7 million) are second only to Syrians (6.7 million) and ahead of South Sudan (2.3 million) (UNHCR – The UN Refugee Agency 2019). The causes of conflict are usually highly complex and go back a long way in history. It is usually cultural-ethnic, religious, economic, political, humanitarian, social or environmental crises and incidents of unrest that drive people from their communities. Relevant macropolitical events in this context are the international arms trade, labour shortages in Germany and other European countries (as a pull factor), international terror and organised crime (especially drug production, drug trafficking), but also globalisation and the associated global trade structures, which usually unilaterally channel most of the profits to the industrialised countries. In addition, millions of people are currently being displaced from their home regions because of the exploitation of resources.

The main escape route for refugees from Afghanistan is via Iran to Turkey and across the eastern Mediterranean Sea in boats or ships of various sizes. Greece and Turkey are ***the*** places of refuge for refugees from Afghanistan, where they usually stay for a longer period of time before they reach Switzerland, Sweden, Austria or Germany as their destination country.

The overland route leads through Eastern European countries such as Bulgaria, Romania, Serbia and Hungary to reach Austria. The following graph (Fig. 7.1) shows that the entire Mediterranean Sea is the largest flight route of refugees to Europe (Fig. 7.2).

Afghanistan as Part of a Global Discourse Formation

Without being able to go into any kind of depth here: Central Asian Afghanistan was and is directly affected by global processes and is an integral part of recent global history, and Germany is also directly involved by way of its military-political commitment. After the inhumane terrorist attack on the World Trade Center in 2001, attributed to the Saudi-born Osama bin Laden, an equally inhumane war against the then radical Islamic Taliban government in Afghanistan has been waged for 20 years now (and continues to this day), illegal under international law (Ganser 2016). The Taliban had initially gone down in recent Afghan history as peacemakers after ending the extremely bloody civil war in Afghanistan between 1992 and 1996, before committing more and more human rights violations on a large scale themselves (Rashid 2010; Sahrai 2018).

Many of the current international military conflicts are framed by a discourse that proclaims a new war of faith in which the civilised, progressive, modern (Christian) Western world is fighting the battle on behalf of humanity against the backward, uncivilised barbaric Muslim world (as formulated in Huntington 2002; more intelligently formulated but with the same thrust Bellaigue 2018; critically, e.g., Hall 1994a; Souza 2008). This bipolar discourse formation conveys the idea that *the* Islamic world is terrorising the West, so that the war in Afghanistan, Iraq, or Syria is a pre-emptive security measure to victoriously combat global terror. With the confusing idea that German democracy is being defended in the Hindukush, former

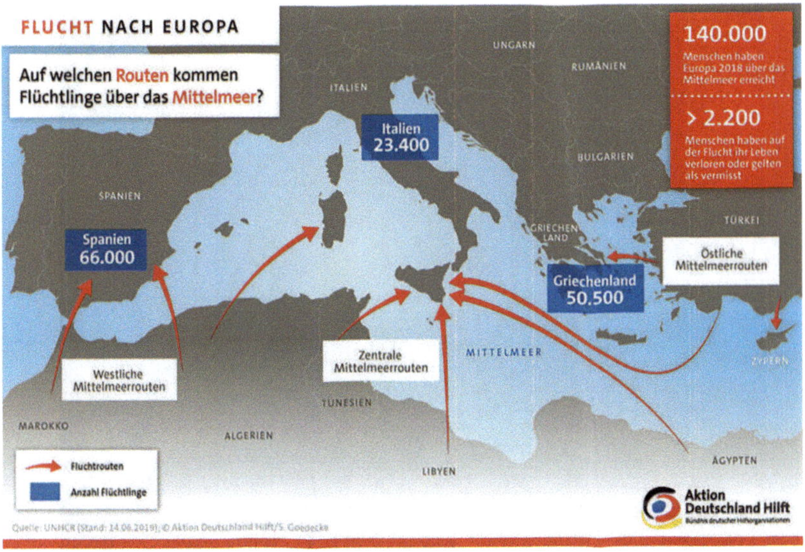

Fig. 7.1 Escape to Europe. (Source: Aktion Deutschland hilft 2019)

Social Democratic (!) Defence Secretary Peter Struck shaped and at the same time divided the opinions of the majority of people in Germany (cf. on this, among others, Weiss 2008).

Terror, it seems, has long since arrived not only on our own doorstep, however, if we consider recent events of terrorist and suicide attacks, including in Madrid (2004), London (2005), Oslo (2011) Paris (2015) and Berlin (2016). The public conclusion is quickly drawn that terrorist attacks are linked to and attributable to the influx of refugees, especially from the Islamic world.

With her famous words "We can do it!", that attracted much international attention, and the knowledge of which demonstrably moved Afghan people to set out for Germany, the former German Chancellor Angela Merkel initially succeeded in setting a counterpoint to the largely xenophobic European discourse. However, her efforts to create a welcoming culture quickly failed for a number of reasons (including internal party resistance, fears of European neighbours, CSU tactics, the increasing strength of right-wing populist movements not only due to nationalist tendencies but also due to increased social inequalities). The success of right-wing populist movements such as the AFD in the wake of the refugee crisis, attributed for

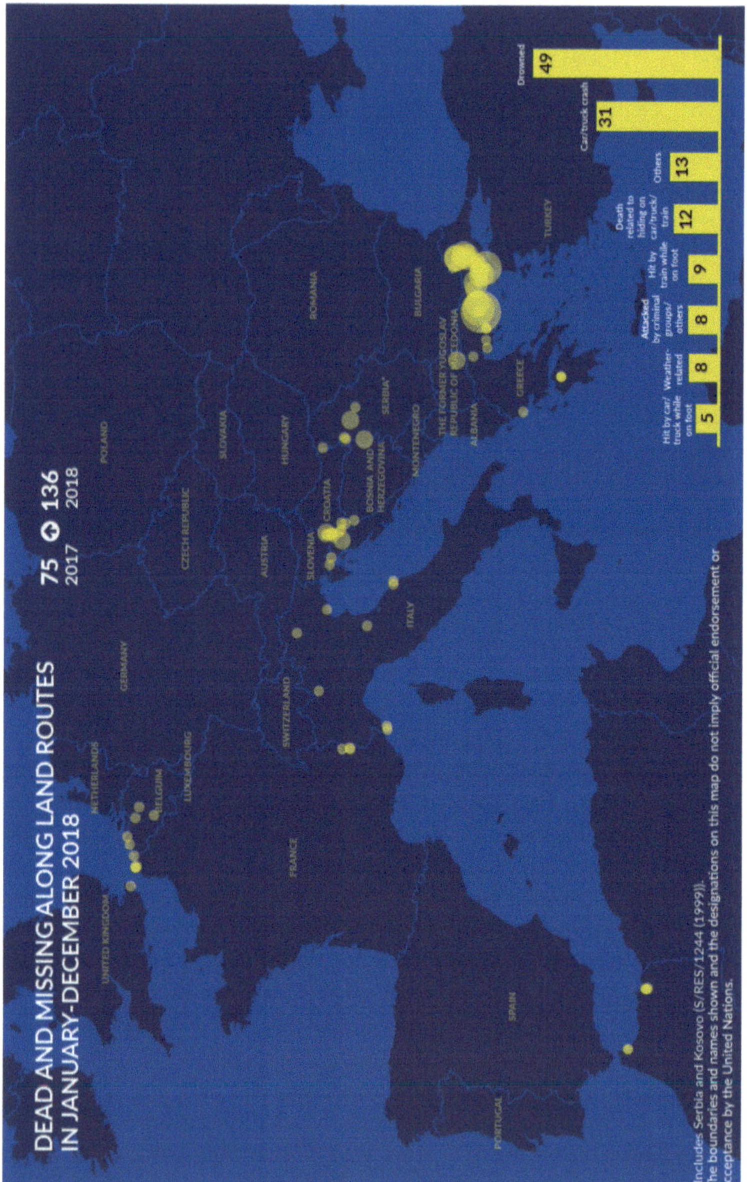

Fig. 7.2 Source (United Nations High Commissioner for Refugees (UNHCR) 2018)

strange reasons to Angela Merkel, quickly disappointed the hopes and expectations of refugees on the one hand, but also those of the resident population.

Nevertheless, the challenge that will remain for the foreseeable future is to offer reasonable prospects to the people who have immigrated to Germany in recent years. This is because in the past 4–5 years, especially from 2015 onwards, there has been a large increase in refugees in Germany. According to statistics from the Federal Office for Migration and Refugees (Bundesamt für Migration und Flüchtlinge (BAMF) 2016), with 31,382 people seeking asylum in Germany, Afghanistan was in fourth place behind Syria, Albania and Kosovo, (recently, the number of Nigerians* and Eritreans in Germany has increased particularly strongly, largely unnoticed by the mass media). According to international reports, the high number of refugees from Afghanistan since 2015 is linked to the Taliban's conquest of large parts of Afghanistan and their significant resurgence (UN Secretary-General (UNSG) 2016, p. 4). Recent developments show that, regardless of the actual cause, the security situation has deteriorated rather than improved, despite recently held democratic elections (see, among others, United Nations, General Assembly Security Council (UNGASC) 2019). It can therefore be assumed that Afghan people will continue to make their way to Europe and try to build a better and safer life here.

According to UNHCR statistical data, in 2018 alone at least 2200 people died or are considered missing on the overland route to Europe (Milz and Tuckermann 2018). However, as UNHCR also suspects, the actual numbers of dead and missing people are far higher (United Nations High Commissioner for Refugees (UNHCR) 2018). The following chart illustrates the quantitative dimensions of refugee deaths and differentiates further between the various causes of death:

The rising death toll of 2017–2018 dramatically illustrates that the countries concerned in Europe are closing their borders more strictly to refugees and are condoning the deaths of people as they flee. The flight of Afghan people to Europe already starts with (sometimes fatally) dangerous situations, including displacement, violence, exclusion, discrimination, in early stages of flight or during the (usually involuntary) stay at stopovers or in refugee camps. The majority of people fleeing Afghanistan are in Iran and Pakistan. Iran and Pakistan each share over a 1000 km of land borders with Afghanistan, which is why the first stop for refugees is often these two (or one of these two) countries. The relationship between Afghanistan and the two neighbouring countries is generally regarded as difficult, conflict-ridden and very complex (cf. e.g., Fischer 2014; Jalilvand 2014), and the situation of Afghan refugees in Pakistan and Iran as problematic. In Pakistan, for example, children and young people of Afghan origin in particular are abducted by the police (!), robbed, and even arrested or killed without reason. In discussions with refugees from Afghanistan, these stories are repeatedly brought up. In Iran, too, the resident Afghan minority is exposed to significant repression and discrimination.

In a study of Afghan returnees from Pakistan and Iran, Mamiko Saito describes the situation based on qualitative interviews with those who returned to Afghanistan as follows:

> Bullying and social exclusion of refugees in all cases of population displacement are common; however, different connotations were observed in the experiences of respondents between the two neighbouring countries. In Pakistan some, if not all, of the non-Pashtun respondents have experienced political discrimination based on stereotypes held by some Pakistanis (often Pashtun Pakistanis) of Afghans from the northern regions. [...] However, the perceptions of Afghans in Iran (as reported by respondents) tend to be more linked to a cultural hierarchy, despite the fact that many Afghans who left for Iran also shared religious beliefs as Shia followers. A sense of shame in relation to being Afghan, more commonly observed among refugees in Iran, is another reason cited for refugees keeping a low profile in public. Respondents universally became highly nervous in reaction to the terms of abuse 'Afghani' or 'Afghani kesafat'-literally meaning dirty Afghans and implying that they have no culture, no manners, no understanding, and that they are rural people who are backward, barbarian and illiterate. Fitting in with this, however, many respondents indeed saw Iranians as more cultured, educated, mannered and wealthier than Afghans – at the same time as they held Afghan nationalist sentiments. (Saito 2009, pp. 25–27).

The flight of people with a migration background from Afghanistan, usually via paid smuggling gangs, from Pakistan usually via Iran further on via Turkey and the various routes to Europe, often takes not only months but years. In view of these difficult and sometimes life-threatening circumstances and daily socio-structural tensions, it is therefore not surprising that there is hardly an Afghan family in Germany in which no member has ever experienced murder, rape, robbery, abuse, unlawful arrests or violence of some kind.

Clearly, the macrostructural phenomena just described provide specific frameworks that cannot be classified as conducive to health for refugees from Afghanistan. In addition to the experiences associated with flight (see the following section), these certainly include the fact that Afghanistan is not officially classified as a civil war country and that deportations to Afghanistan have been enforced since 2018. Furthermore, an Islamophobic (on top of a generally visible xenophobic) background discourse is being conducted in Germany, but also in Europe as a whole, which places Muslim life practices, naturally taken for granted by refugees, under the suspicion of not being compatible with a will to integrate socially in the destination country. The following section will focus on the direct connection between flight and health.

7.3 Flight and Displacement and Health Consequences

Worldwide, studies from Germany, Switzerland, Canada, Australia, Pakistan, or the USA show that many refugees struggle with war, flight, and/or violence trauma, and have been doing so not only since the so-called refugee wave in 2015 (Perren-Klingler 2000; Kassam and Nanji 2006; Alemi et al. 2014; Clark-Kazak 2017; Slewa-Younan et al. 2017; Unger 2017). The Federal Office for Migration and Refugees (BAMF), in co-operation with the Institute for Employment Research (IAB) and the Socio-Economic Panel (SOEP), presented a research report in 2016 in which a total of around 4500 refugees were asked about the causes, motives and risks of fleeing (Rother et al. 2016; see also Milz and Tuckermann 2018; Biakowski et al. 2016; Etzold 2019). When people or groups of people (have to) leave their homeland, there are complex motives such as poverty, danger to life, exclusion, political persecution, discrimination on the basis of religious or ethnic affiliation. Most of the refugees are minority groups, such as the Yazidis from Syria and Iraq, Roma (mainly) from Eastern Europe or Christianized groups from Iran to name just a few arbitrary examples that apply especially to the refugees in Germany. A quantitatively large group of the immigrants who have suffered violence, repression and persecution in recent years are refugees from Afghanistan. The collective term Afghans is not entirely unproblematic because Afghanistan (as in Syria or Iraq) is a multi-ethnic state comprising heterogeneous groups such as Pashtuns, Tajiks, Hazara, Uzbeks, Baluchis and Turkmen.

But regardless of which specific ethnic (minority) group these people belong to in their Afghan homeland and for what reasons they have had to leave their country, their family, their possessions behind, they first have one thing in common: flight! This is associated with insecurity, fear (of violent attacks), illegal residence in transit countries (i.e., countries in which the refugees only stay temporarily before arriving in the destination countries[1]). Not only the situation in the home countries is often life-threatening (or economically desperate), but also the flight to Europe itself.

[1] At the beginning of the flight, for refugees from Afghanistan it is usually Iran or/and Pakistan; at the end of the flight and before arriving at the destination country, it is Turkey or Greece. This is mainly true for those fleeing by land (and later by sea).

Arrival in the Destination Country

Once they have arrived in their destination country, the relief is initially great and Afghan refugees can breathe a sigh of relief. At least their lives are no longer in immediate danger. Initially, they are housed centrally in federal and state reception facilities, where they are housed together with other people in a small space (9 square metres per person) without the possibility to cook for themselves and with limited freedom of movement. They are then assigned to a location anywhere in Germany and can apply for asylum. The procedure usually takes several months to years until the first hearing and at least another 6 months until the decision is announced. Many Afghans' applications for asylum are rejected, so they have to appeal and are threatened with deportation. It is clear that the hardships of flight will at some point make themselves felt. Hence, the consequences of traumatisation and other psychological problems gradually set in. The duration and nature of these can vary from person to person; the way in which they are coped with depends above all on their own experiences before and during the flight. But it also depends strongly on age and gender. For example, a small child does not perceive the dangers as consciously as an adolescent or an adult does. The coping and processing mechanisms are correspondingly heterogeneous. This has not only been the case since the wave of refugees in 2015 (for more on this, using Switzerland as an example, see Achermann et al. 2006). Rather, the processing of individual (or family) flight experiences depends not least on the individual, socio-structural and/or socio-demographic characteristics, the accessible resources and the corresponding (coping) strategies. A common result of refugee experiences that can manifest itself sooner or later are states of depressive and psychosomatic anxiety, often not visible to outsiders or to the institutions and responsible authorities of the host society, especially since the "stranger", especially in Germany, is at the same time observed with an "alien" gaze, so that everything that is "different" about the stranger is explained or legitimised by them being a stranger (i.e. frequently with regard to culture, ethnicity and/or religion), rather than by potential health impairment. Apart from experiences of discrimination in the country of destination, there are therefore additional distortions of observation, perception and interpretation on the part of the host society, which will not leave the refugees alone and continue to be a burden (often for a long time). Consequently, social (mis)constructions of external observation, exclusion and isolation can occur. Using the example of migrants, Christian Ulbricht shows how and for what reasons such constructions arise (Ulbricht 2017). Even before the traumas of flight, violence and persecution are (or can be) processed, or at least simultaneously with such coping processes, refugees are confronted with new challenges that cause their problems and burdens to accumulate and, above all, further damage their

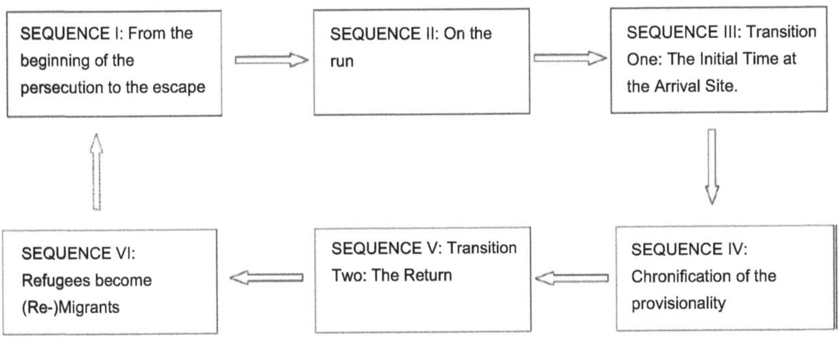

Fig. 7.3 Six potentially traumatic sequences in the context of flight and forced migration. (Source: Zimmermann 2012, p. 45)

mental health even further. Or, with reference to Aaron Antonovsky's model of Salutogenesis (Antonovsky 1987): on the continuum between "healthy" and "ill", there is a shift towards the "ill" pole.

In this context, David Zimmermann has developed the helpful concept of sequential traumatisation, which can be used to appropriately represent the different types of traumatisation potential. Figure 7.3 illustrates the model.

The aspects that can play a role in refugees nevertheless mastering their everyday lives and being considered "objectively" or medically (at least initially) "healthy" will be taken up and discussed again at some later point (Achermann et al. 2006). Even though there is an obvious and clear connection between flight, migration and probable health burdens, for the projected health literacy research we decided in advance (after due consideration) not to openly address possible traumatisation, but to react only spontaneously, if their flight was brought up by the accompanied young people themselves. The reasons for this restraint are various: The first reason relates to the fact that our focus is more on the successful coping with everyday life under difficult conditions, the second reason is that we did not want to further deepen traumas that may not exist or have not yet come to light by actively addressing them. Thirdly, and finally, we are not trained therapists who can directly contribute to trauma recovery through our fieldwork and monitoring, even if we wanted to. We rather hoped for implicit therapeutic effects through stabilisation by keeping the adolescents' company, thus consistently and, from our point of view, successfully signalling appreciation and interest. We will take up this topic again at the end of the case study.

First of all, after these general remarks on Afghanistan, on flight and on the connection between flight and health, we would like to focus on the age group of young people themselves.

7.4 The Young People Accompanied

The situation of young refugees with an Afghan migration background in Germany is the focus of this case study. Within the framework of the BMBF project ELMI (E-Health Literacy and the Health of Minorities), we were able to accompany young refugees for 9 months, once or twice a week. The target group were refugee youths between 14 and 17 years of age who are currently residing in Germany.

The young people were continuously exposed to hardships during their flight. When they are asked about the reasons for their flight, terms and phrases such as "(lack of) security", "staying without official papers" and "no prospects of building a life" often come up; depending on whether they talk about fleeing from Afghanistan or from Iran and Pakistan. Once in Germany, social integration rarely goes smoothly. Since a large number of young refugees are traumatised by violence, war or at least flight and apply for asylum without a clear prospect of staying, the basic conditions for a good health situation are rather suboptimal, even if other (infectious) diseases are not prevalent. Apart from these difficult and health burdening conditions, the acquisition of the German language makes an unproblematic successful integration more difficult. In addition, there are the circumstances of constantly being in a foreign country without permanently valid papers, sometimes illegally, sometimes only tolerated for a short time, and living under constant fear of violent attacks by xenophobic groups. This situation is completely alien to young people of the same age from and in Germany.

All these unfavourable circumstances also apply to the young people we accompanied, who will now be presented in more detail. First of all, some "objective" data on Seleman, Bari and Tamim[2] will be mentioned, before results from the ethnographic field research will be presented and subsequently discussed.

Seleman, 15 Years Old, Monitoring Period: 2 Months

Seleman, whom we were unfortunately only able to accompany for 2 months, as he then moved and left the city, had come to Germany with part of his family in 2014. He himself, his parents and an older sister had fled to Germany together. One sister

[2] All names have been changed to anonymize and protect participants.

lived in England, one lived in Berlin, the latter now lives with them near Frankfurt. An older brother had previously been on the run without the family before coming to Germany, that is, as an unaccompanied minor, probably 17 years old at the time. During their flight, they only had a longer stay or stopover of about 6 months in Turkey before they reached their destination country.

Seleman is interested in boxing and was in a boxing club at the time of the ethnographic observation phase. In addition to school and additional language courses, he took guitar lessons from a German boy. The first impression during the observation suggests a teenager very eager to integrate. In the meantime, he is even said to participate in boxing matches and tournaments despite the integration process being interrupted by the move to another city.

Bari, 17 Years, Monitoring Period: 9 Months

Bari was still 17 years old at the time of the field study and has been living in Germany since 2015. His father had emigrated to Iran over 40 years ago, at that time still single. Furthermore, during a visit to their home, the father told us that at that time the political and other relations between Afghanistan and Iran had been much more relaxed than today. So, Bari was born in Iran and has never seen Afghanistan. He has two sisters and two brothers. His parents, one brother and one sister, both married, came to Germany together with Bari's sister-in-law and brother-in-law. The other two siblings are currently still living in Iran and are also married. Together with a local Iranian, the family ran a shoemaker's shop (that also did leather processing) in Iran. It was possible for the children to attend school, but the fees became so high from the 5th grade onwards that they had to drop out and only worked as helping family members in the shoe shop. Accordingly, their written language skills are low even in their mother tongue. Especially for the older siblings, some of whom are over 30 years old, it will take a lot of effort to compensate for their low literacy skills, while Bari, the youngest sibling, who lived in Iran until he was 16 years old, is not that far behind in terms of school attendance and should have a better chance of acquiring German as a second language.

Contact with family members living in Iran, a sister and a brother, both married with children, is intact and, at the time of the fieldwork, regular. However, Bari told me at some later point, already after the ethnographic field phase, that the frequency of contact has decreased significantly since a year ago, not least since he dropped out of school to start vocational training in a discount food store. The loss of free time due to vocational training probably plays a crucial role here.

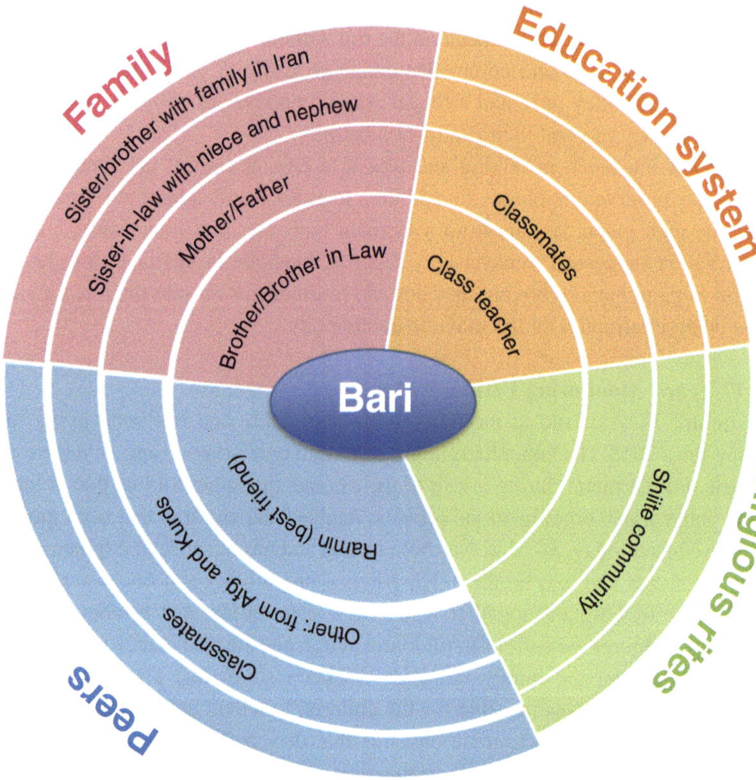

Fig. 7.4 **Bari's** social network

The following figure (Fig. 7.4) shows a sociogram that was created during the field research and operationalizes the importance of people or groups of people in Bari's everyday life through their proximity to the centre. The closer a person is to the centre, the more important and present he or she is for Bari, for example, when it comes to coping with stress or the like.

In Bari's case, some of his classmates are also his peers and close friends.

Tamim, 15 Years, Monitoring Period: 6 Months

Tamim also came to Germany with only part of his family at the end of 2014. A younger brother and an older sister came with their parents. Two of his brothers had come to Austria shortly before, one of them is said to be a very good drawer. I only

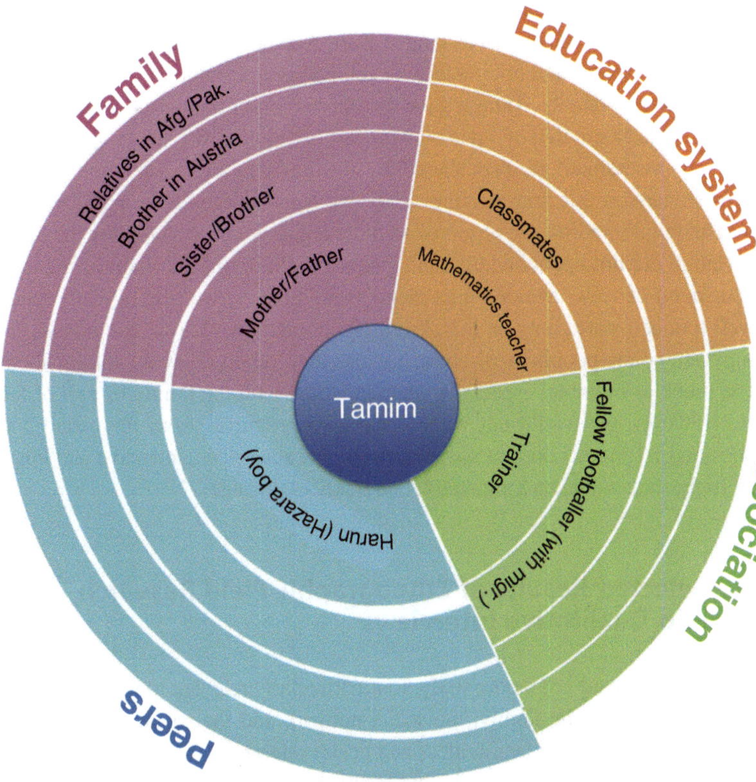

Fig. 7.5 Tamim's social network

learned about the other brother later, after the field phase, and Tamim mentioned him only in passing. Before arriving in Germany, the family lived for a few years in Islamabad, the capital of Pakistan. After that, practically while fleeing to Europe, they spent about a year in Turkey. Tamim is an avid club football player and during the field period he started to take an interest in playing the guitar. The following figure (Fig. 7.5) shows Tamim's network map, featuring some clear differences to Bari's sociogram, especially in the "peers/friends" setting.

Tamim is in a football club and regularly takes guitar lessons. However, his peer group and circle of friends are not as established as Bari's. This may be due to his younger age. This may be due to his younger age, because close friendships may well be established in the next few years, but – in terms of socialisation history – Tamim has been in Germany just as long as Bari. Another explanation for his rather limited social networks and not yet fully developed peer group may lie in Tamim's rather reserved personality. Tamim gave the impression of being rather shy during monitoring, at least not that of a person who was outgoing and actively approached others. This assessment is also shared by Tamim's mother, who pointed out Tamim's shyness at our first meeting. Since we cannot exclude the possibility of violence and flight trauma, the observed shyness may have been caused by the flight itself. Tamim did not openly address the topic of flight during our monitoring and, from our point of view, avoided it as much as possible, so we cannot really make any well-founded statements on this. From ethnography we know that at least the accompanied young people themselves, but also their relatives, avoid talking about flight as much as possible; especially when they fled with the family or part of the family. However, we would not want to derive a prognosis from the extent and composition of Tamim's current social network, because close, intensive and long-lasting friendships develop comparatively quickly at this age.

7.5 Selected Results of Ethnographic Field Research and Qualitative Interviews

In the context of the ethnographic study, four particularly relevant topics recurred in the context of health: the family, the social network and the social capital of the young people (Sect. 7.5.1); health ideas and health references (Sect. 7.5.2); the role of smartphone use (Sect. 7.5.3) and other health-related competences (Sect. 7.5.4). In the following, we will present these topics on the basis of the empirical findings obtained and reflect on them with regard to the fundamental questions addressed by the ELMI project. Since one of the young people remained in touch with us even after the end of the field phase, we will briefly describe the further development of his case, as it became known to us.

7.5.1 Overall Assessment of the Network: Differences, Deficits and Social Capital

If the social network of the adolescents – illustrated in the two sociograms, but clearly evident in everyday observation – is examined more closely, the strong connection to the family, but also to the extended family and circle of relatives, becomes clear in all three adolescents we accompanied. In principle, this is regarded as an important health-promoting resource for young people, as a specific form of social capital (Hartung 2011, 2014).

The importance of the parents to Bari was not entirely clear during the course of the fieldwork, but the importance of other family members in everyday life was evident since communicated. The older brother and brother-in-law are the people Bari spends the most time with when he is in the dormitory. They often sit together and smoke a shisha, barbecue, or play a ball game when the weather is nice. On weekends, they are often outside, making a small fire and spending the whole night like this.

The position or role of Tamim's father is clearly weakened compared to the importance of his mother when it comes to dealing with stress and/or coping strategies. However, Tamim's mother is visibly of paramount importance, playing the most important role in his everyday life, at least over the entire course of the ethnographic field phase.

From the ethnographic observation as well as the interviews and the many conversations with the young people, it became clear again and again, directly and indirectly, how important the relationship to the family is. It represents the prime frame of reference on which the young people (can) draw. The family and the "extended circle of relatives"[3] can thus be seen as a resource that helps the young refugees to cope with everyday challenges such as stress. As will be illustrated in the following sections, family and the well-being of relatives makes for the 'social well-being' of the young people themselves. Contact with relatives who – in the case of the accompanied young refugees – are in Afghanistan, Iran or Pakistan is an essential part of everyday communication practice, which is thus essentially international in nature. Thus, transnational relationships have a special significance in the lives of refugees. It is thus possible that positive or negative events in the lives of relatives who are in a country other than Germany still have a strong effect on their everyday life and can thus be directly or indirectly associated with their health. We are not talking about a bereavement that is mourned for a few weeks; rather, a constantly ongoing "malaise" that can accompany and preoccupy the refugees for years, even for a lifetime. However, as already emphasised, despite visible problems, the young refugees cannot only be described and understood as

[3]In Afghan family constellations, the "extended circle of relatives" includes not only uncles, aunts and cousins, but also the relatives of the wife/husband, sister-in-law/brother-in-law, etc. The term also includes relatives who reside in another country, but who may nevertheless be significant for everyday life.

disadvantaged and endowed with only a limited capacity to act. They have competencies that partly result directly from family resources and partly from successful skill appropriation and coping processes in the destination country.

The observations during and after the ethnographic field phase, especially in the dormitory setting, clearly showed that the family environment provides the most significant orientation for the young people; from our point of view, the peer group takes only second place. This reveals a difference, albeit to varying degrees, to the autochthonous population and to some extent also to young people with a migration background but without a refugee background: the source of available resources for action of young people with a refugee background is predominantly the family; this is different for young people in the comparison group, who because of their better language skills in German (or English) also have much easier access to institutionally available resources. These include ("good") schools as well as youth centres or libraries. The lack of German language skills visibly leads to restrictions in the choice of available resources for action. Social capital therefore plays a particularly prominent role because neither cultural nor economic capital is available to the young people and the resulting options for action are therefore limited from the outset (Lin 1999; Burt 1982, 2000; Lin 2017).

Another difference between the refugee youths and the average peer group, which has visible consequences for the well-being of the youths and presumably also for the available social networks themselves, is their living situation in terms of accommodation: the refugee dorm. The situation in the dormitories is problematic simply because of the thin walls that cause a permanent acoustic overload. The televisions and (not even loudly raised) voices of the adjacent housing units can usually always be heard in one's own room. This became abundantly clear during the many familial visits during monitoring. A possible direct consequence is the insomnia reported by the young people, which is then associated with limited or no performance at school and/or in vocational training. None of the three accompanied adolescents had a room to themselves, a circumstance that applied to everyone living in the dormitory. Accordingly, the conditions for inclusion and integration (which are necessary in this age group) are limited and get in the way of learning at school, developing a prospect for life and the future, and the right to privacy – which is normally widespread and much promoted in Germany.

During our field research, it was very noticeable that the refugees from Afghanistan, despite the massive shortage of space for (possible) visitors just described, redesigned one room as a guest room. In Afghanistan, there is traditionally a large room that is hardly used in everyday life, except when there are visitors. Such "guest rooms" or "guest reception rooms" are usually only carpeted and covered with mattresses, and there is often a cupboard where crockery is stored.

Gradually, new styles (depending on class and interests) and furnishings were added as supplements, such as: musical instruments, television, bar or refrigerator, games, etc. At one boy's parents' house, the room is furnished with a huge table, a bed, a couch, a TV, and a closet, which has the pragmatic advantage of enabling the host to quickly store away items of any kind, for a "guest (reception) room" must be as empty and clean as possible. This is how Afghan refugees make do, yet still try to transfer cultural habits and norms, such as the hospitality that is held in very high regard in Afghanistan, albeit with great compromises, into their everyday practice and the cramped spatial environment.

With regard to the situations described and the living situation in general, especially in the dormitory setting, as well as the strong integration into family (meso) structures, it is clear that these result in great restrictions and deficits for the young people on the one hand. On the other hand, it would be completely wrong to view the three accompanied youths as complete victims of structural adversities. In the following section, opportunities and existing scopes for action are made visible.

7.5.2 Health Perceptions and Health References

At the beginning of the field phase, I asked the two boys a little about health and what they thought it meant. There came the following answer: "Health is kind of everything; of course, family is always important because you're not alone and there's always someone supporting you when you have problems." Seleman (14 years), (meeting 18/6/2016: lines 33–36).

> ... Most of the time, when my family is doing well, I'm doing well. But when my family is not well, I don't feel well either. Bari (17 years), (meeting on 6/18/2016: lines 39–43).

As in various situations, whether observed in action or expressed in words, the overriding importance of the family is again in evidence here. An excerpt from a focus group interview with four adolescents, including Bari and Tamim, once again reveals the mother as an important health support. Tamim explains in this context, "...And otherwise I sit with my mother and talk to her a little bit, sometimes that helps too." (Focus Group 1, June 2017; B1: Z. 393–394).

Previously, in order to reconstruct potential coping strategies in everyday life, Tamim was asked what exactly he does in stressful situations to make himself feel better. Our interpretation goes in the direction that Tamim does not feel the constant and omnipresent pressure to integrate, perform and compete as much when he spends time talking to his mother as he does in other settings, such as school or with peers. Social structures, environments, and conditions that constantly express expectations (and offer recognition only by way of performance) can trigger stress or intensify it.

Lack of sleep is another common problem and was not only addressed in the focus group interviews, but was evident almost consistently throughout the field phase. At almost every meeting, at least one of the two adolescents was exhausted and tired, regardless of the time of day. To what extent traumatization and prior (unprocessed) events play a role, we could not clearly establish from either the ethnography or the (focus group) interviews. However, recent sleep research shows that refugees, especially those with unresolved residence status, are among the high-risk groups for poor sleep, even when they are not traumatised (Wettstein 2018).

The two young people reported virtually nothing about experiences of discrimination that directly affected their health. Only once did Bari briefly mention how difficult school is for him at the moment, since he has changed schools and has classes together with Germans. He started to mention the class atmosphere and interrupted his sentence; he didn't know how to express himself. I asked him if there was such a thing as competition in the class among his classmates. I also asked him if there were any classmates he could talk to if he had problems understanding. He just nodded and said that they don't really help you or sometimes it seems as if they don't want to. Since we intentionally and explicitly did not refer to the educational institutions in our ethnography, but wanted to be present in the life worlds of the young people and therefore did not conduct classroom observations, it is not possible to assess these statements. Bari had nothing to complain about the teachers themselves. On the other hand, Tamim often remarked that his mathematics teacher did not teach so well. Here, too, it is not possible to assess the quality of teaching and thus the significance of Tamim's statement. At the same time, when we talked about the relevance of mathematics and about Bari's good knowledge of it, Tamin remarked that he did not like the subject at all.

In this thematic context, however, it should also be noted that both during the ethnographic monitoring and in the interviews, it became clear how difficult the young people found it to talk openly about certain topics, at least with me. Overall, the young people were very reserved when it came to addressing anything that potentially carried negative connotations. This was also evident in the context of possible experiences of discrimination. These almost never became an issue in the ethnographic monitoring, and if they did, then the boys never directly addressed discrimination even verbally. They conveyed the feeling that they simply want to be perceived and accepted as just normal young people here.

7.5.3 Digital Everyday Life, Digital Health Literacy and Its Ambivalence

The original research question of the ELMi project was to find out more about digital health skills among young people with a migration background and limited socio-economic resources. In the course of the field research, the focus shifted somewhat to everyday coping in general, because the inclusion of young refugees meant that mobile phone use was no longer the priority research interest. Nevertheless, we do not want to exclude the area of digital health literacy among refugee youth in this case study but present the results in this section.

The original research interest arose from the insight (expressed in Sect. 3.4 already) that children and adolescents grow up in a situation where there is no longer a scarcity of information, so that digital health literacy is very closely linked to the critical evaluation and assessment of available health information (Chinn 2011; Paakkari and George 2018; Wharf Higgins and Begoray 2012). It is also clear that digitalisation in the area of health literacy is seen to have enormous potential, particularly from a health policy and health economics perspective (see, inter alia, Lawson 2010; Lyles et al. 2015; Spahn 2019). However, it is also clear that, especially for adolescents, the digital world, i.e., social media and smartphones, and ubiquitous internet access are not things they have to "connect" with their everyday practices and health routines as they are an integral part of adolescents' life world, anyway. "If there is one thing that defines the current generation of teenagers, it is the degree to which they are always 'connected' – spending vast amounts of time online and on their gadgets, using social media, surfing the web, watching YouTube videos, Tweeting and using apps." (Wartella et al. 2015, p. 1; a German study argued analogously a few years earlier: cf. Rager and Sehl 2008).

If it is true, then, that young people's lives today are totally permeated by digital media, and we do not doubt this description for a moment, then the isolation of a digital sphere of action among young people is questionable overall, and determining young people's digital health skills *becomes identical* with the observing their everyday lives. This also applies to the young refugees from Afghanistan we accompanied.

Smartphone Use by the Accompanied Young People

Among the Afghan refugees, at least at first glance, no particular (or direct) differences or new findings can be observed regarding the use of new media compared to peers of other social and/or ethnic origins. Only the particularly frequent use of certain apps such as Viber, WhatsApp, Imo, among others, for communication with people in other countries is striking. Overall, it can be deduced from the observation and conversations during the monitoring phase that (1) fears, worries, reading news (about the security situation in the home country as well as about normal social conditions), (2) playing (online) games, (3) overcoming language barriers, and (4) communicating with peers and relatives are among the main motives for smartphone use. In addition to communication within peers (e.g., as "entertainment"), these communication apps are used in particular to maintain contact with the "homeland", for example with relatives living in Afghanistan, Iran or Pakistan. The everyday practice of using translation tools (German-Dari/Persian) to overcome everyday language barriers is explained by Tamim in a focus group interview:

> Yes, yes, if I don't understand something, then I translate. German to Persian, or Persian to German. Uh, the verbs and stuff. I have an app my phone, on my phone and if I don't know something, like um, what's that and stuff, I translate, and I don't know like that (thinking), what that's called, I don't know. And I use this app. It says yeah, what comes from sie or er or and so. He uses so many verbs in German and stuff, and I don't understand. (Focus Group 1, June 2017; B3: Z. 318–323).

The unsurprising, ordinary usage behaviour we observed is consistent with the existing research in which the media usage of young people with a migration background is compared with that of autochthonous young people.

> In the synopsis of the results, one cannot speak of a gap between the media use and media competence of young migrants on the one hand and their peers in the overall population on the other. However, it can be noted that there are quite obviously some peculiarities in the selection of content and the intensity of the use of mass and individual media among young migrants that are typical for their respective migration backgrounds. (Trebbe et al. 2010, p. 8).

In the course of the ethnographic research, it becomes apparent that their ways of using new media is strongly oriented towards the young refugees' (situational and contextual) needs and requirements. Thus, it can be said that media and computer *literacy* are present, but to a limited extent and depending on the everyday activities and needs of young refugees.

On the other hand, it should not be ignored that their very limited written German language skills also clearly limit the digital health literacy of adolescents, despite the use of the translation app mentioned above. During the observation period, none of the three adolescents was able to independently and deliberately search for health information in German on the Internet and to comprehensively understand the information; not to mention the selection of trustworthy and less trustworthy content and websites, which, after all, denotes the key competence of eHealth literacy. Nevertheless, in our view, it would be misguided not to attribute any digital health literacy skills to the three boys. Although they would be sure to score low in eHealth literacy performance tests due to their deficits in the German language alone, and although the test fairness would also be clearly limited in the self-report, e.g., the eHeals instrument by Norman and Skinner, everyday observations show that the three boys are definitely tech-savvy and can operate many functions of a smartphone, including games, communication and translation apps. In this respect, they are in any case competent with regard to sub-elements of Norman and Skinner's eHealth *Literacy* Model, such as *Computer & Media Literacy*. In addition to these digital health competencies, which are certainly lower overall than those of the young people born here, there are also unhealthy aspects to smartphone use itself.

The Everyday Ambivalence of Smartphone Use

In the course of the ethnographic research, it became very clear at some points that smartphone use is also associated with aspects that are detrimental to health. In the following, these aspects will be compiled. At first, these were some not very dramatic statements about stress experienced due to lost online games. Later, however, the statements became somewhat weightier.

The following two statements are from Tamim, who describes the conditions under which he feels particularly stressed out.

> For example, I get more stressed when I lose a game. Sometimes I'm also restless because of the family . . . (doesn't go into it further). What often keeps me busy is also my mobile phone and the games (computer). And sometimes, when I'm stressed, it's also because of the game (computer). And just when I lose football games, I am also stressed. (Focus group 1, June 2017; B3: Z. 379–383).

When asked about the frequency of such situations, Tamim answers: "Yes, so it's not so often that it's every day. Maybe it's more often on the weekend. I worry about this and that, but when I do, it's usually on the weekend. I don't know exactly what I'm worried about, but it's just the way it is. I think then, what's happening now, what's happening now." (Focus group 1, June 2017; B3: Z. 397–400) When I asked Tamim further what he did in situations of worry or stress, he remarked, ". . . It helps when I'm with my friends. Then we get busy with our phones." (Focus Group 1, June 2017; B3: Z. 403–404).

Finally, during the focus group, Tamim voiced a point that was indeed critical in terms of digital health skills, when he referred to massive sleep problems. The reason given, by Tamim himself, was the above-average use of the smartphone. Since he had received his smartphone back from repair, he communicated and played with it until he fell asleep, even during the week when he had regular school lessons.

After he was asked how important his mobile phone or the internet was to him, he gave the following answer:

> Yeah, not 99%, but 90% certainly. Because when I don't have it, it's good. For a while I didn't have it, then the weather was also nice, then my sleep was also good, and I didn't have any illnesses or headaches. And since I have had the mobile phone, illnesses have also started. A lot (...) keeps me very busy. And when I sit like that, I don't learn much of what we are taught in school. Then somehow my head doesn't work properly and I can't concentrate properly. Actually, I don't want the phone to be with me much. But that it keeps pulling me like a magnet, that's another matter. (Focus group 1, June 2017; B3: Z. 213–220).

This statement first of all features two very different dimensions with regard to general health competencies. *On the one hand, it* becomes clear that Tamim has a reasonably well-developed health awareness, at least with regard to his own body. Not only does he notice negative changes in his body and in his everyday life, but he also reflects on the possible causes of perceived health impairments. *On the other hand,* Tamim openly mentions loss of control and powerlessness – vis a vis new media and the digital world. These are signs of the clearly adverse health effects of smartphone use. Although WHO recently included internet addiction in its updated ICD-11 catalogue of diseases (WHO 2019), we would rather be cautious than rashly make a clinical diagnosis here. In our view, one explanatory cause for Tamim's problematic smartphone use is his lack of an established peer community, which, it is true, is usually activated digitally, but also seems to act as a regulator at the same time (here, further studies would be helpful to examine this connection in more detail).

Compared to Tamim, Bari has a larger circle of friends and acquaintances and, despite similar smartphone habits and similar living conditions in many respects, he has a greater scope of actioned and freedom in his spare time; but monocausal explanations that focus only on the role of peers are certainly far too simplistic, not least because the reverse conclusion does not work: "only" having a great number of acquaintances and friends does not mean being protected from addictive or risky behaviour, digital or otherwise.

7.5.4 The Identification of (Possible) Health-Related Competences

The "category" of possible health-relevant competencies initially refers to the theoretical presupposition of the ELMi project that cultural, religious, cognitive and social prior knowledge or previously acquired competencies of the refugees in the destination country or the "host society" are not necessarily visible. On the one hand, however, these play a major role in the refugees' (partly isolated) everyday practice. On the other hand, we saw and still see potential in building on the *(previously acquired)* competences of refugees, in order to acquire *necessary competences,* thus doing justice to (e-)health literacy. This approach is based on findings of ours, which (i.e., findings) emerged through the study of Salutogenesis. In practice, it offers opportunities that combine and expand the socio-culturally different scopes of action. A simple example is multilingualism. It simply expands the options for communication and interaction. Moreover, it helps to cope with everyday challenges or, as shown in example (1), is used to solve the problems of others. Additionally, we wondered whether there (could) be further observations regarding (refugee-specific) competencies outside of linguistic-verbal communication. Refugee-specific competencies, if any, could only be guessed at and not made directly "visible", with the exception of refugee-specific coping strategies, as discussed earlier. Nevertheless, three examples are worth mentioning separately because they at least point to potentials and skills that can serve refugees (generalised in this case) as a stepping stone to get (direct or indirect) access either to educational resources (1. and 3.) or to the world of work (2.):

Overview

1. *Keen perception (meeting 10.12.2016: lines 45–50)*

During a meeting in my apartment (present were a student assistant with an Afghan migrant background, Tamim, Bari and me), Bari showed amazing powers of observation while playing cards. After showing us several card tricks (most of which we didn't know), he watched as the rest performed some. While the three of us didn't or barely saw through his tricks while watching (even when he slowly demonstrated them, with explanations), he in his turn was able to copy our tricks directly.

Bari had already acquired logic and mathematical skills in his father's shoemaker's shop, where he worked at the cash register. There he also acquired manual skills, as shown in the second example.

Overview

2. *Craftsmanship (meeting 25.6.2016: lines 33–45)*

On that day we (i.e., Seleman and his sister, Bari and me) visited an international summer festival. There were food stalls, a music stage and many handicraft and painting activities. When we stopped at a craft stall, Bari once again showed his quick intuitive understanding of the craft. Here is an excerpt from my field notes:

> [...] Eventually we got there and it all looked very colourful. We walked once through the crowd to the other end where there was a stage set up with costumed toddlers aged 3–4. S(eleman) spotted a side street in the middle where something was going on. Bari confirmed.
>
> We decided to go there. Once there, we saw many stalls offering various craft & painting activities for children. We got interested in a stall where you could make your own bracelet. I asked the youngsters if they would like to do something like that. They looked but shook their heads. Fortunately, a woman came along shortly afterwards and asked us about it. She knew better how to get the young people to sit down and join in.
>
> B(ari) understood the technique of braiding several bracelets together quite quickly. When I asked him about it, he told me that he had had experience with it here and there in Iran (where he grew up), including in his father's shoemaking shop. [...]

And finally, one last example, which we assume reveals possible everyday health-relevant competences. Assistance and support due to multilingualism are another aspect that is underestimated or neglected in refugees (but also migrants in general). Due to their lack of German language skills, it is not uncommon for young people to have their cognitive or social skills ignored. The following excerpt shows, however, that they can still communicate interactively in everyday situations.

Overview

3. *Multilingualism as mediation (Meeting 10.12.2016: lines 25–30)*

While the food was cooking, we passed the time by playing cards. We started with Fiscot, a card game that is often played in Afghanistan. B[ari] cheats all the time. But does not even try to hide it. T[amim] notices it too and seems amused. He doesn't seem to care either. The student assistant didn't know the game. The boys try to explain it to her. B[ari]'s Persian or hieratic accent often makes it difficult for us to understand him. Again, T[amim] helps, and translates some terms into Dari.

These comparatively simple and everyday incidents are intended to illustrate by way of example that the young refugees certainly have competences for action that they could use in the destination country, for example to build up and expand necessary (digital) health skills, but also to engage in supporting other people. Especially with regard to vulnerable youth, the advocacy dimension is still a completely underestimated factor in health literacy development. Rather untypically for our line of argumentation so far, the examples are at first sight more closely related to the cognitive competence pole (examples 1 and 3) than to the social one. However, if one reflects further, embedding them situationally and contextually, one can see what social interactions can result from them. This is somewhat similar to board games, which require cognitive skills from the players, but enable collective social interactions. Occasions such as the ones quoted above allow for social interaction, and likewise for the development and expansion of health skills (and resources), transcultural exchange, learning processes, or in short: they would, if properly employed, have a broader potential for social integration and inclusion.

After the completion of the project, the contact with Bari has been strengthened. Through conversations with Bari, we have also been able to learn a little more about Tamim. We would like to briefly present these updates.

7.5.5 Further Developments After the Official End of the Field Phase

Unfortunately, I lost contact with Seleman completely after his move. I do know, however, that he now participates in boxing matches and tournaments. How he has been doing at school or health wise is unknown to me at present.

During the observation phase, positive and ambivalent developments were recorded. One of the refugee boys, the older Bari, changed school types with the chance of a secondary school diploma or higher due to his very good performance in mathematics.

Unfortunately, Bari had great difficulties with the change of schools, as the workload and the associated expectations were suddenly much too high and Bari was not able to catch up in time on his language skills in particular, and there were no reasonable supporting measures taken on the part of the school either. His school grades dropped drastically, so that he had to drop out of secondary school due to excessive pressure to perform and competition. This example shows above all the German education system's detrimental effect on health. Most recently, Bari had accepted a training position in retail. During this time, he got engaged, which can be interpreted as a positive development in the private and family sphere. At the same time, he has since dropped out of the training, which makes a permanently precarious educational and professional biography quite likely in the future (should he be allowed to stay in Germany).

From Bari we also learned that he has now made good progress in playing the guitar and can already play some famous pieces well. Unfortunately, in contrast to Bari, there is hardly any contact with Tamim. Therefore, there is not much to report about him at this point. After a short and coincidental meeting with Tamim and his mother I was able to find out that Tamim is not well at the moment.

These updates lead us to the final section of the case study, where the impressions, difficulties, challenges and findings of this ELMi sub-project will be discussed in more detail and placed in a slightly broader context.

7.6 Discussion

Overall, there are positive things to report from our ethnographic research project, even or maybe especially with regard to health literacy and digital health literacy in particular. Both are weakly developed among the young people, would they be measured by the usual procedures. However, if we look at the young refugees' everyday life and their resulting needs and requirements, it becomes apparent that they have, for example, the necessary competences to organise their leisure time, to maintain contact with family abroad as well as to overcome everyday language barriers. On the one hand, new media, especially smartphones and new types of apps, harbour risks and dangers, such as addiction; this could also be recorded during the monitoring. However, it also became clear how much even simple computer and media skills (use of translation tools) make for interactive creative scope, and in this respect the digital world is indeed not at all abstract, but actually instrumental in expanding the options in the everyday life of young refugees. Therefore, if one takes into account the socio-cultural as well as the situational contexts and the experiential aspect of knowledge (cf. on this, for example, Gilstad 2014; Samerski 2019), one can hardly deny young refugees (digital) health skills despite their probably very low scores on traditional health literacy scales. Language deficits are not the only, but the main obstacle to the young refugees' making use of media resources (non-fiction books, Internet, documentaries, etc.) for themselves, for example, in order to supplement experiential knowledge through the informative acquisition of knowledge.

As for the young refugees from Afghanistan, the close connection between general media skills and digital health literacy is particularly clear, for example in the use of general smartphone functions such as downloading apps (games and translator tools) despite low language skills. Accordingly, they can prove in everyday life that they have health literacy, even if their literacy in the (written) language of the host country is still weak. General health awareness, which, in the first instance, is independent of somebody's education and digital health literacy level, certainly also plays a crucial role here. Still, the young refugees' health-related use of new media, for example the deliberate search for information on the German-language Internet, leaves a lot to be desired. This does not mean, however, that the accompanied young people do not make use of other (social or "analogue") sources to get information about health topics. Thus, family and friends, but also older people from the circle of acquaintances, often serve as advisers the young people can exchange information with.

This aspect leads to the overriding importance of the family for the young people. In this ethnographic study, we wanted to accompany adolescents in their extra-institutional everyday life and in their leisure time, and we met families (the same applies to the case study on girls with a Turkish migration background, cf. Chap. 6). In particular, the family provides a kind of basic orientation and support needed to find one's way in everyday life, to master everyday challenges, and to develop coping strategies. Using Tamim as an example, both aspects could be shown when he spoke of his mother, with whom he spends a lot of time outside of school.

We were unable to encounter the idea of a (compulsory) replacement or substitution of the family by the peer group either in male refugees or female adolescents with a migration background who were born here. From our observations, it follows from our perspective that a concept of Family Health Literacy – yet to be developed – would make sense, which focuses not only on the obvious association of families with young children (see the following Sect. 8), but also includes families with (also adult!) adolescents.

In the age group studied, and this applies to all social strata, there are still many options and possibilities open to change behaviours and circumstances (or to influence them on one's own initiative), to adapt, to improve and to shape them in a way that promotes health – an expanded concept of Family Health could take its cue from any and all of these aspects. As to the latter point, the various academic disciplines concerned, such as (social) psychology, health education, educational sciences, social work and sociology should be called upon to work on such a holistic concept. Particularly crucial with regard to refugees is the question of how health potentials and (digital) health competences or health resources previously acquired (for example, from other settings and cultures), which the young people have drawn upon so far, can be transformed, as smoothly as possible, for use in the target society. Precisely because the young refugees are still in the developmental phase, in linguistics as well as in other respects, much can be done even in the area of primary prevention. The host society plays a special role here, because it has the power to ensure the successful inclusion of refugees through targeted health promotion. They would have to ensure access to the necessary resources on the one hand, but also that access is facilitated or can be adapted (low threshold).

Limitations

Of course, reflection on the limitations of the present ethnographic study is also part of a concluding discussion section.

The fact that flight was not a voluntary option for most refugees usually only becomes apparent over a longer period of time. The ethnographic study as well as the qualitative (focus group) interviews therefore served rather to reconstruct contexts of meaning, which, however, always remain dependent on the applicable as opposed to the proprietorial interpretation. Within the framework of the research project, a verification of the causes of flight was hardly possible – we did not want to copy the symbolically negatively charged official procedures here in any way; this applied equally to the actual situation during the flight. Nor did we on our part want to deal extensively with the topic of flight and the experiences connected with it, first because we are not trained therapists, and second because the young people we accompanied are happy if they can forget those experiences (for the time being) and concentrate on the challenges in the destination country.

It must also be acknowledged that the observation of the refugees' everyday actions and the challenges facing them during the ethnographic research phase should indeed be considered more strongly in the light of the results of international studies and reports such as those by the UN (UNGASC 2019), UNHCR (2017a, 2017b) and UNSG (2016). The reference back to the international state of research, as well as to the increasing sociological and socio-pedagogical research on flight and finally to the multitude of literature worth reading, produced in the environment of activists (cf. among others Milz and Tuckermann 2018) must be reserved for further publications.

Our ethnographic study was designed as a milieu study from the very beginning. The number of just two young refugees accompanied over a period of 9 months naturally belies the fact that we conducted conversations and interviews with around 25 people, conducted another insightful and in-depth focus group at the end of the field phase. Moreover, the material from the field research is relatively comprehensive. Nevertheless, a methodological question remains in the room, which is not easy to answer: *If a cognitivist understanding of health literacy is inadequate for the reasons explained in chapters two, three and four, and at the same time the understanding of health literacy is to be led out of the constriction in the care process, how exactly does health literacy anchored in the lifeworld express itself?* This question has a methodological aspect in the narrower sense and a theoretical-normative aspect. We will only briefly discuss the methodological aspect here and save the discussion of the theoretical-normative dimension for the final chapter.

If we assume that quantitative test theories do not measure actions, but rather readiness to act, attitudes, and (always biased) reports about past actions, then the fundamental transformation problem of this type of research remains the relationship between (general) attitudes and (actual) actions. This transformational relation is then further dealt with by more or less plausible social psychological or sociological theories of action. However, if one proceeds ethnographically, as we have done, and as is very often called for in the health literacy debate, especially with respect to the target group of children and adolescents (as for example in Bröder et al. 2017; Okan et al. 2017a, 2015; Zamora et al. 2015; Pitt et al. 2019; Pinheiro et al. 2021), then the same problem arises from the other side. What do you even see when you look methodologically differently and observe actions directly rather than measure attitudes? In particular, the question arises if one places oneself, as we do here, in the Salutogenesis tradition. Then the question becomes more pointed: *How can Generalised Resistance Resources be pinpointed in observed actions, what do you know a "strong sense of coherence" by? From our point of view, qualitative Salutogenesis research, to which this overall study is only a first contribution, urgently needs to be developed at a fundamental level.* In the relevant handbook of Salutogenesis, the contribution on the measurement of the sense of coherence does not think beyond the classic ideas (Eriksson and Mittelmark 2017). In our view, considerably more progress could be made here if the call originating from health literacy research itself to analyse the lifeworlds of those involved (in part even in a participatory manner!) were combined with what would then be fruitful qualitative Salutogenesis research, which could go a long way here, especially when guided by interventionist and health-promoting intentions (cf. on this also the comments in the final chapter).

Health, Health Literacy and Health Socialisation in Swiss Families with Young Children and a Latin American Migration Background

8

Abstract

The topic of immigration or migration has been regularly in the spotlight in Switzerland, too, and is characterised by ambivalences. *On the one hand,* there are repeated country-wide discourses and mass media productions about cultural differences, different values, especially with regard to gender relations, and questions about social integration into the country with its strong federalist democratic tradition. Debates that became known far beyond the borders of Switzerland were the so-called minaret ban (NZZ, https://www.nzz.ch/zunehmende_empoerung_ueber_minarett-verbot-1.4089840#register, 2009), the ban on face coverings (so-called "burqa ban") introduced in individual cantons since 2016 (Krummenacher, *Neue Zürcher Zeitung,* 2017), and the large-scale discussion about the correct observance of school welcoming rituals (Gerny, https://www.nzz.ch/schweiz/aktuelle-themen/religionsfreiheit-haendedruck-wird-in-baselland-zur-pflicht-ld.84599, 2016).

8.1 Introduction

The topic of immigration or migration has been regularly in the spotlight in Switzerland, too, and is characterised by ambivalences. *On the one hand,* there are repeated country-wide discourses and mass media productions about cultural differences, different values, especially with regard to gender relations, and questions about social integration into the country with its strong federalist democratic tradition. Debates that became known far beyond the borders of Switzerland were the so-called minaret ban (NZZ 2009), the ban on face coverings (so-called

U. H. Bittlingmayer et al., *Health Literacy From A Health Ethnology Perspective*, https://doi.org/10.1007/978-3-658-42348-3_8

"burqa ban") introduced in individual cantons since 2016 (Krummenacher 2017)[1] as well as the large-scale discussion about the correct observance of school welcoming rituals (Gerny 2016). Beyond such discourse events, grouped around individual particularly emotionally charged topics, Switzerland, *on the other hand,* is traditionally a particularly well-functioning multi-ethnic society. The two largest groups of foreigners living in Switzerland are people from Italy and Germany. Of all OECD countries, the proportion of foreigners in the permanent resident population is the second highest (behind Luxembourg) at 25% (Statista 2018) and the proportion of people with a migration background in the population group aged 15 and over was just under 38% at the end of 2018, of which only one fifth were second generation (Schweizerische Eidgenossenschaft – Bundesamt für Statistik 2019b).

The migrant group of people living in Switzerland with a Latin American migrant history or corresponding migration background, which is the focus of the ELiS project, very rarely appears on mass media. They play only a minor role in public perception and are considered well integrated throughout Switzerland. This comparatively quiet integration goes hand in hand with the fact that knowledge about this migrant group in Switzerland is very low. In the Switzerland-wide measurement of health literacy, for example, parts of the migrant population are attested a lower level of health literacy, although the number of cases is too small to arrive at reliable statements in the individual migration groups (Schweizerische Akademie der Medizinischen Wissenschaften 2015). The results obtained by our study can contribute to significantly increasing knowledge about the Latin American migrant group in Switzerland with regard to health, health perceptions and health-relevant everyday actions as well as health literacy. In addition, the ELiS project used an intergenerational perspective, focusing on families with young children. In this context, one motive was to advance the concept of family health literacy, which has so far remained very vague in the literature, conceptually and empirically with regard to migrant families.

In the following, we will provide a frame for this case study with findings on the general topic of migrant health in Switzerland, because Swiss data on people of Latin American origin is indeed very thin on the ground (Sect. 8.2). This is followed by a closer look at the target group of people with Latin American roots (Sect. 8.3).

[1] A nice detail here is that the majority of violations of the ban on hooding, which was first introduced in Switzerland back in 2016 in the canton of Ticino, are somewhat different than probably intended. "According to the authorities, there were fewer than 50 incidents there in the first 2 years. In 90% of those cases, hooded football fans broke the law." haz/kle (afp 2018).

Next comes a detailed description of the data available for the case study and the methodology used for this project (Sect. 8.4). Key findings from the ethnographic study are then presented and linked to further considerations from education and health research (Sect. 8.5). The case study is then wrapped up with a short conclusion and an outline of open follow-up questions (Sect. 8.6).

8.2 The Health of Migrants in Switzerland

Within the framework of Health 2020, the health policy priorities of the Federal Council, improvement on equal opportunities in the health system was identified as an important field of action (Bundesamt für Gesundheit 2013a). All people should have the opportunity to be as healthy as they possibly can. However, the report identifies several vulnerable groups for whom this can be more difficult and who should consequently receive special attention in healthcare. The migrant population is included among these vulnerable groups (Bundesamt für Gesundheit 2013b). The health of migrants has been the subject of increasing interest in Switzerland for some time, as evidenced by the fact that the Federal Statistical Office (FSO) has already carried out the Health Monitoring of the Migrant Population (GMM) twice. This revealed what is known elsewhere as the "healthy migrant" effect: Migrants who have only been in the host country for a short time have better health than the native population, even when controlling for age (Bundesamt für Gesundheit 2012). The frequently observed health advantage of migrants over natives is explained by selection effects: only people who are in good health take up migration (Fennelly 2007; Sahrai 2009; Spallek and Razum 2008b). At the same time, however, the GMM showed that with the increase in the length of stay in Switzerland, health status declines and migrants show poorer health after a longer stay than the native population (Bundesamt für Gesundheit 2012; Guggisberg et al. 2011). Importantly, it was also found that in the migrant population, women are more impaired than men in all health status variables, but especially mental health. These gender differences are often/generally explained by socioeconomic factors – lower levels of education and lower employment rates among migrant women than among migrant men – as well as by low social capital; however, none of the presumed relationships could be statistically confirmed (Moussa and Pecoraro 2013).

The findings on health status and behaviour in the migrant population are very heterogeneous, as are the living situations of the migrant population (Kaya and

Efionayi-Mäder 2007).[2] The Swiss Health Survey shows very similar results to the GMM, and the following point is particularly highlighted: *Socioeconomic status plays a very significant role in the health of migrants in Switzerland. The higher the level of education and the better the employment situation, the better the state of health (Andreani et al.* 2014*; Bischoff and Wanner* 2008*).*

The strong associations between health status and socioeconomic variables such as educational attainment and financial situation in the migrant population suggest that similar mechanisms prevail as in the native majority population and that social disadvantage is directly associated with health disadvantage. Certain groups in the migrant population are also at greater risk of socioeconomic disadvantage than natives. For example, the at-risk-of-poverty rate[3] was 9.9% in 2014 for the population without a migration background and 15.3% for the population with a migration background (Bundesamt für Statistik 2016). These figures have continued to rise in recent years, reaching 12.1% for the native population and 18.8% for the population with a migration background in 2017 (Bundesamt für Statistik 2019). The proportion of the permanent resident population with a migration background who report having difficulty making ends meet is also significantly higher (18.1%) compared to 7.5% of the population without a migrant background (Bundesamt für Statistik 2016).

However, socioeconomic factors alone do not explain health inequalities, neither within the native population nor between native and migrant populations (Sahrai 2009; Schenk 2007). Equally important are ethno-cultural factors which, among other things, shape a person's or group's resources for action and (health-related) practices (Bittlingmayer and Sahrai 2010). Different health concepts can also be associated with differences in health behaviour and thus indirectly with health status (Faltermaier 2001; Kizilhan 2009; Obrist and Büchi 2008).

[2]In this respect, at least in social science research, the meaningfulness of the entire category of migrant or migration background as a statistical catch-all for all persons not considered natives has been called into question; see Chaps. 3 and 4 in this book for more detail on this; the problem, to which Albert Scherr, Ulrike Hormel or Paul Mecheril, for example, continually point, becomes at least latently virulent again at this point.

[3]Regarding the at-risk-of-poverty rate, the Swiss Federal Statistical Office specifies the following: "This indicator, recommended by the EU, measures the risk of social exclusion and the importance of income inequality between different population groups. A higher at-risk-of-poverty rate in a given population group indicates that this group does not have the same participation opportunities in various areas of social life as the rest of the population." Schweizer Bundesamt für Statistik (2019).

Another explanatory approach considers health differences between the migrant and the autochthonous population caused by stress experience in connection with the acculturation that follows migration. It is assumed that there is a specific stress situation in which people with a migration history find themselves and which can additionally shape their state of health. The process of integration into a new, initially foreign environment places high demands on those affected and their coping strategies. Intercultural psychology uses the term "acculturation stress", i.e., the totality of interpersonal, material-instrumental and political-social stressors that are rooted in acculturation and can potentially influence the health of migrants (Berry 1992; Berry et al. 1987; Susan Caplan 2007). As shown in the GMM, experiences of discrimination and limited labour market participation, among other indicators of acculturation stress, play a role in the health of the migrant population in Switzerland (Bundesamt für Gesundheit 2012). When considering theories of acculturation and acculturation stress, it is important to note that migration is not seen as a negative stressor only. Contact with a new culture and society can be equally enriching and a resource for shaping identity to people with a migration background; at the same time, immigration also changes the receiving society itself, so that social integration is described as a "two way process" in migration and transnationalism research (cf. e.g. Kymlicka 2000, 2013, cop. 2007), in political theory (cf. e.g. Peters 1993) or by international organisations such as the United Nations and even the OECD.

Other health resources are social support and control beliefs, i.e., the conviction that one can shape one's own life in a self-determined manner. The GMM shows that the influence of these two variables on the state of health is stronger among migrants than among the native Swiss population. In addition, migrants who speak a Swiss national language show a better state of health (Guggisberg et al. 2011; Bundesamt für Gesundheit 2012). Factors that are regarded as indicators of integration thus have a very clear influence on the health of migrants.

In the context of health inequalities, the multi-perspective view of the 'social determinants of health' is gaining importance (CSDH 2008; Marmot 2005) and is also strongly recommended for the study of migrant health. In summary, in studies investigating health in the context of migration, it is important that "health disadvantages of migrants are always analysed taking into account socio-economic *and* ethno-cultural factors" (Sahrai 2009, p. 88; emphasis added).

Official (health) statistics generally do not take sufficient account of the diversity within the migrant population in terms of socioeconomic status, origin, duration and status of residence, etc. (Razum et al. 2011). In Switzerland, for example, only the largest immigrant groups are included separately in the evaluations, if at all. The above-mentioned health monitoring of the migrant population (GMM) in 2010 can be cited as an example. Only people from Turkey, Portugal, Serbia, Kosovo, Somalia and Sri Lanka were examined. The justification for limiting the GMM to certain nationalities was that "a representative survey of the entire migrant population would have been beyond the scope of what was possible" (Bundesamt für Gesundheit 2012, p. 11). There is still a need for research here in order to adequately cover those groups that have hardly been studied to date. These include, among others, Latin American migrant groups in Switzerland, which have received little attention in the research so far. The next section will focus on people living in Switzerland with a Latin American migrant history or migration background.

8.3 People from Latin America in Switzerland

To direct the analytical focus on Latin American migrants is not entirely unproblematic, as we are thus implicitly lumping people from very different countries of origin together into one virtual group. Historical, political and cultural differences between the countries of Latin America do not seem to support the idea of a uniform "Latino culture" among immigrants from this region of the world, which after all encompasses two continents. Although this kind of group construction is often made, such an approach threatens to promote cultural stereotypes, especially at the thematic interface of family, health and culture (Hunt 2005; Hunt et al. 2004).

In fact, the ELiS study was originally intended to focus only on people with a Colombian migrant background. The background for this preliminary determination was the ethnographer's good field knowledge of the Colombian community. However, during the difficult recruitment phase (described in Chap. 5), we then discovered to our own surprise that people from Latin America, spanning from Argentina to Mexico, who live in Switzerland identify as the Swiss Latino community.

By way of an explanation, Spanish as their common first language is particularly emphasised by the people with a Latin American migration history. With regard to the area covered by our study (Basel and the surrounding region), this is also reflected organisationally. For example, in Basel, the education department of the Spanish embassy offers Spanish language courses at the adult education centre free of charge. However, this only applies to families in which at least one parent has Spanish citizenship. For this reason, migrants from Spanish-speaking Latin America founded the parents' organisation "FOLC Hispanoamerica" (Fomento de la lengua y cultura hispanoamericana – Promotion of Hispanic Language and Culture) in Basel and organised for themselves meeting places and play groups in which the Spanish language is promoted and transmitted. These organisations unite different people and especially families, who can thus experience and cultivate linguistic and cultural aspects of their origin in the country of immigration. The organisational offer in the cantons Basel-Stadt and Basel-Landschaft also includes "GGG Basel" (Gesellschaft für das Gute und Gemeinnützige) with the integrated contact point for migrants and the competence centre for integration, as well as the contact point 4055 – Kontaktstelle für Eltern und Kinder (Contact point for parents and children), which is open every Wednesday as an integrative Latin American meeting point for parents with preschool aged children.

The fact that language is so much at the centre is in conformity with early considerations by Max Weber on the construction of ethnicity, which emphasise language as a supremely relevant, though not exclusive, cultural asset. Commonly held religious beliefs are also specified by Weber, and this again applies, as Catholicism predominates in all of Latin America, although occasionally linked to other traditions such as especially liberation theology (Weber 1972, 237 ff.). This process can be described as moderate self-ethnicization in the sense of the construction of a "social belonging" and group affiliation, by which crucial identity resources are created in the country of immigration. We have pragmatically taken up this self-description in the context of ELiS and expanded our target group from Colombian families with young children to families with young children who have Latin American roots. This did not affect the central project goal, i.e., to obtain as comprehensive a picture as possible with regard to the factors shaping the way in which the families studied deal with health in everyday life, and how these factors interact.

Specifics of the Latino Community in Switzerland

People with Latin American roots residing in Switzerland are heavily underrepresented in social and health science research and, as already mentioned, are not specifically reported on in most Swiss statistics. According to Bolzman, Carbajal and Mainardi, one of the reasons for this is that for a long time it was assumed, in a way similar to the first generation of German guest workers, that these groups were only planning short stays and would soon return to their countries of origin (Bolzman et al. 2007). Likewise, in the public perception, other migrant groups are seen as more exotic and/or have come more into focus, e.g., because of their status as asylum seekers or because of the assumed "cultural distance". On the other hand, many Latin American migrants stay in Switzerland illegally (so-called sans-papiers or undocumented migrants) and as low a profile as possible due to their precarious residence status, which considerably limits social and health research on them.

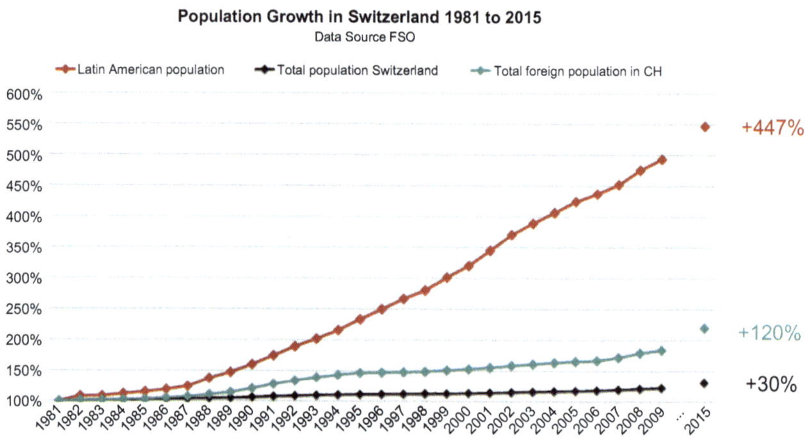

Fig. 8.1 Data according to the Federal Statistical Office, Switzerland. (Source: author)

From a public health perspective, however, we believe that there are important reasons for focusing more research on Latin American groups in Switzerland. First of all, there is a heavily disproportionate growth of the Swiss resident population with Latin American roots compared to the total population and compared to the foreign resident population (see Fig. 8.1 below). More specifically, at the end of 2018, 54,730 people from Latin America and the Caribbean were resident in Switzerland – representing approximately 2.5% of the total population with a migrant background. Of these, 63% were women. At the end of 2018, 3693 people of Latin American and Caribbean origin resided in the cantons of Basel-Stadt and Baselland.

It is of particular relevance for family health literacy research, that Latin American migration to Switzerland often takes place as "family migration", i.e., in the course of marriage to a Swiss woman or man or to a person of foreign origin already living in Switzerland. A large proportion, around two thirds, of Latin American immigrants are female, which contradicts the traditional view of migration as a male phenomenon (Riaño 2012) and which, considering the findings of the GMM on the comparatively greater health burden on migrant women, hints at a potentially increased health burden in this migrant group. A significant proportion of immigrant Latin Americans are considered "highly skilled", i.e., have an above-average level of education (Pecoraro and Fibbi 2010), which is generally considered a protective factor for health. However, as Riaño notes (Riaño 2003, 2011a, b; Riaño and Baghdadi 2007), the economic integration of Latin American migrant women in

Switzerland is considerably hampered by restrictive visa requirements and residence regulations, as well as the non-recognition of Latin American educational qualifications by authorities and employers (we will return to this in Sect. 8.5). Despite the above-average level of education of this migrant group, this repeatedly leads to various forms of disadvantage for those affected, from employment significantly below qualification to non-participation in the (primary) labour market (Goguikian Ratcliff et al. 2015). If professional integration is possible, there are nevertheless still high stress factors: the high qualitative and quantitative demands in the work environment are experienced as challenging (Tejada and Kwankam 2007), and women from Latin American countries cite the difficulty of reconciling family and professional obligations in Switzerland as an additional burden, as childcare places outside the family are rare (Tejada 2010). According to Riaño (2007, 2011a), cultural prejudices and difficulties in learning the German language also make it difficult for Latin American migrants to integrate into (German-)Swiss society.

Taken together, this results in a multitude of stress factors for Latin Americans living in Switzerland, which potentially affect their health. Due to the Latin Americans not being identified by official statistics, there are hardly any figures so far that confirm or refute whether the health risk factors to which Latin Americans in Switzerland are exposed are actually associated with health restrictions and poorer health outcomes. Against this backdrop, comprehensive ethnographic research is an obvious option if more is to be found out about this specific, statistically elusive group.

8.4 The Theoretical Approaches and Methodology of the ELiS Study

This section briefly outlines the overarching theoretical approaches of salutogenesis and the setting approach that we used as a basis for the ELiS study. This is followed by a presentation of the data collected.

A Salutogenic Perspective on Migrant Health

The virtual absence of pathogenetic health data on the Latin American migrant population in Switzerland opens up the possibility of looking at their health from a lesser-known perspective: Aaron Antonovsky's (1985, 1997) salutogenesis (Mittelmark et al. 2017). Rather than a sick-health dichotomy, salutogenesis assumes a continuum on which a person moves between the poles of "health" (ease) and "ill health" (dis-ease) throughout their life. In this context, the two poles are only heuristics that are never found in full expression in reality (Franke 2016). When considering a specific case, the salutogenic paradigm focuses on the following question: what factors contribute to a person moving in one direction or the other on the continuum? In contrast to quantitative cross-sectional data on health status, as collected in monitoring studies, a salutogenic approach is concerned with the broader context. In order to be able to answer the question about the factors due to which a person moves in one direction or the other on the continuum, in-depth knowledge about the history and life circumstances of a person or group is required: "Salutogenesis (...) compels us to examine everything of importance about people who are ill" (Antonovsky 1985, p. 37). *In this respect, a salutogenic perspective and an ethnographic or health anthropological approach are very closely related to each other.*

A salutogenic perspective on the health of Latin American migrants in Switzerland can also be supported by the core statement of the Ottawa Charter on Health Promotion: "Health is created and lived by people in their everyday environment: where they play, learn, work and love" (WHO Europe 1986, p. 4). The importance of the lifeworld and (everyday) culture for health has been repeatedly emphasised, for instance in connection with the setting approach to health promotion (Altgeld 2008; Rosenbrock 2015a). However, studies on the production of health in everyday life are rare. How health is lived in everyday life cannot be satisfactorily surveyed with questionnaires. Instead, a qualitative approach is best suited, which strongly emphasises active participation in, and observation of, the daily lives of those studied. In this sense, the primary aim of the present study is to work out, within the framework of an ethnographic research perspective, how health is produced in the everyday lives of Latin American migrants in Switzerland. The family as the primary instance of socialisation (Hurrelmann 2006; Hurrelmann and Bauer 2015) as well as the place where social inequalities get reproduced (Abel et al. 2009; Bauer and Vester 2015; Lareau 2003; Schwinn 2015) has been chosen as the primary unit of observation.

The Family as a Setting

The setting approach is considered one of the most important strategies for implementing health promotion (Altgeld 2004b; Rosenbrock 2005). "Health is created and lived by people in their everyday environment: where they play, learn, work and love" (WHO Europe 1986, p. 5). This aspect is also echoed by the WHO in the context of health literacy: "To reach target populations, initiatives to build health literacy are best grounded in settings of everyday life" (WHO Europe

2013, p. 90). Attributing great significance to settings in the context of health promotion and health education draws on a lifeworld-based understanding that embeds health in people's everyday lives (Altgeld 2008; Hartung et al. 2011, 2009).

In the context of health socialisation and health education, the family plays a very special role. As a rule, the family is the first and, biographically, most important instance of socialisation, because it is here that the foundations for later life are laid at an early age (Grundmann 2011; Erhart et al. 2008a; Grundmann et al. 2003; Bauer 2012a, b; Hurrelmann and Bauer 2015). However, the family is also the central hinge between society and the individual (Hoffmeister 2012) because it is through the family that not only behaviours, but also social status and the possession of social, economic and cultural capital are inherited (Abel et al. 2009; Bourdieu 1982; Lareau 2011, 2006; Vester 2009). From this perspective, it can be understood as a "place" where social and (ethnic) cultural lifestyles are reproduced intergenerationally. Depending on ethnic and social background, everyday culture in families also differs, this includes parenting ideas, division of labour, health behaviour, etc. (Grundmann et al. 2003; Grundmann 2006; Grundmann and Wernberger Angela 2015; Otyakmaz and Karakaşoğlu 2015). Therefore, as part of habitus formation (Bourdieu 1982), health behaviour, understanding of health and illness, and attitudes towards and knowledge about prevention and health promotion, among other things, are shaped in the family (Ohlbrecht and Schönberger 2010; Perrig-Chiello and Höpflinger 2003; Schnabel 2001b). The family also plays a key role in imparting health literacy, as the resources of the family or the parents are crucial in determining the resources that are passed on to children. Although the importance of the family for health is unanimously emphasised both from the perspective of the socialisation of adolescents and as a place of social support with a positive effect on health (Bauch 2010; Schnabel 2001b; Sting 2007), studies that examine everyday health activities in families are very rare.

Despite the reproduction of inequalities and the health inequalities visible in socio-epidemiological data, a large proportion of vulnerable families are able to cope with life under very difficult living conditions and to bring up their children in a largely healthy way[4]. The central aim of the ELiS project is to avoid the common

[4]Socio-epidemiological data show statistical associations and correlations which are significant, but which must not be interpreted deterministically. This must be mentioned in this context, because especially in the case of vulnerable groups, deterministic statements are often made about the respective groups on the basis of statistical correlations, for example that children in families with few economic resources are more frequently overweight. It is always

deficit-guided view of vulnerable groups (see in detail Chap. 4). *Instead, the families' existing competencies and resources are to be examined and made visible from an ethnological perspective of difference.* Such an approach should not and will not hide structural inequalities and disadvantages as well as existing difficulties. Rather, it is primarily a matter of perceiving people from vulnerable groups, in the tradition of cultural studies (Hall 1994b; Willis 1979), as actual agents and describing their health competence in the context of their everyday actions (Huschke 2013, 2015).

Addressed Research Desideratum

Programmes and measures in the field of prevention and health promotion that aim at strengthening health competencies, e.g., parent education programmes or school-based life skills programmes, often face difficulties in trying to reach vulnerable groups (Bauer 2005; Bauer and Bittlingmayer 2005; Hurrelmann et al. 2013; Kickbusch 2009; Stutz Steiger 2011). This is mainly due to the fact that in the day-care sector, better resourced day-care centres are more easily reached and within programmes implemented in the day-care centre, parents of migrant* groups are reached less easily (Sahrai 2010c; Hartung et al. 2010). In schools, the situation is similar: Larger schools that rank higher in the formal educational hierarchy are more easily reached by extracurricular teaching programs than are schools that educate children and adolescents in the lower levels of the hierarchy (Bauer 2005; Bittlingmayer and Sirch 2006). In order for vulnerable groups or "hard-to-reach" groups to be more easily reached by health promotion programmes and to strengthen health literacy, there have been repeated calls for greater inclusion of the living environments, culture and everyday settings of the groups concerned:

> Health literacy benefits from diversity. Health literacy initiatives work best when they customize approaches based on understanding the diversity of how individuals and communities approach health. The roles of family, social context, culture and education need to be factored into the development of all health literacy messages and proposals. (WHO Europe 2013, p. 23).

Despite this widely accepted claim, *there have been few studies in the field of health literacy and health promotion that examine how different groups conceptualise health and live health in their everyday lives, what resources and competencies they have to address health-related problems in the family, and how parents strengthen*

a question of relational values, and the majority of children in these families lie within the socially accepted normal range.

health literacy in their children. The ELiS project addresses this desideratum of health literacy research. Ethnography is the only method that can be used to study health literacy as an everyday practice in the lifeworld of vulnerable groups (Papen 2009 argues along similar lines; see also Walters and Papen 2008). In contrast to the usual methods of researching health literacy, which start at the level of attitudes or self-reports and deduce social practice from them, the ethnographic approach aims to directly observe everyday actions and behaviour.

Research Design and Methods

The ELiS project was designed as a qualitative-explorative field study based on an ethnographic approach. Ethnography can be defined as a "methodologically plural contextual research strategy" that aims to explore social lifeworlds and social practices (Breidenstein et al. 2015, 41 f.). An ethnographic approach is concerned with "lived cultural practices" (Willis 2000, xiv) and cultural meanings attributed to them. In ethnography, researchers aim to understand the ways in which those studied view their world and gradually come to understand the inherent logic of the field. The aim of ethnography is to directly observe everyday actions and social practice and reconstruct them as embedded in their context (Breidenstein et al. 2015). Working in the field, which is characterised by observation and simultaneous participation in situations of the everyday life of the investigated, enables the gradual appropriation and understanding of the counterpart's lifeworld: "By at least approximately adopting the interpretations of the members of a particular (...) social group, which often requires an intensive engagement with this unit, it is possible to 'understand' it and to 'explain' its rules" (Girtler 2001, p. 40). By moving away from self-reporting, ethnography makes it possible to examine health and health literacy more closely as an everyday practice in the lifeworld of vulnerable groups. In contrast to mere questionnaires, surveys, or even qualitative interviews, ethnological research can methodically distinguish between normative statements, attitudes and actual behaviour in everyday life (Bittlingmayer and Sahrai 2010).

The main method used in the ELiS project was participant observation. This was supplemented by ethnographic interviews and informal conversations as well as document analysis. The ethnographic work in the families was flanked by guided expert interviews with people who are well acquainted with the culture of origin of the families studied or who offer professional support for families in vulnerable situations. In addition, other data sources such as publicly accessible or private documents, audio and video material, etc. were consulted as needed. In the ELiS project, too, reference was made to the principle attributed to Clifford Geertz (1973) that "everything is data". The particular strength of the ethnographic approach lies in its openness, which allows research questions, methods and types of data to be continually adapted to the circumstances in the field (Christensen 2004). This helps the researchers' efforts to understand behaviour and underlying interpretations "whilst ensuring that they are not treated as discrete and divorced from the policies, actions and interventions of outsiders" (Parker and Harper 2006, p. 3).

Documentation of participant observations was primarily through the writing of field notes, diaries, and memos (Emerson et al. 2011; Walford 2009). Reflection on and questioning of one's own perceptions and constructions was also part of the overall research process (Laine 2000; Graneheim et al. 2001; Oeye et al. 2007).

Sampling

According to international consensus, early childhood is defined as ranging from 0 to 8 years (Irwin et al. 2007). The ELiS project focused on families that could be considered vulnerable or disadvantaged in various dimensions and had at least one child in this age group, in order to trace the processes and socialisation motives of family health literacy. We defined a family as a community spanning at least two generations, in which the relationships between individuals are characterised by emotional closeness and intimacy, and where there are high expectations regarding the durability of these bonds (Ecarius et al. 2011). The entire socio-ecological environment of the family was included in the empirical work, but the research focused on the nuclear family setting, i.e. situations in which the child or children were present and spent time with at least one parent.

The measures of vulnerability or disadvantage are not clearly determinable and cannot be defined in general terms. For inclusion criteria, we first assessed the educational level (not higher than compulsory school leaving certificate or equivalent) and/or the employment situation (no earned income, precarious employment or single parent) of the parents or parent. When considering the level of education, we made explicitly sure whether recognition of the acquired educational title was guaranteed in Switzerland. As already mentioned, it is extremely difficult to obtain recognition for Latin American educational qualifications in Switzerland, and a sole focus on acquired degrees is not sufficient for assessing possible social disadvantage.

Field Access and Recruitment

Since Latin American migrants in Switzerland are well connected through social networks (Riaño 2003, 2011b), the first step in recruiting families with a Latin American migrant background was to contact clubs/societies in which they had joined together. We got in touch with them by letter and sent them flyers in Spanish.

Furthermore, project flyers were distributed at the Contact Point for Parents and Children 4055, a neighbourhood and family centre that offers a meeting place especially for Latin American families. In some cases, the project was presented directly to the participating families at one of the meeting points by a project employee. The project was also made known through the Spanish-speaking parishes of Basel-Stadt and Basel-Land. The pastor in charge allowed a presentation of the research during Sunday mass and also approached potentially suitable families directly. In addition, personal networks and the networks of gatekeepers were used to recruit participants. For the most part, contacts were made through third parties who themselves belonged to the community or were close to it. In an ethnographic study from Germany on Latin American migrants, it was shown that the recommendation by acquaintances to participate in a research project is the most effective way of recruitment (Huschke 2013). After initial contact with a few interested people, the participants recommended the ELiS project to their friends, and contact was made via telephone calls and social media – primarily WhatsApp or Facebook. The target group, which was originally to be confined to the Colombian community, was expanded in the course of recruitment in favour of the Latin American community in the study area, as there were too few Colombian families with young children in the study area overall and the Latin American community also forms a key frame of reference for Colombian families. The reasons why, with regard to the substance of our study, this seemed permissible to us have already been explained above.

Data Acquisition and Data Evaluation

In ethnographic research, the data collection, data analysis and interpretation stages are strongly intertwined, the boundaries between perception, description, analysis and interpretation are fluid (Becker 1958; Geertz 2003; Schatzman and Strauss 2005). Experiences were put in writing already during the field phases and thus processed for the first time (Scheffer 2002). Likewise, events in the field were continuously analysed in order to plan the further progress of the field phase in a meaningful way. The process understanding of grounded theory was accordingly applied to data collection and analysis: The structuring of the research object was not done a priori but emerged from the material in the course of our work (Flick 2014). Evaluations were carried out circularly in several phases (Lamnek 2005), while observation categories were formed from the beginning, which formed the foundation for the first evaluation steps (Whyte 2005). These were then gradually supplemented with new categories and modified until theoretical saturation was achieved (Glaser and Strauss 2010). In ethnographic work, the confrontation of data with theory also occurs partly in parallel with data collection.

As complex interdependence between inequalities and disadvantages on several levels was to be expected in the ELiS project, an intersectional analysis perspective on the object of research was considered useful.

> Intersectionality is understood as a perspective and an analytical view that illuminates, in a non-essentialist and inequality-critical way, the interplay of different, socially effective and hierarchically organised constructions of difference (starting from the triad of race, class and gender) and the associated structural relations of inequality and domination, and asks about the consequences of their mutual interplay. (Riegel 2012, p. 2; cf. in more detail on intersectionality Chaps. 2 and 4).

The analysis of the interdependence of inequalities based on different attributes such as social status and ethnocultural origin[5] provides a sensitive picture of the opportunities that open up to the families or family members studied in their everyday lives and the diverse effects this has or can have on their health-related actions. It also enables a critical examination of the circumstances under which (health) competencies of the individual or the family system have developed and thus promotes the adoption of a difference perspective on these competencies. Intersectional analyses have been rare in health research on migrant groups, but their implementation is strongly recommended (Abraído-Lanza et al. 2016; Acevedo-Garcia et al. 2012; Viruell-Fuentes et al. 2012).

Data Collected and Use of Data for the Case Study

In accordance with the perspective described above that in principle everything can be considered relevant data, very different sources were identified and used in the ELiS project. Figure 8.2 gives an overview of the entire available data pool.

Of the twelve interviews conducted, one was with a Colombian woman who was married to a Swiss man and had no children, one was with a Colombian woman with a Latin American husband whose children were 10 and 12 years old at the time of the interview, and one was with an unmarried Colombian man with no children. All three interviews served for early field exploration and establishing contact with

[5] It is important, especially with an intersectional analysis perspective, not to assume a priori categories of difference, which are then searched for in the material. Similarly to the process of understanding of grounded theory, it makes sense to work with categories of difference that emerge inductively from the data (Winker and Degele 2010). Consequently, this project does not restrict the analysis to the constructions of difference mentioned in the text.

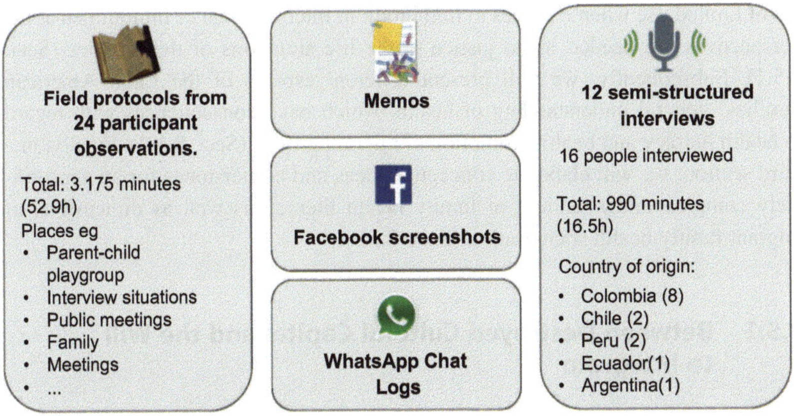

Fig. 8.2 Available data pool ELiS project

families from our target group and are selectively included in the analysis (approximately in Sect. 8.5.1). Two families were accompanied ethnographically, one of them more intensively than the other. In addition, observations were carried out in different settings such as a playgroup or in sports courses, and field notes were drawn up.

Available data consisted not only of the field notes, which were created as memory notes after meetings at different locations, and guided interviews, but there were also the recordings of WhatsApp chats or Facebook posts relevant to the project. It should not be concealed at this point that the ELiS project was terminated prematurely due to the ethnographer's change of jobs. In consequence, a lot of primary data remained unprocessed. Against this background, we limit the presentation of results in this chapter of the book primarily to the analysis of the interviews and selected observation notes. A complete documentation and analysis must be reserved for further publications. In the following section, we will now present some key findings on the health perceptions and health literacy of Latin American families with young children living in Switzerland.

8.5 Considerations of Health-Related Framing and Family Health Literacy in Families with Young Children and a Latin American Migrant Background

In this section, we will now present key findings from our study. To this end, in a first step we will adopt a social structure analysis perspective and assess the available resources for action. As will be shown, traditional stratification indicators are of limited use when it comes to immigration. Intersectional or multidimensional perspectives are needed to do justice to the life situations of the families (Sect. 8.5.1). Subsequently, we will present different aspects of the Latin American families' general understanding of health, which have consequences with regard to health literacy and health promotion of migrant groups (Sect. 8.5.2). Finally, in a third section, we will elaborate conceptual ideas and cornerstones for an appropriately complex understanding of family health literacy as well as dimensions of migrant family health socialisation (Sect. 8.5.3).

8.5.1 Between Destroyed Cultural Capital and the Will to Integrate

The traditional models of social structure analysis still form the basis for health reporting by the WHO and most countries. As a rule, a stratification index is used, which is composed of the dimensions of school education and vocational training, current occupation(s) and income (usually household income). More complex models also take into account immigration history, migration background, gender, age or dependence on social transfer income in regression models. However, statistical modelling should not be confused with the real penetration of structural dimensions. This quickly becomes clear in the case of the families with a Latin American migration background that we are looking at.

In particular, the cultural capital acquired in the country of origin is often subject to drastic devaluation in the country of immigration. From the specific educational perspective of adult education, people who do not know the written language of the country in which they live and love are called functionally illiterate, regardless of how many other written languages they know (Grotlüschen and Riekmann 2012; Grotlüschen and Buddeberg 2020).[6] This devaluation process has been called the annihilation of cultural capital (Sahrai et al. 2011). In Switzerland, the recognition of immigrants' foreign educational and university qualifications is handled in a restrictive manner, and in our sample the destruction of cultural capital has been a consistent experience.

This experience of having your employment history shattered can also be clearly identified as a stress factor from a health science perspective. One mother, for

[6]The only exceptions are people who are active in specific parts of the economic, artistic or scientific field and who can read and write English. In the German-speaking world, much less effort is expected from such people than, for example, from mothers raising children at home.

example, has two degrees and relevant professional experience in these fields, neither of which has been recognised. She then completed a short training course to become a playgroup leader in order to gain a professional foothold in Switzerland. Another mother studied design and worked in the fashion industry, only to find herself working in a furniture warehouse after immigration. In some cases, the professional fields remain the same, but the position in the hierarchy changes. For example, a civil engineer worked as a construction worker after his engineering degree was not recognised, and a hotelier's daughter with a degree in tourism worked as a clerk in a hotel.

It is surprising that this massive devaluation of educational qualifications and professional experience is hardly ever openly criticised in the interviews. In most cases, the approach is comparatively pragmatic. Typical, for example, is the statement of a woman who also has two degrees and now works (among other things) as a part-time language teacher:

> [...] since last year I have been teaching Spanish (.) in an organisation [name of organisation]. It's paid, and it's only one group a week. So, it's really very little what I get, but it's interesting because I'm already in the Swiss job market. It's not the job I would have wanted. But as a teacher it's not bad either. (Interview 006: 00:16:34–00:17:04).

The motif of destroyed cultural capital also has a special gender-specific dimension. It is true that the lack of recognition affects both genders equally and without any discernible differences; the women in our sample had very good and, without exception, academic professional positions in their home countries, for example as lawyers or as executives in the tourism industry, and there was no recognition or successful transformation of their previous titles and professional positions. But in the context of immigration to Switzerland and with regard to the care of young children, it is explicitly emphasised several times that *Switzerland* is perceived *here, on the one hand, as a special family option space.*

Thus, in at least one case, it is considered a strong privilege by a mother to be at home with the children as a mother and to be able to focus appropriately on motherhood with young children. This assessment must be understood against the backdrop of Latin American countries where it is often economically necessary for mothers of young children to integrate into the labour market.

A Chilean mother of two, one of whom was born in Chile, reports, "And we were very happy working in our jobs until we became parents. And in Chile it was almost impossible to combine fatherhood, motherhood and work." (Interview 009: 00:15:28–00:15:40) In this case, the decision to migrate to Switzerland (which was structurally facilitated by the fact that the man had an emigrated Swiss great-grandfather and thus a Swiss passport) was a calculated rearrangement of the work-family-life balance. The perspective was that the social security systems in Switzerland would make it possible to focus on raising children, at least some of the time, and to have a close-knit family life. A Colombian mother describes something very similar, characterising the time with her children as particularly valuable and unique.

> This [time with children; author] is a moment because it's just a moment. I don't know, because other mothers might say, 'No, I've had my baby and I use a day-care centre.' I couldn't do that. I spent my seven years with my kids raising them. There would have been a choice because I have my job and my languages, but I didn't have the strength to put my child in other hands. And I said I'm not going to go to work just to give the money I earn to other strangers to take care of my own child. (Interview 003: 00: 19:04–00:19:56).

However, this motif of privileged family life is highly ambivalent, because *on the other hand* it also happened in one case that the pregnancy of a hitherto childless woman, who according to her own statement in a conversation had already given up the desire for motherhood, must be regarded in exactly the opposite way: i.e., as a consequence of the barred access to the labour market. Motherhood is then a kind of "way out" in order to have legitimate employment and not "just" be her husband's wife, although this was not communicated openly.

Overall, it is by no means the case that families with a Latin American migration background are unanimous in their praise of conditions in Switzerland with regard to gender relations there. For example, the women complain about their particularly difficult access to the Swiss labour market, to which the men often have better access simply because they have Swiss roots or are Swiss themselves, and the women face language barriers in the course of "love migration". As a reminder, around two thirds of Latin American immigrants to Switzerland are women. Here, gender-specific inequalities in the structure of the world of work have an impact on relationships, which can even lead to the devaluation of women within the family. For example, a Colombian woman who immigrated to Switzerland as a "love migrant" and who previously worked in Colombia as a lawyer for a private company says the following: "My husband sometimes says to me: 'Oh, you and your 5% job!' I know it's meant as a joke, and he doesn't mind that I don't make more money. But still, it always leaves a bitter aftertaste. I would so love to work more or go back to university." (Observation record 007a, lines 28–31).

Finally, with regard to the gender dimension, it should be noted that Latin American women do indeed observe strong differences between the machismo in their home countries and the behaviour of Swiss men. However, the difference is not understood and experienced as a categorical one, but rather as a gradual one: in Switzerland, machismo is also observed, but it is much more implicit and indirect, and it is identified, for example, in the disparity in the occupation of leadership positions, especially in business.[7]

A Chilean couple expresses the discrepancy between expectations and reality with regard to gender equality:

> Switzerland needs to change this aspect, because in this respect it is far from other European countries, so to speak. With equal opportunities for men and women. Very far away! For me it was super surprising because I would have never imagined it. [...] Because from South America, they see Switzerland as the most developed European country and not a more traditional one. Very open, they imagine that. So, they imagine that labour laws and equality for women are super. And then you see that they're not. That it's not like Germany, France or Spain, let alone Sweden, Finland and all that. Then you say, 'uff, why?' And of course, you find that the income is so good that one person in the house working is enough. (Interview 010: 00:27:17–00:28:14).

The (gender-specific) destruction of cultural capital, which in part leads to considerable difficulties in gaining a foothold in the Swiss labour market, particularly in connection with "love migration", and the clearly perceived deficits in gender equality within Swiss society meet with a strong will to integrate in almost all the Latin American families in our sample.[8] It is important to note here, first of all, the distinction made by one Hispanic-Swiss family between, on the one hand, those women who "only" accompany their husbands in their labour migration and return to their home country after a few years; and, on the other hand, those who have Swiss roots themselves or are in a relationship with a person from Switzerland and whose migration project is geared to a permanent life in Switzerland from the outset. From this perspective, the second group is more willing to integrate.

> The thing about Hispanics – I'm there working. There are two groups: Those who are with a person from Switzerland or are Swiss expatriates like us. Well, they come here and they're going to stay forever. Then they are more worried about integration because they are going to stay. Their children will grow up here, they have chosen

[7] A classic indicator to make such structural gender gaps visible is the gender pay gap; this decreased in Switzerland from 18.4% in 2008 to 17% in 2016 but was still slightly above the OECD average (16.1% in 2014); Statista (2017); EuroStat and Statista (2014).

[8] Of course, a positive selection in our sample is likely due to our recruitment strategies. People who learned about the research project and allowed themselves to be interviewed or accompanied by us probably are disproportionately successful with their integration.

> to live here. And then there are all the expats [experts recruited from abroad; author's note] who [work] at Novartis, Roche for two or three years and then go back. 90% of my friends are expats. And these people have a different approach. The women have more resources, but on the other hand they don't have so much time because they come here to let their husband work all day [...], so they are with the children all day. (Interview 009: 00:05:47–00:06:45).

We cannot map this sharp differentiation on the basis of our data, because the group of recruited experts alluded to in this interview passage are mainly families from Spain and not from Latin America.[9] Our sample is clearly dominated by "love migrants" and Swiss expatriates. However, this internal differentiation is worth mentioning because it contains an implicit and latently held normative perspective and divides the Latin American community in Switzerland into those who have, in a sense, fully embraced Swiss society and those who are only temporarily in Switzerland and who therefore do not (have to) take social integration as seriously as the group of permanent immigrants. From the perspective of health science, this would place precisely those under particular integration and acculturation stress who are planning their future life in Switzerland, while the "temporary" ones, in contrast, would be at an advantage because they still have the choice of returning.

In fact, almost all of the people we interviewed and accompanied emphasised a very strong willingness to adapt to Swiss society and stressed the need for personal change. Typical, for example, is the statement by one mother: "Then I think you have to adapt here. They can't expect the environment to adapt to them. Otherwise, they better stay where they were." (Interview 010: 00:44:50–00:45:06) In another mother's statement, the willingness to adapt is directly linked to health: "But you have to try to adapt to this country and to the place where you are, so that you are well. Because the more you are always against it and limit yourself, then you will always find problems. And the more you suffer and the more you get sick." (Interview 003: 00:13:03–00:13:29) In several statements, this attitude involves explicit distancing from people who are described as not being adequately willing to integrate. For example, from a mother who strongly distances herself from other Latin Americans: "I'm not like other people I know from Colombia or other

[9]The group of Spaniards living in Switzerland, as EU nationals, benefit on the one hand from the free movement of persons, and on the other hand from the recognition of most educational qualifications, especially since Bologna. The conditions for this group of migrants are therefore quite different from those for migrants from Latin America. From Latin America, in the classic sense of "expats", you can only come to Switzerland if you are highly specialised, e.g., with a PhD. A "simple" university degree is not enough.

countries, sad about [leaving home] and saying: ‘I can’t get used to it, the language is difficult, the climate, this and that’.” (Interview 003: 00:12:40–00:12:58).

The fact that adapting to (German-)Swiss society is not easy, however, is clearly stated by all, the aspect most frequently brought up being the difficulty of learning the standard German language and the local dialect. Here, once again, a limit to integration is found in the ability to speak or at least understand not only High German but also Swiss German. It is repeatedly pointed out that it is very difficult for Latin Americans to learn German – in contrast to English, for example, or French, another national language in Switzerland.

At the same time, however, Switzerland is described as a special country that has a great deal to offer and in which the quality of life is significantly higher than in Latin American countries. Not only are the existing social security systems emphasised, but Switzerland is also described as a comparatively quiet country that also has great resources with regard to health produced in everyday life:

> They are better off in Switzerland than in any other country – people really appreciate having time for their hobbies. And they take care of them. I think that’s great because it makes them healthier than in many other countries. You don’t get to see a lot of obese people here, and not a lot of mentally ill people either. [. . .] People feel good because they have time to enjoy their family and the lifestyle is not so stressful. (Interview 010: 01:04:52–01:05:45).

With a view to this construction of Switzerland as a calm and low-stress country with a very high quality of life and many advantages, we have now come close to the subject area of health itself. In the next section, the general understanding of health of families with a Latin American migration background will be traced.

8.5.2 The Understanding of Health in Families with a Latin American Migration Background

Health references, health behaviour – especially concerning nutrition – as well as the general understanding of health in families with a Latin American migration background are of course not uniform, but heterogeneous in many respects. Nevertheless, several overarching motifs can be identified with regard to the general understanding of health, which are surprisingly homogeneous and bring the attitudes towards health in this group very close to the salutogenic view. In the vast majority of interviews, in response to our question about what health is, it was spontaneously stated that individual health involves more than not currently having any illnesses.

First of all, it is very often emphasised that health must be linked more strongly to mental or psychological health than to just physical infirmities. One interviewed mother works her way towards a more complex understanding of health in her answer:

> Good health to me is – obviously you think health is absence of disease. So, the healthy person who has no disease. That's a first concept that can come to mind, but health goes far beyond that [...]. So, for me, health is divided into physical health and emotional health. Both are equally important. (Interview 002: 00:53:45–00:54:15).

The aspect of well-being is very closely linked to health in several interviews. One father states the following:

> Mmm, for me it [health] is not just the absence of disease. I, the word I associate with health is well-being. [...] Yeah, like it's broader than just being sick; but as comprehensive health: feeling well, happy, relatively satisfied with life and with what you're doing; mentally and physically. It [health] is not just reduced to physical health, but mental health. Well-being is the word I associate with it. Feeling good, being healthy. (Interview 010: 00:55:06–00:55:57).

Furthermore, health and well-being are very explicitly linked to an integral social dimension: In response to a question, noted with surprise, about what it generally means to the interviewees to feel well, it is first expressed that this is a very difficult question, only to continue, "No! [emphasised]. For me [emphasised] to feel good? For Nicolle [her daughter] to feel good. [...] That Nicolle is in good health. For Carlos [husband] to be well, for me to be well. Because when we are all well, everything works." (Interview 004: 00:25:08–00:25:24).

This social dimension – as we have explained in more detail in the theoretical chapters – has not been sufficiently reflected in the conceptualisation and measurement of health literacy to date. However, it plays a very important role in the perspective of families with a Latin American migration background. As with the Afghan and Turkish adolescents in the other two case studies, their own well-being is linked to the fact that those close to them are also doing well. One's own well-being is even defined by and made to depend on the well-being of the people closest to oneself. An appropriate concept of family health literacy cannot avoid taking this fact into account.

Apart from the emphasis on mental health and the consistent presentation of comparatively holistic conceptions of health, as well as the emphasis on the social dimension of one's own health, there are three further motifs that bring the health understandings and conceptions of families with a Latin American migration background into close proximity to the salutogenic understanding of health. Firstly, the special importance of psychological and psychosomatic factors for their own state of health is pointed out. In the case of a mother of two, this goes as far as to border on esoteric positive thinking approaches and the conscious mental effort to avoid "bad" thoughts and feelings in order not to become mentally ill. In several interviews – implicitly and explicitly – stress-theoretical arguments are put forward and stress is recognised as a cause of illness, although stress does not (officially) represent an illness.

Second, in many interviews, health and well-being are associated with a balanced relation between, for example, work and leisure, available time with family, balanced diet (sweets yes, but not too much), and the word "balance" alone appears explicitly in a health context in more than half of the interviews.

Thirdly, it is clearly recognized that illness and health are not polar and categorical opposites, and this is made plausible in an interview with an example from the interviewee's own environment. The starting point for the following quotation from a Latin American couple interviewed together is the question of whether health is also possible within illness.

> Yes, I think so. I think because there are people who have, for example, a diagnosis of 'X'. Okay, that person has cancer, but that doesn't mean she can't feel healthy and feel good. Because the cancer might not stop her from doing all the things she wants to do because they're on their meds. [...] For example, Martin [husband] is hypertensive. He has high blood pressure. And because he takes his medication [...] he doesn't feel bad and he can work and do whatever he wants. [...] And when he fills out these forms, he has to declare high blood pressure. But that doesn't mean he doesn't have a well-being. Therefore, there can be a well-being within the illness. (Interview 010: 01:10:46–01:11:42).

Even though we have a positively selected group of families in our sample with regard to cultural capital, the understandings of health are still strikingly sophisticated. The definitions given by our interviewed and observed families are in fact very close to what can be found in the 1985 WHO-Ottawa Charter. The health dimensions of physical, psychological and social well-being expressed by the WHO can be identified in almost every interview. In addition, the frequently expressed understanding of health as balance, as dependent on stress factors, and compatible with illness are, in our view, very close to the salutogenic understanding of health.

From our point of view, there are two possible interpretations that can explain the closeness of the interviewees' health understandings to the WHO understanding and to salutogenesis. The first and simple explanation is, of course, that the interviewees are familiar with the approaches and have a high degree of public health expertise.

Then, for example, the distinction between experts and laypersons in the field of health could not be maintained (Faltermaier et al. 1998a), because the persons we interviewed would then technically be experts themselves. It is not impossible that such original knowledge exists, but against the background of the academic professions of law, tourism, economics or engineering, it is not particularly likely.

It seems much more plausible to us that a salutogenic perspective and the multidimensional WHO understanding of health are themselves very close to people's basic intuitive ideas and are thus deeply anchored in common good sense. If this interpretation is correct, this would have consequences for public health interventions and for the conception of general health literacy, because from the outset we would expect social actors to be much more competent in health and there would be many more points of contact – especially in the context of family health literacy – if the strict division between public health experts and public health laypersons were mitigated in advance.

In the following section, we will present some basic motivations for a family health literacy approach and for a somewhat broader perspective on health socialisation.

8.5.3 Family Health Literacy and Migrant Family Health Socialisation

Finally, in order to link the material presented so far with Family Health Literacy and then, in a final step, to broaden the perspective to include motifs and dimensions of a more comprehensive family health socialisation, a number of links can quickly be found, which can be derived, for example, from the explored understanding of health alone. It is quite possible that the awareness of a social dimension to health is favoured by the presence of young children, whose vulnerability is often visible in everyday life (although, against the background of the other two case studies, similar ideas also got mentioned by migrant young people). But there is no doubt that there is a clear and consistent awareness of the social dimension of health and thus of health literacy in the families with a Latin American migration background that we researched.

What Could Family Mean in a Family Health Literacy Concept for Migrants? We have criticised above (cf. Chaps. 2, 3 and 4) that, although the necessity of starting from the lifeworlds of children, adolescents and families has repeatedly been emphasised, this demand is then institutionally bent in the context of increasing family health literacy and the focus yet again directed towards health-promoting day-care centres and schools, i.e. institutions which, in a Habermasian or Husserlian understanding, are certainly not to be counted as family lifeworlds in the narrower sense. Therefore, the next step is to ask what exactly comes into view when one accompanies families ethnographically and wants to gain knowledge on the basis of a lifeworld analysis of the conditions and opportunities for realisation of family health literacy among specific migrant groups.

First of all, even in such a small group of Latin American immigrants, there are internal differences which the parents interviewed and accompanied vehemently insisted on. This included, for example, the complaint of an immigrant Swiss expatriate who thought that family support services for immigrants are very undifferentiated. He describes his experience as follows:

> So, when these experts [in parent education and health] go to parents and make recommendations and say, 'Before such an age, nothing, because it damages the brain.' [...] Sometimes they assume that parents don't have enough knowledge; and that's a big mistake! When they give these lectures to foreigners, they are meant for an uneducated audience. So, you have to see what audience you have in front of you. [...].
>
> So, you have to see first, 'what kind of migrant am I facing?' [...] And I know when you do that in other parent education programs and you give it to the experts, you look at what audience you have in front of you first, for sure. But when they're designed for immigrants, they all come in the same way, like all immigrants are the same. (Interview 010: 00:16:05–00:16:30 and 00:17:45–00:18:15).

Moreover, throughout the empirical material, internal differentiations are repeatedly drawn, for example between Latin American families who are very serious about social integration in Switzerland (according to their self-description, all the people in our sample) and people who constantly complain about Switzerland and the Swiss, or, as shown, between people who permanently relocate their centre of life to Switzerland, and those who are merely temporary labour migrants.

The second finding from the field points to the fact that (as in the other two case studies) it is by no means immediately clear what family is and who counts as family. The classic ethnological insight that kinship is not biologically determined but socially constructed is clearly confirmed here (cf. e.g., Schnegg et al. 2010). A reduction of family to the parent-child dyad does not capture the reality of families with a Latin American migration background; the understanding and everyday practice of family is more comprehensive. One married couple emphasises the special importance of families, which includes three siblings (or sisters-in-law and brothers-in-law) living in other cities in Switzerland and their children; two other brothers of the husband live (again) in Colombia, the wife's family lives in Miami, except for two other brothers living in Colombia.

On the relevance to everyday life, they state:

> [Wife:] Well, we're always in contact. I have contact with my father [Wife's father living in Miami] every day. And with my brothers. And we always go to Miami a lot and stuff. And always Isabel [husband's sister-in-law] [...] and the nephews come here. [...] [Husband:] But the relationship is good. [Wife:] It's very good. [Husband:] We have often, we are in contact. [Wife:] That is, by phone. Or they come and we go, however; we have dinner or a barbecue. Yeah, we always get together for birthdays. Sometimes even if it's not a special occasion, we always try to meet to keep in touch." (Interview 004: 00:18:03–00:18:52).

The wife of another family states the following in this regard:

> It's like that in Latin America, we call ourselves family down to the second uncle. [...] I have a second-degree aunt who lives in Sweden, but I talk to her more often than I talk to my cousin [who lives in Switzerland]. So, I have an aunt in Sweden, I have family in the US, I have a cousin also in Spain who lives in the same place as my cousin. [...], that's what I have in terms of family, in the US, Spain, Sweden. (Interview 007: 00:20:54–00:21:29).

These comparatively low-key descriptions of the high importance attached to the family and, at the same time, of family groups in the migrant population, some of which are ramified internationally, certainly should have consequences with regard to a possible family health literacy concept. First of all, with regard to the social dimension of health and well-being described above, it must be taken into account that events occurring far away from one's own centre of life, such as the illness of a relative living abroad, can also have an impact on one's own well-being. A concept of family health literacy that only refers to the nuclear family would not be complex enough. The educational reformatting of life-world health literacy in particular does not do justice to this more complex form of family and focuses too strongly on the parent-child dyad.

On the other hand, it should not be underestimated that, due to large-scale and, above all, international family networks, very different national discourses on health-related topics such as vaccinations, dental care, advice on health-oriented forms of behaviour (diet, exercise, sport), compliance, patient autonomy or health-oriented parenting styles can come into play, which also have an impact on everyday family routines and situation assessments. Technically speaking, families with intact international family networks generally have a larger information base for dealing with health issues than do locals, because the exchange about the issues takes place in the light of very different healthcare systems and public discourses.

This is an argument in favour of a complex concept of – at least immigrant – Family Health Literacy. Our plea for conceptualising families that is as complex as possible within a Family Health Literacy concept is confirmed by the observation of a Latino immigrant woman who was confronted with cultural differences of Eritrean mothers in the context of a call on parents to read books aloud to their children and to visit libraries with children. She reports that the whole effort to attract families to libraries to boost domestic reading time failed because Eritrean families were very close-knit and their mothers and children formed such a noisy unit that, from the perspective of Eritrean mothers, they would disrupt the usual library routine and therefore would certainly not be welcomed (Interview 009: 00:00:15–00:02:18) From all that has been said in this section, it follows that an adequate, lifeworld-anchored concept of Family Health Literacy, at least in the case of migrant parents resp. those with a migrant background, must from the start be based on a very broad understanding of "family", in order to make customised offers for health literacy promotion that are actually compatible with everyday practice.

Migrant Health Socialisation

These descriptions ultimately point to the question of how and to what extent immigration societies should deal with cultural differences, which integrally include different notions of family and everyday family routines, in the context of health promotion among migrant families with young children in general and Latin American families in particular. This topic is relatively complex and is associated, on the one hand, with the danger of exaggerating and essentializing cultural differences between groups of different origin. On the other hand, ignoring cultural differences goes hand in hand with continuing to fail to reach parents and young children adequately with meaningful health promotion interventions (see also Chap. 4). This is particularly problematic with respect to health and health literacy promotion, as it also ignores the ambivalences and the *double cultural reference spaces of children and their parents,* and thus precisely those life worlds which most approaches aim to address.

The fundamental experiences of migrants and their children include above all the difficulties in learning the German language and the Swiss dialect. All the families we interviewed and accompanied report on the diverse experiences of language acquisition, which also often have negative connotations, of course especially those families who permanently resettle in Switzerland. One Latin American mother, who has a Master's degree and worked for 8 years in the public sector in the social field, describes language learning as being within her self-attributed sphere of competence, so does not believe that it presents her with insurmountable difficulties; but at the same time, language acquisition is linked to the devaluation of previous professional expertise and the uncomfortable feeling of the coerciveness of the naturalisation measures. "That is, learning German and fulfilling all the requirements they demanded [referring to naturalisation] was not so difficult emotionally. But the idea that you have to do it persisted: 'Okay, I'm starting from scratch, I'm illiterate in this language.' And I'm going to be on the other side now." (Interview 009: 00:22:10–00:22:38).

The acquisition of the German language is described by all families as a necessity for integration into Swiss society. In the following, we document in more detail passages from an interview with a Latin American "love migrant" and her experiences, motivations and self-observations, in order to highlight differences in health-related socialisation between autochthonous Swiss families and families with a Latin American migration background, which can be derived from the self-evident availability of the national language (or one of the national languages) alone. From the interview, a direct analogy emerges between immigrant and educationally disadvantaged groups, whose sharply contrasting experiences – divided as they are between their socialisation in working class or peasant families and the demands placed on them by educational institutions – Bourdieu so forcefully described (Bourdieu 1992, 2001). For all immigrant families and families with an immigrant background, the question arises of how to deal with their own cultural heritage. In many assimilation theory considerations, both cultural affiliations are played off against each other, especially with regard to migrants with little schooling, ultimately in the way of a zero-sum game. The following interview excerpt must be read as a statement by a woman who is extremely willing to integrate and who is very involved in the area of social commitment.

> And I always try – to talk to Manu [older son, 3 years old at the time of the first interview] more than to Sandra [daughter, about one and a half years old at the time of the interview], because she is still very small, about Peru, about their family, the culture, so that he feels that Peru is always there for him. He knows Peru. He went to Peru when he was one year old; Sandra didn't: with Sandra we want to go [incomprehensible.] and Manu when he is five, six years old. But it's important because when someone talks to them about Peru; their mother is from Peru and they need to know the culture and what people are like in Peru, right? Mama [the interviewee's mother] talks to Manu a lot in Spanish. [...] And Sandra hasn't had any contact with Peru. But I also tell her [about Peru] and I also think she understands. Because it's important. For me it's important that they know my origin, the origin of oneself. There are people who say 'no, no, don't tell them about there, just tell them about here'. I don't. I think that my origin is also part of their origin. [...] So, it's important that they have that too.

> [...] That they know their culture (.) and Spanish! Especially Spanish! (Interview 007: 00:25:17–00:26:52).

This desire for intergenerational transmission of knowledge of one's own cultural origins as well as the social valorisation of one's own cultural identity as a Peruvian (Hall 1994b), however, encounters, in the early educational institution, an adaptive behaviour by which the complete social integration of the child is to be guaranteed and the difference to other parents and children, for example, minimised.

> Only when I'm in kindergarten, for example, I speak German with him. Because, so people don't think, 'What is she saying to him right now?' It's better, so he can socialise too: in kindergarten, German; in my house, Spanish; and in the park, something. He speaks Spanish very well. [...] I talked to the kindergarten teacher and she told me he never speaks Spanish, only German. And so, it's very good, the difference between German and Spanish. (Interview 007: 00:28:48–00:29:21).

Somewhat later in the interview, the mother explicitly points out that her children must know different cultural worlds and also themselves represent them. At this point, too, however, the will to integrate into the host society is emphasised at the same time:

> [...] the customs of the country you're in – in Latin America, for example [...], people drink in the street. They get together. Here [in Switzerland] you won't see that. And you're not supposed to. I don't plan to drink in the street with my friends because they don't do it here. So, I have to do what I see. And teach that to my kids, too. In Peru, he [Manuel, her son] will realize that it's his other [emphasises] culture. In Peru, you see them out on the street drinking and laughing. The kids play in the street, maybe half naked because it's hot. It's normal there. Here, they don't like to see it. But I respect that because it's a different [emphasises] culture. And there are a lot of people who don't understand that and want to practise the customs of their country here. And that, I think, is not adapting to the culture here. (Interview 007: 00:42:13–00:43:16).

The last quote from the interview deals with the socialising task, specifically mentioned by the mother, of imparting competences to her children to be able to reflect their knowledge of the two heterogeneous cultures in their repertoire of actions in a way that is appropriate to the situation. In other words, the mother considers it a very conscious part of her educational task to enable the children to appropriately balance the cultural reference spaces.

> I want to, [...] tell them that in Peru there is a different way of life. That their family from there could do things that could make them [their children] feel bad. So, they don't feel bad and he [the son Manuel] is also not shocked when my family does

> something. [...] And sometimes, when he does something or I do something with him, I tell him, 'You do it here, at home, in the closest family circle, but don't do it with other children'. Because it's different, isn't it. Like, kissing, hugging. It's not like that here. I don't want him to be shocked by that. So, I don't want my child to be numb either. [...] So, I want to teach him that it's good to have contact with people, but only with the closest ones; not with everybody, but with the ones that are closest to you. It's good because you have to see that families are different in Latin America. [...] And that's one of the things I want to inculcate in them, that they be loving, that they treat people respectfully, that they be tolerant, because it's a different [emphasises] world, it's a different mentality. (Interview 007: 00:49:20–00:51:49).

The motif that emerges here is momentous for the health socialisation of migrant children. They grow up with specific experiences of difference – emphasised more or less strongly by the parents and presented as more or less compatible – of being members of a social minority. With regard to the Peruvian mother's statement, there are at least some areas of the child's cultural reference spaces that fall outside the framework of the majority culture's ideas of what is normal and that can only be acted out in a protected family setting.

With regard to health literacy and the health literacy development of children and families, a healthy development of children thus becomes dependent on competencies that aim at a prudent handling of cultural differences and at first sight have little overlap with health literacy. On closer examination, however, devaluing the everyday practices of cultural minorities has great potential for harming identity and personality development or – in salutogenic terms – enormous potential for coping with a wide variety of everyday situations. For, navigating between different cultural contexts and frames of reference (without wanting to overstretch cultural differences here) is from the outset very close to the balance models favoured by Aaron Antonovsky, Klaus Hurrelmann, Peter-Ernst Schnabel and other health researchers.

Moreover, this connection adds another component to the concept of family health literacy. We have already argued several times for employing a broad understanding of health literacy and have made the competencies dependent on social determinants at an early stage. With regard to health inequalities, and based on these considerations, the key question arises to what extent a society is able, in Will Kymlicka's sense, to create multicultural institutions and spaces in which cultural differences at the everyday level and at the institutional level can be acted out not as deficits but as actual differences (Gerdes 1996; Kymlicka 2000, 2013, cop. 2007). Whether a society is permeated by cultural racism in everyday life and in its institutions and cultural differences are perceived as threatening to one's survival, or whether migrant people or migrant backgrounds and their cultural differences are considered a normal part of the contemporary society of a specific territory, must have significant implications for how problematic identity constructions of minorities are (Hall 1994b). In the case of family circumstances, (early) child health is thus directly affected by the extent to which parents or parental units can unproblematically invoke multicultural identity components in their parenting. Thus, a concept for strengthening family health literacy among migrants would, at least in our understanding shaped by health promotion and salutogenesis, be directly linked to questions of dealing with cultural differences in society as a whole.

8.6 Conclusion

This case study had two overarching objectives. On the one hand, the group of Latin American migrants, which had hardly been researched in Switzerland, was to be examined more closely and a contribution made to understanding this community. On the other hand, within the framework of health literacy research, an ethnographic study was to be carried out focusing on families with young children, in order to meet the frequently voiced demand to consider the living environments of vulnerable groups more closely. Parents with a Latin American migration background were interviewed and accompanied for this purpose.

In particular, it became clear that families with a Latin American migration background have a surprisingly differentiated and holistic understanding of health, which comes close to the salutogenic model and which, in our view, can be considered a particularly promising starting point for interventions – for example, in the context of strengthening family health literacy. Furthermore, it became clear that it doesn't make sense for a family health literacy concept appropriate to these families (and yet to be developed) to refer to notions of the family as a local two-generational context, because this perspective has little to do with the ideas and practices of migrating Latino families. Finally, it also became clear that questions about overall social integration and how to deal with cultural differences – and the people who represent them! – have a significant impact on health socialisation and health literacy development and must be considered an important factor in family health literacy.

We are aware that the sample we were allowed to ethnographically accompany has an academic bias and that no statements can be made here about the entire Swiss Latino community and its health (competence) perceptions and practices. Compared to the families we accompanied, for example, the "Sans Papiers" who immigrated from Latin America are considerably more vulnerable in many dimensions. Nevertheless, we believe we have identified some overarching patterns that can serve as further guidance for future studies. The particular vulnerability of the families we accompanied, it became clear, lies for the most part much less in the traditional area of available socio-economic resources for action, which were described by all families as clearly sufficient. It lies above all in processes of lacking acceptance and appreciation of cultural differences and considerably restricted access to the labour market. In this respect, the important result to be derived from the study, in our opinion, would be that health research and health literacy research urgently need to deal with the theory and practice of multicultural societies and integrate the insights thus gained into public health.

Part III

Outlook

9 What Do You See When You Look Differently? On the Insight Potential of Ethnographic Health Literacy Research

Abstract

The study presented here is first of all a project report of a study carried out within the framework of a larger BMBF network for research into the health literacy of children and adolescents (www.hlca-consortium.de) (cf. also Zamora et al., *Präv Gesundheitsf* 10(2), pp. 167–172, 2015). The basic idea of the ELMi and ELiS projects was to ethnographically research the health literacy of young people with a migration background, later in a sub-project with their own flight history and of migrant families with young children.

The study presented here is first of all a project report of a study carried out within the framework of a larger BMBF network for research into the health literacy of children and adolescents (www.hlca-consortium.de) (cf. also Zamora et al. 2015). The basic idea of the ELMi and ELiS projects was to ethnographically research the health literacy of young people with a migration background, later in a sub-project the HL of adolescents with their own flight history, and finally that of migrant families with young children. This basic idea itself was motivated by two points: *First, in* 2014, when we developed the projects (and partly even to this day), the state of research on health literacy of children and adolescents (in German-speaking countries and internationally) was (and still is) to be described as very poor and incomplete (Zamora et al. 2015; Okan et al. 2015; Bröder et al. 2017; Bröder and Carvalho 2019). This situation, which the numerous papers from the HLCA consortium have made a visible contribution to changing, has now changed significantly and the body of research has grown considerably – we have presented the

U. H. Bittlingmayer et al., *Health Literacy From A Health Ethnology Perspective*, https://doi.org/10.1007/978-3-658-42348-3_9

current state of research on health literacy in children and young people in detail in Chapter Three. *Second,* the existing models of health literacy were, and in our view still are, too much rooted in cognitivism and based on a problematic decision-theoretic model that constitutively links action with finding, understanding and applying information, thus ignoring both social situatedness (regardless of age, regardless of context) and the largely preconscious structure of everyday actions (Schütz 1971; Schütz and Luckmann 2003; Goffman 2008; Bourdieu 1982, 1979). In this study, with regard to research on health literacy, we wanted to address what Ullrich Bauer (2019a, p. 577) calls the "challenge of an extended concept of context", "which should rather focus on the entire range of social embedding".

To this end, we elaborated the basic cognitivist tendencies of health literacy definitions and models in the second chapter and then concentrated on highlighting the limitations and theoretical implications in the fourth chapter (pioneering work has been done here above all by Papen 2005, 2008, 2009). Finally, in the fourth chapter we outlined a "negative-dialectical model of health literacy", which takes up (but does not resolve) the tension between health literacy deficits, which can hardly be denied and are linked to social and health inequalities, on the one hand, and a difference perspective on the other.

We have thus formulated a theoretical claim that cannot be smoothly taken up and implemented empirically. In the fifth chapter, we then placed this theoretical claim somewhat deeper *within* the framework of methodological considerations and linked it to the *question of what exactly comes into view in the attempt to look differently,* i.e., ethnographically, at *the health competences* of refugee male adolescents from Afghanistan, of girls with a Turkish migration background and of families with a Latin American migration background and young children. We do not want to conjure up any new insights in the concluding review that are not already apparent in the case studies presented, nor do we want to simply repeat what has been unfolded in chapters six through eight. Rather, we want to include here three more motifs that seem to us particularly worthwhile following up on. First, we want to take another look at the relationship between "analogue" and digital health literacy among young people (Sect. 9.1). We will then revisit the concept of family health literacy (Sect. 9.2). Thereupon, the concluding thoughts will once again present a generalised perspective which, in our view, ties in with the theoretical considerations and the ethnographic case studies from the ELMi/ELiS projects (Sect. 9.3).

9.1 The Relationship Between Analogue and Digital Health Literacy Among Young People (with a Migration Background)

The health literacy concept began its triumphant march out of the confines of the care system in the slipstream of the major literacy studies in the 1990s (Nutbeam 2000; Okan 2019a, pp. 24–25). From here, the concept has continued to expand, shedding more and more of its care-related corset and extending the subject matter of health literacy to lifeworld and nasospatial domains (Nutbeam 2000, 2008; Kickbusch 2002; Sørensen et al. 2012a). At the same time – in addition to the enormous increase in health-policy decision makers' appreciation of the health literacy approach in the last 10 years (cf. for example WHO Europe 2013; The Scottish Government 2014; Saboga-Nunes et al. 2019; cf. also the contributions in the third part in Okan et al. 2019a) – two further developments took place – on the *one hand,* in the course of the review of health inequalities, target groups were identified that should be addressed with health literacy promotion programmes in order to reduce health inequalities. In the case of older people, a catch-up development strategy is pursued; in the case of children and adolescents, the focus is primarily on prevention. *On the other hand,* a *simultaneous* specialisation, differentiation and expansion of the health literacy concept took place, which despite some conceptual efforts (cf. e.g., Sørensen et al. 2012a) has not yet been theoretically caught up with.

The contradictory development of a *simultaneous expansion and specialisation of* health literacy refers, for example, to concepts developed later, such as food literacy, diabetes literacy or eHealth literacy, which are intended to transfer health literacy to more specific fields of application and represent specialisation and differentiation. In the case of eHealth Literacy, however, this is at the same time an extension, because eHealth Literacy, according to the standard model by Norman and Skinner still in use today (but also according to more recent models), is itself based on Health Literacy and in this respect represents an extension (Norman and Skinner 2006; Soellner et al. 2014). In general, the relationship between "analogue health literacies" and digital health literacies was defined in such a way that "analogue health literacies" potentially limited the option space of digital health literacies. "The full potential of e-health to improve users' health, however, may be limited by users' health literacy" (Mackert et al. 2014, p. 517).

On the basis of our two ethnographic case studies, we believe that the previous definitions of the relationship between health literacy and eHealth literacy in young people need to be revised. This is because the traditional notion of adolescents using their smartphones separates this unit of action from the rest of their everyday activities on the grounds that, after all, action takes place in the digital world. In fact, smartphone use in the everyday lives of adolescents (and not only adolescents) is not structured in a way that makes it a conscious and intentional decision to leave the analogue world and enter the digital world in its place. If, therefore, health literacy is not to be limited exclusively to the area of health care, and lifeworld dimensions are to become part of health literacy, then this is quite consequential. For in the context of everyday life activities, also in contrast to the educational-institutional field of action such as school, the two dimensions (analogue/digital) are inseparably intertwined. A separation into health literacy and digital health literacy can therefore perhaps still work as an analytical separation. But the theoretical adherence to two different areas of competence within adolescent lifeworlds seems arbitrary and no longer convincing. This is probably the kernel of truth contained in the otherwise somewhat problematic generationalised description of (children and) adolescents as *digital natives*.

The feedback from the digitalised living environment is particularly important for the behaviour and emotional states of the young people. We know from the field studies that, for example, messages from the WhatsApp group of the mosque community had immediate consequences for the behaviour of the two girls of Turkish origin. In the case of the Afghan boys who had fled, communication with family members who had remained in other countries was particularly emotionally stressful because, in the context of the poor security situation, conversations with uncles, aunts, cousins repeatedly mentioned the oppression of those who had not (yet) fled, leaving those who had (successfully) fled with a mixture of worry and a guilty conscience. This feedback obviously have health-promoting or harmful consequences, but they can no longer be meaningfully linked to a description of health competence that is differentiated into analogue and digital. It remains to be seen to what extent this interconnection observed in members of ethnic minorities is also found in other social groups – from our point of view, however, it can be assumed that the young people we observed do not differ greatly from their peers *in this respect.*

9.2 Family Health Literacy (Narrow and Broad)

A second motif, which we will explore in more depth in this final section, relates to the concept of family health literacy, which plays an exceedingly marginal role in the very large number of publications on health literacy in recent years. This is somewhat surprising, above all, because the health sciences generally agree that the family is the most important institution in the context of health socialisation, and that patterns of preference, lifestyle elements and behaviours acquired at an early age can only be corrected with great difficulty in the course of later life (cf. the instructive study by Bauer 2012b; cf. for the health literacy context, e.g. Okan 2019b). Paradigmatically, already in the early 2000s Peter-Ernst Schnabel stated in a book on the connection between health and the family "that no more important and suitable instance of intervention exists than the family for achieving a maximum of health-securing effects with much less effort than that which must later be expended in school or at work." (Schnabel 2001a, p. 13) But Schnabel was and remains one of the very few sociologically oriented public health researchers who systematically dealt with the family as a health resource.[1]

Overall, it can be stated that *the family and family health have largely faded from the focus of public health while at the same time their fundamental importance have been widely acknowledged.* This is not only a phenomenon of health literacy research in the narrower sense; even in the relevant overarching health science studies, the description of family contexts of action remains strangely superficial and unsubstantial (for example, in Dippelhofer-Stiehm 2008; Hurrelmann and Richter 2013, pp. 182–185). From a public health perspective, the family comes into view primarily as a transmission belt of health inequalities, as a socialisation instance in which more or less resources for action are available for the health development of the next generation (Hurrelmann and Richter 2013).

At this interface between socialisation and inequalities, the family is well and specifically connectable in the context of health literacy research, since it can be critically noted with reference to it that, especially in childhood, health literacy can only with difficulty be understood as an individual endowment. In this context, we already pointed out in the third chapter that the concept of health literacy in children and adolescents remains dependent on the overall family situation (Bauer 2019a argues similarly). Furthermore, we pointed out there that while families are dealt with as a particularly important resource for the development of children's health

[1]Even in the impressive International Handbook of Health Literacy Research, there is no contribution that deals decidedly with the family or family health literacy; cf. Okan et al. 2019a. Nor is there any reference to the family in an overarching perspective in the otherwise very strong book by Thomas Hehlmann, Henning Schmidt-Semisch and Friedrich Schorb on the sociology of health; cf. Hehlmann et al. 2018. Finally, even in relevant anthologies on the sociology of youth, there is often not a single contribution that determines the relationship between adolescents and their families; cf. e.g. Mansel and Klocke 1996; or Riegel et al. 2010 – to pick out just a few quite arbitrary examples.

literacy, the promotion of family health literacy is subject to institutional diversion. Instead of strengthening families themselves and directly, strategies to strengthen family health literacy focus on educational institutional settings such as dayc-are centres and schools, hoping to reach families via indirect effects (Okan et al. 2017b; Simovska et al. 2012; Paakkari 2015; Paakkari and George 2018; Maier and Felder-Puig 2017). We would also, towards the end of our study, again explicitly *argue for a direct conception of Family Health Literacy* that, at the theoretical level, takes appropriate note of the insights of socialisation research, family sociology, childhood and health liter*acy* research, and, at the conceptual level, catches up with the life-world reference and the dialectic of deficit and difference. *This would be a narrow understanding of Family Health Literacy,* which from our point of view would have to be elaborated reasonably urgently and for the necessity of which the case study of Swiss families with young children and Latin American migration background provides sufficient arguments from our point of view.

At the same time, we consider such a Family Health Literacy concept for families with young children as a reference group to be insufficient, but in need of specific expansion. Based on our two case studies with adolescents, the importance of family in general and particularly for health during adolescence became very clear. Without wanting to overgeneralize here, it seems to us that the motif of detachment from family during adolescence is the central focus in the relevant sociological studies of adolescence. In one of the early standard works on this subject, Bernhard Schäfers (1998, p. 123), for example, states that the "processes of distancing and detachment of the adolescent from the family of origin, which, according to their duration and significance, are an essential criterion for adolescence as a life phase in general". The notion of youth as a definable phase of life and a sociological subject area with its own problems on the one hand, and the late revenge of an individualisation thesis eagerly taken up in youth research, which proclaimed the declining importance of family and milieu of origin on the other, are two possible explanations for the surprising absence of the family as an analytical framework in the sociology of youth.

The increasing importance of the peer group in the course of socialisation remains quite unaffected by this, as long as it is not linked to the paradigm of familial detachment, which is problematic in our view. After all, in our two ethnographic studies on adolescent health literacy, peers also play a very visible health socialisation role. However, family socialisation influences are not substituted, but simply complemented. As trivial as this may sound on the one hand, the doubling of socialisation effects (as opposed to replacement or substitution) is very consequential when it comes to adolescent health promotion or health literacy promotion. For it follows from these considerations that it is not particularly useful to identify adolescents as an isolated target group for any intervention or promotion programme. Instead, the ongoing intergenerationality must be taken into account, even while conceding the enormous increase in the importance of peers. For this reason, we argue for a comprehensive – and certainly yet to be properly developed – concept of family health literacy that is not limited to families with young children, but also addresses families with adolescents as well – and addresses them directly.

The final section will address some existing research gaps and further implications for interventions meant to increase the health literacy of families, children and adolescents.

9.3 Concluding Remarks

From the theoretical considerations and from the case studies presented, it follows that the first perspective to be pursued further is that of an intergenerationally based health competence research which closely follows the paradigm of socialisation research. In this context, the salutogenic question must be at the centre of how exactly generalised resistance resources develop, how the sense of coherence works in practice, how socialisation conditions for success or family compensation possibilities can be identified.

Along the lines of the critique of the lonely and well-informed health decision-maker (Bittlingmayer and Bauer 2007b), ethnographic studies should be expanded that take the social embedding of health literacy and health action (Bauer 2019a) seriously in an appropriate manner. A reference study for such an endeavor would be the work of Annette Lareau (2003), who followed families in their everyday lives and elaborated the differently situated socialization-relevant mechanisms of action in the reproduction of social inequality. For the health sciences, it would make sense to cooperate much more closely with social work, also in research and development projects, since a tradition of ethnographic family research has been established here for some time, the subject area of both sister disciplines overlaps strongly, and social work has an urgent need for clarification of a health science perspective. Another interesting ethnographic reference study was provided by Alice Goffman (2014) who, in order to gain a proper understanding of disadvantage, moved to a deprived and stigmatized African-American dominated neighborhood in order to gain from there better insights into the working mechanisms of racism, social domination, and oppression. This approach might also be appropriate in exploring more precisely the health options (present or absent) of stigmatized neighborhoods. Such ethnographic studies, in the urban sociological tradition of the Chicago

School, could be expanded in German public health. In perspective, however, it would also seem appropriate for the health sciences to reflect on their multidisciplinary heritage in order to cooperate more closely with other disciplines such as social and human geography, architecture and urban planning, or, as already mentioned, social work. As an overarching goal, a kind of Interdisciplinary Materialism of Health Research could be established, in which theoretical reflection, empirical research and applied practical intervention development would be integral parts of the common project of developing a healthy society.

Part of the perspective on a healthy society would certainly be the large-scale equipment of the population with health literacy. However, the normative approach would turn most of the previous health literacy concepts upside down. At the moment – especially among families, children and adolescents – health literacy works in a sense inversely. Inverse production of health means that it is not the food industry that switches production to healthy food, but individual health literacy is needed in order not to risk illness; or that it is not the working conditions that are organized in as stress-free (and family-friendly) a way as possible, but the population, suffering from work compression (while structural unemployment remains high), books additional yoga courses in order to maintain employability. In current models, high health literacy is inscribed with an equally high degree of asceticism. To exaggerate but slightly, someone proves to be particularly competent in health *if he or she does not exhaust the incomprehensible range of goods and services available in industrialised countries.*

Because it has not been possible in the last 30 years to implement the great motto of the WHO Ottawa Charter, "making the healthier choice the easier choice!", responsibility for individual health has been shifted to the individuals. This criticism has been voiced many times (cf. among others Schmidt 2008, 2017; Brunnett 2009; Kühn 1993; or from a socio-epidemiological direction Pickett and Wilkinson 2015; Wilkinson 2005; Wilkinson and Pickett 2010) and is anything but spectacular. However, a health literacy concept could be spelled out from here, at least theoretically, in which health literacy is aligned with a critique of society and domination structures. The path to a changed social (and industrial) practice is of course easier with a broader theoretical concept: "It requires [...] many innovations of family, educational, labour market, housing, social and tax policy scope, introduced in a roundabout way via alternative projects with imitation value, in order to make actual health a reality in the form of living and working contexts designed to be conducive to health" (Schnabel 2001a, p. 11–12). However, in view of current national and international conditions, we believe that it is still worthwhile to remember the objectives of the Ottawa Charter and to make efforts to implement them, however limited they may seem.

Appendices

U. H. Bittlingmayer et al., *Health Literacy From A Health Ethnology Perspective*, https://doi.org/10.1007/978-3-658-42348-3

References

Abel, Thomas (2008): Measuring health literacy: moving towards a health – promotion perspective. In: *International journal of public health* 53 (4), S. 169–170. DOI: https://doi.org/10.1007/s00038-008-0242-9.

Abel, Thomas; Abraham, Andrea; Sommerhalder, Kathrin (2009): Kulturelles Kapital, kollektive Lebensstile und die soziale Reproduktion gesundheitlicher Ungleichheit. In: Matthias Richter und Klaus Hurrelmann (Hg.): Gesundheitliche Ungleichheit: Grundlagen, Probleme, Perspektiven. Wiesbaden: VS Verlag für Sozialwissenschaften, S. 195–208.

Abraído-Lanza, Ana F.; Echeverría, Sandra E.; Flórez, Karen R. (2016): Latino immigrants, acculturation, and health: Promising new directions in research. In: *Annual review of public health* 37, S. 219–236. DOI: https://doi.org/10.1146/annurev-publhealth-032315-021545.

Abrams, Mary Ann; Klass, Perri; Dreyer, Benard P. (2009): Health literacy and children: introduction. In: *Pediatrics* 124 Suppl 3, S262–4. DOI: https://doi.org/10.1542/peds.2009-1162A.

Acevedo-Garcia, Dolores; Sanchez-Vaznaugh, Emma V.; Viruell-Fuentes, Edna A.; Almeida, Joanna (2012): Integrating social epidemiology into immigrant health research: A cross-national framework. In: *Social Science & Medicine* 75, S. 2060–2068. DOI: https://doi.org/10.1016/j.socscimed.2012.04.040.

Achermann, Christin; Chimienti, Milena; Stants, Fabienne (2006): Migration, Prekarität und Gesundheit. Ressourcen und Risiken von vorläufig Aufgenommenen und Sans-Papiers in Genf und Zürich. Neuchâtel: Swiss Forum for Migration and Population Studies (SFM) (Etudes du SFM, 41).

Ackermann Rau, Sabine; Sakarya, Sibel; Abel, Thomas (2014): When to see a doctor for common health problems: distribution patterns of functional health literacy across migrant populations in Switzerland. In: *International journal of public health* 59 (6), S. 967–974. DOI: https://doi.org/10.1007/s00038-014-0583-5.

Adorno, Theodor W. (1966): Negative Dialektik. Frankfurt am Main: Suhrkamp.

Adorno, Theodor W. (1973): Studien zum autoritären Charakter. Frankfurt a.M.: Suhrkamp.

U. H. Bittlingmayer et al., *Health Literacy From A Health Ethnology Perspective*, https://doi.org/10.1007/978-3-658-42348-3

Aktion Deutschland hilft (2019): Flucht nach Europa. Retrieved from (https://www.aktion-deutschland-hilft.de/de/mediathek/infografiken/infografik-fluchtrouten-nach-europa/, last checked on 26.06.2019).

Alanen, Lena (1988): Rethinking Childhood. In: *Acta Sociologica* 31 (1), S. 53–67.

Alemi, Qais; James, Sigrid; Cruz, Romalene; Zepeda, Veronica; Racadio, Michael (2014): Psychological Distress in Afghan Refugees: A Mixed-Method Systematic Review. In: *J Immigrant Minority Health* 16 (6), S. 1247–1261. DOI: https://doi.org/10.1007/s10903-013-9861-1.

Alternative für Deutschland (2018): Islamkonferenz 2018: Der Islam gehört nicht zu Deutschland! AfD- Fraktion im Bundestag. Retrieved from https://www.afdbundestag.de/islamkonferenz-2018-der-islam-gehoert-nicht-zu-deutschland-afd-fraktion-im-bundestag/.

Altgeld, Thomas (2004a): Expertise. Gesundheitsfördernde Settingansätze in benachteiligten städtischen Quartieren. Retrieved from https://www.gesundheit-nds.de/downloads/altgeld.settingexpertise.pdf.

Altgeld, Thomas (2004b): Expertise: Gesundheitsfördernde Settingansätze in benachteiligten städtischen Quartieren. Landesvereinigung für Gesundheit Niedersachsen e.V. Hannover.

Altgeld, Thomas (2008): Gesundheitsfördernde Settingarbeit als Schlüsselstrategie zur Reduktion von gesundheitlichen Ungleichheiten. In: Ullrich Bauer, Uwe H. Bittlingmayer und Matthias Richter (Hg.): Health Inequalities. Determinanten und Mechanismen gesundheitlicher Ungleichheit. Wiesbaden: VS Verlag für Sozialwissenschaften, S. 511–529.

Andreani, Tanja; Berrut, Sylvie; Gazareth, Pascale; Hauri, Dimitri; Kaeser, Martine; Lieberherr, Renaud et al. (2014): Gesundheitsstatistik 2014. Bundesamt für Statistik. Neuchâtel.

Andresen, Sabine; Möller, Renate (2019): Children's Worlds+. Eine Studie zu den Bedarfen von Kindern und Jugendlichen in Deutschland. Gütersloh.

Antonovsky, A. (1987): Unraveling the mystery of health. How people manage stress and stay well. 1. ed. San Francisco: Jossey-Bass (The Jossey-Bass health series).

Antonovsky, Aaron (1985): Health, stress, and coping. San Francisco/London: Jossey-Bass.

Antonovsky, Aaron (1997): Salutogenese. Zur Entmystifizierung der Gesundheit. Hg. v. Alexa Franke. Tübingen: dgvt Verlag (Forum für Verhaltenstherapie und psychosoziale Praxis, Band 36). Retrieved from https://d-nb.info/952269910/04.

Appleton, Sarah; Biermann, Sam; Hamilton-Bruce, Anne; Piantadosi, Cynthia; Tucker, Graeme; Koblar, Simon; Adams, Robert (2015): Functional health literacy is significantly associated with risk factors for stroke in a population sample. In: *International journal of stroke: official journal of the International Stroke Society* 10 (3), E23. DOI: https://doi.org/10.1111/ijs.12425.

Australian Bureau of Statistics (2006): Health Literacy, Australia. Retrieved from https://www.ausstats.abs.gov.au/Ausstats/subscriber.nsf/0/73ED158C6B14BB5ECA2574720011AB83/$File/42330_2006.pdf, last checked on 05.04.2018.

Babitsch, Birgit (2009): Die Kategorie Geschlecht: Theoretische und empirische Implikationen für den Zusammenhang zwischen sozialer Ungleichheit und Gesundheit. In: Klaus Hurrelmann und Matthias Richter (Hg.): Gesundheitliche Ungleichheit. Grundlagen, Probleme, Perspektiven. 2., aktualisierte Aufl. Wiesbaden: VS Verlag für Sozialwissenschaften/GWV Fachverlage GmbH Wiesbaden, S. 283–299.

Babitsch, Birgit; Götz, Nina-Alexandra; Zeitler, Julia (2017): Gender und Gesundheit. In: Monika Jungbauer-Gans und Peter Kriwy (Hg.): Handbuch Gesundheitssoziologie, Bd. 19. Wiesbaden: Springer, S. 1–19.

Baker, D. W.; Parker, R. M.; Williams, M. V.; Clark, W. S.; Nurss, J. (1997): The relationship of patient reading ability to self-reported health and use of health services. In: *Am J Public Health* 87 (6), S. 1027–1030.

Baker, David W. (2006): The meaning and the measure of health literacy. In: *J GEN INTERN MED* 21 (8), S. 878–883. DOI: https://doi.org/10.1111/j.1525-1497.2006.00540.x.

Baker, David W.; Gazmararian, Julie A.; Williams, Mark V.; Scott, Tracy; Parker, Ruth M.; Green, Diane et al. (2002): Functional health literacy and the risk of hospital admission among Medicare managed care enrollees. In: *Am J Public Health* 92 (8), S. 1278–1283. DOI: https://doi.org/10.2105/AJPH.92.8.1278.

Baker, David W.; Williams, Mark V.; Parker, Ruth M.; Gazmararian, Julie A.; Nurss, Joanne (1999): Development of a brief test to measure functional health literacy. In: *Patient Education and Counseling* 38 (1), S. 33–42. DOI: https://doi.org/10.1016/S0738-3991(98)00116-5.

Baker, David W.; Wolf, Michael S.; Feinglass, Joseph; Thompson, Jason A. (2008): Health literacy, cognitive abilities, and mortality among elderly persons. In: *Journal of General Internal Medicine* 23 (6), S. 723–726. DOI: https://doi.org/10.1007/s11606-008-0566-4.

Bauch, Jost (2010): Gesundheit als sekundäre Zweckmäßigkeit von familialen Alltagsroutinen. In: Heike Ohlbrecht und Christine Schönberger (Hg.): Gesundheit als Familienaufgabe. Zum Verhältnis von Autonomie und staatlicher Intervention. Weinheim/München: Juventa, S. 176–190.

Bauer, Ullrich (2005): Das Präventionsdilemma. Potenziale schulischer Kompetenzfördeurng im Spiegel sozialer Polarisierung. Wiesbaden: VS Verlag für Sozialwissenschaften.

Bauer, Ullrich (2012a): Das sozialisationstheoretische Paradigma. In: Ullrich Bauer, Uwe H. Bittlingmayer und Albert Scherr (Hg.): Handbuch Bildungs- und Erziehungssoziologie. Wiesbaden: VS Verlag für Sozialwissenschaften, S. 473–490.

Bauer, Ullrich (2012b): Sozialisation und Ungleichheit. Eine Hinführung. Wiesbaden: Springer VS.

Bauer, Ullrich (2019a): The social embeddedness of health literacy. In: Orkan Okan, Ullrich Bauer, Diane Levin-Zamir, Paulo Pinheiro und Kristine Sørensen (Hg.): International Handbook of Health Literacy. Research, practice and policy across the lifespan. Bristol: POLICY Press, S. 573–586.

Bauer, Ullrich (2019b): The social embeddedness of health literacy. In: Orkan Okan, Ullrich Bauer, Diane Levin-Zamir, Paulo Pinheiro und Kristine Sørensen (Hg.): International Handbook of Health Literacy. Research, practice and policy across the lifespan. Bristol: POLICY Press, S. 573–586.

Bauer, Ullrich; Bittlingmayer, Uwe H. (2005): Wer profitiert von Elternbildung? In: *ZSE: Zeitschrift für Soziologie der Erziehung und Sozialisation* 25, S. 263–280.

Bauer, Ullrich; Bittlingmayer, Uwe H.; Richter, Matthias (Hg.) (2008): Health Inequalities. Determinanten und Mechanismen gesundheitlicher Ungleichheit. 1. Aufl. Wiesbaden: VS Verl. für Sozialwiss (Gesundheit und Gesellschaft). Retrieved from https://www.socialnet.de/rezensionen/isbn.php?isbn=978-3-531-15612-5.

Bauer, Ullrich; Büscher, Andreas (Hg.) (2008): Soziale Ungleichheit und Pflege. Beiträge sozialwissenschaftlich orientierter Pflegeforschung. Wiesbaden: Springer VS.

Bauer, Ullrich; Vester, Michael (2015): Soziale Milieus als Sozialisationstheorie. In: Klaus Hurrelmann (Hg.): Handbuch Sozialisationsforschung. 8., vollständig überarbeitete Auflage. Weinheim: Beltz (Pädagogik), S. 557–586.

Bautista, John Robert (2015): From Solving a Health Problem to Achieving Quality of Life: Redifining eHealth Literacy. In: *Journal of Literacy and Technology* 16 (2), S. 33–54.

Bayaz, Ahmet (2002): Das Türkeibild der Deutschen und das Deutschlandbild der Türken. In: Hans-Georg Wehling (Hg.): Türkei. Politik – Gesellschaft – Wirtschaft. Wiesbaden: VS Verlag für Sozialwissenschaften (Reihe, 4), S. 197–207.

Beck, Ulrich (1986): Die Risikogesellschaft. Aufbruch in eine andere Moderne. Frankfurt am Main: Suhrkamp.

Becker, Howard S. (1958): Problems of inference and proof in participant observation. In: *American Sociological Review* 23, S. 652–660.

Becker, Peter (2006): Gesundheit durch Bedürfnisbefriedigung. Göttingen: Hogrefe.

Becker, Rolf; Beck, Michael (2012): Herkunftseffekte oder Diskriminierung von Migrantenkindern in der Primarstufe? In: Rolf Becker und Heike Solga (Hg.): Soziologische Bildungsforschung. Sonderheft der Kölner Zeitschrift für Soziologie und Sozialpsychologie Nr. 52. Wiesbaden: VS Verlag für Sozialwissenschaften, S. 137–163.

Bellah, Robert N.; Madsen, Richard; Sullivan, William M.; Stridler, Ann; Tipton, Steven M. (1985): Habits of the Heart. Individualism and Commitment in American Life. New York: Perennial.

Bellaigue, Christopher de (2018): Die islamische Aufklärung. Der Konflikt zwischen Glaube und Vernunft. Frankfurt a.M.: S. Fischer.

Bennett, Ian M.; Chen, Jing; Soroui, Jaleh S.; White, Sheida (2009): The contribution of health literacy to disparities in self-rated health status and preventive health behaviors in older adults. In: *Annals of Family Medicine* 7 (3), S. 204–211. DOI: https://doi.org/10.1370/afm.940.

Berens, Eva-Maria; Vogt, Dominique; Messer, Melanie; Hurrelmann, Klaus; Schaeffer, Doris (2016): Health Literacy among different age groups in Germany: results of a cross-sexctional survey. In: *BMC public health* 16, S. 1151. Retrieved from DOI https://doi.org/10.1186/s12889-016-3810-6.

Berkman, N. D.; DeWalt, D. A.; Pignone, M. P.; Sheridan, S. L.; Lohr, K. N.; Lux, L. et al. (2004): Literacy and Health Outcomes: Evidence Report/Technology Assessment, No. 87. In: *AHRQ Publication* (04-E007-2), last checked on 26.03.2018.

Berkman, Nancy D.; Davis, Terry C.; McCormack, Lauren (2010): Health literacy: what is it? In: *Journal of health communication* 15 Suppl 2, S. 9–19. DOI: https://doi.org/10.1080/10810730.2010.499985.

Bermejo, Isaac; Mayninger, Elena; Kriston, Levente; Härter, Martin (2010): Psychische Störungen bei Menschen mit Migrationshintergrund im Vergleich zur deutschen Allgemeinbevölkerung. In: *Psychiatrische Praxis* 37 (5), S. 225–232. DOI: https://doi.org/10.1055/s-0029-1223513.

Bernhardt, Jay M., Brownfield, Erica D. & Parker, Ruth M. (2005): Understanding health literacy. In: Schwartzberg, Joanne C., VanGeest, Jonathan B. & Wang, Claire C. (eds.): Understanding health literacy : implications for medicine and public health. Chicago, Ill.: American Medical Association.

Berry, John W. (1992): Acculturation and adaptation in a new society. In: *International Migration* 30, S. 69–85. DOI: https://doi.org/10.1111/j.1468-2435.1992.tb00776.x.

Berry, John W.; Kim, Uichol; Minde, Thomas; Mok, Doris (1987): Comparative studies of acculturative stress. In: *The International Migration Review* 21, S. 491–511. DOI: https://doi.org/10.2307/2546607.

Beushausen, Jürgen (2012): Genogramm- und Netzwerkanalyse. Die Visualisierung familiärer und sozialer Strukturen ; mit 2 Tabellen. Göttingen, Bristol, CT, U.S.A.: Vandenhoeck & Ruprecht.

Biakowski, André; Halotta, Martin; Schöne, Thilo (Hg.) (2016): Zwischen Kommen und Bleiben. Ein Gesellschaftlicher Querschnitt zur Flüchtlingspolitik. Berlin: Friedrich Ebert Stiftung.

Bilgin, Y.; Doppl, W.; Bretzel, R. (1988): Besonderheiten bei der internistischen Betreuung türkischer Patienten mit koronarer Herzerkrankungen in einer medizinischen Poliklinik (12), S. 354–356.

Bischoff, Alexander; Wanner, Philippe (2008): The self-reported health of immigrant groups in Switzerland. In: *Journal of immigrant and minority health* 10 (4), S. 325–335. DOI: https://doi.org/10.1007/s10903-007-9089-z.

Bittlingmayer, Uwe H. (2016): Strukturorientierte Perspektiven auf Gesundheit und Krankheit. In: Matthias Richter und Klaus Hurrelmann (Hg.): Soziologie von Gesundheit und Krankheit. 1. Auflage. Wiesbaden: Springer VS (Lehrbuch), S. 23–40.

Bittlingmayer, Uwe H.; Bauer, Ullrich (2007a): Aspirationen ohne Konsequenzen. In: *Zeitschrift für Soziologie der Erziehung und Sozialisation* 27 (2), S. 160–180.

Bittlingmayer, Uwe H.; Bauer, Ullrich (2007b): Individualisierte Prävention: Zur Ideologie des a-sozialen Gesundheitsentscheiders. In: Bettina Schmidt und Petra Kolip (Hg.): Gesundheitsförderung im aktivierenden Sozialstaat. Präventionskonzepte zwischen Public Health, Eigenverantwortung und Sozialer Arbeit. Weinheim: Juventa, S. 105–116.

Bittlingmayer, Uwe H.; Bauer, Ullrich; Richter, Matthias; Sahrai, Diana (2009): Die Überund Unterschätzung von Raum in Public Health. Brennpunkt Prekarität, Segregation und Armut im Sozialraum. In: *Deutsche Zeitschrift für Kommunalwissenschaft* 48 (2), S. 21–34.

Bittlingmayer, Uwe H.; Sahrai, Diana (2010): Gesundheitliche Ungeichheit: Plädoyer für eine ergänzende ethnologische Perspektive. Beilage der Zeitschrift Das Parlament. In: *Aus Politik und Zeitgeschichte* (45/2010), S. 25–31.

Bittlingmayer, Uwe H.; Sahrai, Diana (2019): Health literacy for all? Inclusion as a serious challenge for health. The case of disablity. In: Orkan Okan, Ullrich Bauer, Diane Levin-Zamir, Paulo Pinheiro und Kristine Sørensen (Hg.): International Handbook of Health Literacy. Research, practice and policy across the lifespan. Bristol: POLICY Press, S. 689–703.

Bittlingmayer, Uwe H.; Sahrai, Diana; Schnabel, Peter-Ernst (Hg.) (2008): Normativität und Public Health. Vergessene Dimensionen gesundheitlicher Ungleichheit. Wiesbaden: VS Verlag für Sozialwissenschaften.

Bittlingmayer, Uwe H.; Sirch, Ulrike (2006): „Erwachsen werden“ an deutschen Schulen. Eine Implementierungsstudie in den ausgewählten Bundesländern Hamburg, Rheinland-Pfalz und Baden-Württemberg. Bielefeld: Fakultät für Gesundheitswissenschaften.

Bittlingmayer, Uwe H.; Ziegler, Holger (2012): Public Health und das gute Leben. Der Capabilities-Approach als normatives Fundament interventionsbezogener Gesundheitswissenschaften? Berlin (WZB Discussionpaper, SP I 2012–301). Retrieved from https://www.ssoar.info/ssoar/handle/document/46223, last checked on 01.04.2019.

Black, Douglas; Whitehead, Margaret (1992): Inequalities in health. The Black report [and] The health divide. Reprinted. London: Penguin Books (Penguin books).

Blaxter, Mildred (1983): Peter Townsend and Nick Davidson, *Inequalities in Health: the Black Report*, Penguin, London, 1982. 240 pp. £2.50. In: *Journal of Social Policy* 12 (2), S. 284–285. https://doi.org/10.1017/S0047279400012812.

Böker, W. (1977): Zur psychischen Morbidität ausländischer Arbeitnehmer (Gastarbeiter) in der BRD. Bisherige Befunde und Hypothesen. In: *Öffentliches Gesundheitswesen* (39), 720–232.

Bollweg, Torsten M.; Orkan, Okan; Fretian, Alexandra Maria; Bröder, Janine; Domanska, Olga; Jordan, Susanne et al. (2020a, in press): Adapting the European Health Literacy Survey Questionnaire for 4th-grade Students in Germany. Validation and Psychometric Analysis. In: *Health Literacy Research and Practice* 3.

Bollweg, Torsten M.; Orkan, Okan; Pinheiro, Paulo; Bröder, Janine; Bruland, Dirk; Fretian, Alexandra Maria et al. (2020b, in press): Adapting the European Health Literacy Survey Questionnaire for 4th-grade Students in Germany. Questionnaire Development and Qualitative Pretest. In: *Health Literacy Research and Practice* 3.

Boltanski, Luc (1976): Die soziale Verwendung des Körpers. In: Dietmar Kamper und Volker Rittner (Hg.): Zur Geschichte des Körpers. Wien: Hanser, S. 138–177.

Bolzman, Claudio; Carbajal, Myrian; Mainardi, Giuditta (2007): La Suisse au rythme latino. Dynamiques migratoires des Latino-Américains: logiques d'action, vie quotidienne, pistes d'interventions dans les domaines du social et de la santé. Genève: ies éditions.

Bond, Emma; Rawlings, Vanessa (2019): Children as active participants in health literacy research and practice? From rhetoric to rights. In: Orkan Okan, Ullrich Bauer, Diane Levin-Zamir, Paulo Pinheiro und Kristine Sørensen (Hg.): International Handbook of Health Literacy. Research, practice and policy across the lifespan. Bristol: POLICY Press, S. 587–600.

Boos-Nünning, Ursula; Siefen, Rainer Georg (2005): Jugendliche mit Migrationshintergrund und Sucht. In: Hans-Jörg Assion (Hg.): Migration und seelische Gesundheit: Springer Berlin Heidelberg, S. 195–213.

Borde, Theda; Blümel, Stephan (2015): Gesundheitsförderung und Migrationshintergrund. Bundeszentrale für gesundheitliche Aufklärung. Retrieved from https://www.leitbegriffe.bzga.de/bot_angebote_idx-156.htm.

Borzekowski, D. L.G. (2009): Considering Children and Health Literacy: A Theoretical Approach. In: *Pediatrics* 124 (Supplement), S282-S288. DOI: https://doi.org/10.1542/peds.2009-1162D.

Bostock, Sophie; Steptoe, Andrew (2012): Association between low functional health literacy and mortality in older adults: longitudinal cohort study. In: *BMJ (Clinical research ed.)* 344, e1602. https://doi.org/10.1136/bmj.e1602.

Bourdieu, Pierre (1979): Entwurf einer Theorie der Praxis auf der ethnologischen Grundlage der kabylischen Gesellschaft. 1. Aufl. Frankfurt am Main: Suhrkamp (Suhrkamp-Taschenbuch Wissenschaft, 291).

Bourdieu, Pierre (1982): Die feinen Unterschiede. Kritik der gesellschaftlichen Urteilskraft. 1. Auflage. Frankfurt am Main: Suhrkamp Verlag.

Bourdieu, Pierre (1985): Sozialer Raum und Klassen. Leçon sur la leçon. Zwei Vorlesungen. Frankfurt am Main: Suhrkamp.

Bourdieu, Pierre (1987): Sozialer sinn. Kritik der theoretischen vernunft. Frankfurt am Main: Suhrkamp (suhrkamp taschenbuch wissenschaft, 1066).

Bourdieu, Pierre (Hg.) (1992): Die verborgenen Mechanismen der Macht. Schriften zu Politik & Kultur 1. Hamburg: VSA.

Bourdieu, Pierre (2001): Wie die Kultur zum Bauern kommt. Über Bildung, Schule und Politik. Hamburg: VSA-Verl. (Schriften zu Politik & Kultur, 4).

Bourdieu, Pierre (2005): Die männliche Herrschaft. 1. Aufl. Frankfurt am Main: Suhrkamp.

Bourdieu, Pierre; Passeron, Jean-Claude (1973): Grundlagen einer Theorie der symbolischen Gewalt. Frankfurt am Main: Suhrkamp.

Brady, Geraldine; Lowe, Pam; Olin Lauritzen, Sonja (2015): Connecting a sociology of childhood perspective with the study of child health, illness and wellbeing: introduction. In: *Sociology of Health & Illness* 37 (2), S. 173–183. DOI: https://doi.org/10.1111/1467-9566.12260.

Breidenstein, Georg; Hirschauer, Stefan; Kalthoff, Herbert; Nieswand, Boris (2015): Ethnografie. Die Praxis der Feldforschung. 2. überarbeitete Auflage. Konstanz, München: UVK Verlagsgesellschaft mbH; UVK/Lucius (UTB Sozialwissenschaften, Kulturwissenschaften, 3979). Retrieved from https://www.utb-studi-e-book.de/9783838544977.

Brettschneider, Anna-Kristin; Hölling, H.; Schlack, R.; Ellert, U. (2015): Psychische Gesundheit von Jugendlichen in Deutschland. Ein Vergleich nach Migrationshintergrund und Herkunftsland. In: *Bundesgesundheitsblatt, Gesundheitsforschung, Gesundheitsschutz* 58 (4–5), S. 474–489. https://doi.org/10.1007/s00103-015-2129-2.

Britz, Lisa (2007): Bildungssituation von Kindern und Jugendlichen aus Zuwanderfamilien. Retrieved from https://www.bpb.de/gesellschaft/migration/dossier-migration/56491/schule-und-integration?p=all.

Bröder, Janine; Carvalho, Graça S. (2019): Health literacy of children and adolescents: Conceptual approaches and development considerations. In: Orkan Okan, Ullrich Bauer, Diane Levin-Zamir, Paulo Pinheiro und Kristine Sørensen (Hg.): International Handbook of Health Literacy. Research, practice and policy across the lifespan. Bristol: POLICY Press, S. 39–52.

Bröder, Janine; Okan, Orkan; Bauer, Ullich; Bruland, Dirk; Schlupp, Sandra; Bollweg, Torsten M. et al. (2017): Health literacy in childhood and youth: a systematic review of definitions and models. In: *BMC public health* 17. https://doi.org/10.1186/s12889-017-4267-y.

Brodmerkel, Anke (2017): Einwanderungsland Deutschland. Retrieved from https://www.bpb.de/politik/innenpolitik/demografischer-wandel/196652/einwanderungsland-deutschland.

Broeder, J.; Okan, O.; Bauer, U.; Pinheiro, P. (2017): Health literacy in children – towards a child-centered conceptual understandingJanine Broeder. In: *Eur J Public Health* 27 (suppl_3). https://doi.org/10.1093/eurpub/ckx187.138.

Bromand, Z.; Temur-Erman, S.; Yesil, R.; Heredia Montesinos, A.; Aichberger, M. C.; Kleiber, D. et al. (2012): Mental health of Turkish women in Germany. Resilience and risk factors. In: *European Psychiatry* 27, S17-S21. DOI: https://doi.org/10.1016/S0924-9338(12)75703-6.

Brown Stephen L, Teufel James A, Birch David A (2007). Early adolescents perceptions of health and health literacy. In: Journal of School Health. 2007;77:7–15.

Bruland, Dirk; Kornblum, Katharina; Harsch, Stefanie; Bröder, Janine; Okan, Orkan; Bauer, Ullrich (2017): Schüler mit einem psychisch erkrankten Elternteil und die Mental Health Literacy von Lehrkräften. In: *Praxis der Kinderpsychologie und Kinderpsychiatrie* 66 (10), S. 774–790. DOI: https://doi.org/10.13109/prkk.2017.66.10.774.

Bründel, Heidrun; Hurrelmann, Klaus (1996): Einführung in die Kindheitsforschung. Weinheim, Basel: Beltz.

Brunnett, Regina (2009): Die Hegemonie symbolischer Gesundheit. Eine Studie zum Mehrwert von Gesundheit im Postfordismus. s.l.: transcript Verlag (Sozialtheorie). Retrieved from https://www.content-select.com/index.php?id=bib_view&ean=9783839412770.

Bühler-Niederberger, Doris (2010): Childhood sociology – Defining the state of the art and ensuring reflection. In: *Current Sociology* 58 (2), S. 156–164.

Bundesamt für Gesundheit (2012): Gesundheit der Migrantinnen und Migranten in der Schweiz. Wichtigste Ergebnisse des zweiten Gesundheitsmonitorings der Migrationsbevölkerung in der Schweiz, 2010. BAG. Bern.

Bundesamt für Gesundheit (2013a): Die gesundheitspolitischen Prioritäten des Bundesrates. Eidgenössisches Departement des Innern EDI. Bern.

Bundesamt für Gesundheit (2013b): Nationales Programm Migration und Gesundheit: Bilanz 2008–13 und Schwerpunkte 2014–17. BAG, Direktionsbereich Gesundheitspolitik, Nationales Programm Migration und Gesundheit. Bern.

Bundesamt für Migration und Flüchtlinge (BAMF) (2016): Migrationsbericht 2015. Berlin. Retrieved from https://www.bamf.de/SharedDocs/Anlagen/DE/Publikationen/Migrationsberichte/migrationsbericht-2015.html, last checked on 05.10.2019.

Bundesamt für Statistik (2016): Indikatoren Migration und Integration. Bevölkerung nach Migrationsstatus.

Bundesamt für Statistik (2019): Ständige und nichtständige Wohnbevölkerung nach Jahr, Kanton, Bevölkerungstyp, Staatsangehörigkeit (Land) und Altersklasse. Zürich. Retrieved from https://www.bfs.admin.ch/bfs/de/home/statistiken/bevoelkerung/migration-integration.html, last checked on 8.10.219.

Bundesministerium für Arbeit und Soziales (2005): Lebenslagen in Deutschland- Der 2. Armuts- und Reichtumsbericht der Bunesregiereung. Retrieved from https://www.bmas.de/DE/Service/Medien/Publikationen/forschungsprojekt-a332-zweiter-armuts-und-reichtumsbericht.html.

Bundesministerium für Arbeit und Soziales (2017): Lebenslagen in Deutschland. Der fünfte Armuts- und Reichtumsbericht. Retrieved from https://www.armuts-und-reichtumsbericht.de/DE/Bericht/Archiv/Der-fuenfte-Bericht/Der-Bericht/der-bericht.html, last checked on 10.09.2019.

Bundesministerium für Familie, Senioren, Frauen und Jugend (2009): Familienreport 2009. Leistungen-Wirkungen-Trends. Retrieved from https://www.bmfsfj.de/blob/93796/7c7c7f7dadc91c619349be4a54feb17b/familienreport-data.pdf.

Bundeszentrale für politische Bildung (2018): Zahlen und Fakten. Die soziale Situation in Deutschland. Retrieved from https://www.bpb.de/wissen/NY3SWU,0,0,Bev%F6lkerung_mit_Migrationshintergrund_I.html.

Bundeszentrale für politische Bildung; Statistisches Bundesamt (2016): Datenreport 2016. Ein Sozialbericht für die Bundesrepublik Deutschland. Retrieved from https://www.destatis.de/DE/Publikationen/Datenreport/Datenreport.html.

Burt, Ronald S. (1982): Towards a Structural Theory of Action. New York: Academic Press.

Burt, Ronald S. (2000): The network structure of social capital. Chicago Ill.: University of Chicago Paper.

Butler, Judith (2001): Das Unbehagen der Geschlechter. [Nachdr.]. Frankfurt am Main: Suhrkamp (Gender studies Vom Unterschied der Geschlechter, 1722 = N.F., 722).

BZgA (2001): Was erhält Menschen gesund? Antonovskys Modell der Salutogenese – Diskussionsstand und Stellenwert, last checked on 03.02.2018.

Canadian Council on Learning (2007): Health Literacy in Canada. Initial Results from the International Adult Literacy and Skills Survey 2007. Ottawa.

Canadian Council on Learning (2008): Health Literacy in Canada. A Healthy Understanding. Ottawa. Retrieved from https://mips.ca/assets/healthliteracyreportfeb2008e.pdf, last checked on 04.09.2019.

Chang, F.-C.; Chiu, C.-H.; Chen, P.-H.; Miao, N.-F.; Lee, C.-M.; Chiang, J.-T. et al. (2015): Relationship Between Parental and Adolescent eHealth Literacy and Online Health Information Seeking in Taiwan. Retrieved from https://nccur.lib.nccu.edu.tw//handle/140.119/79420.

Chew, Lisa D.; Bradley, Katharine A.; Boyko, Edward J. (2004): Brief questions to identify patients with inadequate health literacy. In: *Family Medicine* 36, S. 588–594.

Chinn, Deborah (2011): Critical health literacy: A review and critical analysis. In: *Social Science & Medicine* 73, S. 60–67. DOI: https://doi.org/10.1016/j.socscimed.2011.04.004.

Chisolm, D. J., & Buchanan, L. (2007): Measuring adolescent functional health literacy: a pilot validation of the Test of Functional Health Literacy in Adults. The Journal of adolescent health : official publication of the Society for Adolescent Medicine, 41(3), 312–314. https://doi.org/10.1016/j.jadohealth.2007.04.01.

Cho, Young Ik; Lee, Shoou-Yih D.; Arozullah, Ahsan M.; Crittenden, Kathleen S. (2008): Effects of health literacy on health status and health service utilization amongst the elderly. In: *Social Science & Medicine* 66 (8), S. 1809–1816. DOI: https://doi.org/10.1016/j.socscimed.2008.01.003.

Christensen, Pia Haudrup (2004): Children's participation in ethnographic research: Issues of power and representation. In: *Children & Society* 18, S. 165–176. DOI: https://doi.org/10.1002/chi.823.

Chung, Seon-Yoon; Nahm, Eun-Shim (2015): Testing Reliability and Validity of the eHealth Literacy Scale (eHEALS) for Older Adults Recruited Online. In: *Comput Inform Nurs* 33 (4), S. 150–156. DOI: https://doi.org/10.1097/CIN.0000000000000146.

Cimasi, R. J.; Sharamitaro, A. P.; Seiler, R. L. (2013): he association between health literacy and preventable hospitalizations in Missouri: Implications in an era of reform. In: *Journal of Health Care Finance* 40 (2), S. 1–16.

Clark-Kazak, Christina (2017): Ethical Considerations: Research with People in Situations of Forced Migration. In: *Refuge* 33 (2), S. 11–17. DOI: https://doi.org/10.7202/1043059ar.

Cleppien, Gabriele; Kutscher, Nadia (2004): Digital Devide und Online-Bildung. In: Hans-Uwe Otto und Nadia Kutscher (Hg.): Informelle Bildung online. Perspektiven für Bildung, Jugendarbeit und Medienpädagogik. Weinheim, München: Juventa, S. 80–96.

Cockerham, William C.; Hinote, Brian P.; Abbott, Pamela (2006): A Sociological Model of Health Lifestyles. In: Claus Wendt und Christof Wolf (Hg.): Soziologie der Gesundheit. Kölner Zeitschrift für Soziologie und Sozialpsychologie. Wiesbaden: VS Verl. für Sozialwiss (Kölner Zeitschrift für Soziologie und Sozialpsychologie Sonderhefte, 46), S. 177–197.

Como, June M. (2014): Health literacy and self-efficacy: Impact on medication adherence and health outcomes in urban cardiology practices. In: *Dissertation Abstracts International Section B: The Sciences and Engineering* 74, 11-B (E).

Connor, Melanie; Mantwill, Sarah; Schulz, Peter J. (2013): Functional health literacy in Switzerland – validation of a German, Italian, and French health literacy test. In: *Patient Education and Counseling* 90 (1), S. 12–17. DOI: https://doi.org/10.1016/j.pec.2012.08.018.

CSDH (2008): Closing the gap in a generation: health equity through action on the social determinants of health. Final Report of the Commission on Social Determinants of Health. WHO. Geneva.

CSU (2018): Meldung. Islam gehört nicht zu Deutschland. Retrieved from https://www.csu.de/aktuell/meldungen/maerz-2018/islam-gehoert-nicht-zu-deutschland/.

Daniel, Ellen (2009): Türkische Familien sind zu dick. Focus Online. Retrieved from https://www.focus.de/gesundheit/ernaehrung/news/tid-14759/uebergewicht-tuerkische-familien-sind-zu-dick_aid_413723.html.

Daniels, Norman (2008): Just Health. Meeting Health Needs Fairly. New York: Cambridge University Press.

Davey Smith, George (2008): Die Bedeutung einer Lebenslaufperspektive für die Erklärung gesundheitlicher Ungleichheit. In: Ullrich Bauer, Uwe H. Bittlingmayer und Matthias Richter (Hg.): Health Inequalities. Determinanten und Mechanismen gesundheitlicher Ungleichheit. 1. Aufl. Wiesbaden: VS Verl. für Sozialwiss (Gesundheit und Gesellschaft), S. 291–330.

Davis, Terry C.; Long, Sandra W.; Jackson, Robert H.; Mayeux, E. J.; George, R. B.; Murphy, Peggy W.; Crouch, M. A. (1993): Rapid estimate of adult literacy in medicine: A shortened screening instrument. In: *Family Medicine* 25 (6), S. 391–395.

Davis, Terry C.; Wolf, Michael S.; Arnold, Connie L.; Byrd, Robert S.; Long, Sandra W.; Springer, Thomas et al. (2006): Development and Validation of the Rapid Estimate of Adolescent Literacy in Medicine (REALM-Teen): A Tool to Screen Adolescents for Below-Grade Reading in Health Care Settings. In: *Pediatrics* 118 (6), e1707-e1714. DOI: https://doi.org/10.1542/peds.2006-1139.

Degenhardt, Louisa; O'Loughlin, Christina; Swift, Wendy; Romaniuk, Helena; Carlin, John; Coffey, Carolyn et al. (2013): The persistence of adolescent binge drinking into adulthood: findings from a 15-year prospective cohort study. In: *BMJ open* 3 (8). https://doi.org/10.1136/bmjopen-2013-003015.

Del Giudice, P. (2017): The IC-Health project: improving digital health literacy in EuropePietro Del Giudice. In: *Eur J Public Health* 27 (suppl_3). https://doi.org/10.1093/eurpub/ckx187.065.

Deutsches Institut für Internationale Pädagogische Forschung (2016): Bildung und Migration- Nationaler Bildungsbericht. Retrieved from https://www.google.com/search?q=Deutsches+Institut+f%C3%BCr+Internationale+P%C3%A4dagogische+Forschung+2016%3A++Bildung+und+Migration-+Nationaler+Bildungsbericht&ie=utf-8&oe=utf-8&client=firefox-b-ab.

DeWalt, Darren A.; Berkman, Nancy D.; Sheridan, Stacey; Lohr, Kathleen N.; Pignone, Michael P. (2004): Literacy and health outcomes: a systematic review of the literature. In: *J GEN INTERN MED* 19 (12), S. 1228–1239. DOI: https://doi.org/10.1111/j.1525-1497.2004.40153.x.

DeWalt, Darren A.; Dilling, Marylee H.; Rosenthal, Marjorie S.; Pignone, Michael P. (2007): Low parental literacy is associated with worse asthma care measures in children. In: *Ambulatory pediatrics: the official journal of the Ambulatory Pediatric Association* 7 (1), S. 25–31. DOI: https://doi.org/10.1016/j.ambp.2006.10.001.

DeWalt, Darren A.; Hink, Ashley (2009): Health literacy and child health outcomes: a systematic review of the literature. In: *Pediatrics* 124 Suppl 3, S265–74. DOI: https://doi.org/10.1542/peds.2009-1162B.

Diemand, Stefanie (2017): Deutschtürken. Der viertgrößte türkische Wahlbezirk. Zeit Online; online available https://www.zeit.de/politik/2017-03/deutschtuerkentuerkei-referendum-recep-tayyip-erdogan-waehler-praesidialsystem

Dilger, Hansjörg; Dohrn, Kristina (Hg.) (2016): Living in refugee camps in Berlin. Women's perspectives and experiences. Institute of Social and Cultural Anthropology at Freie Universität Berlin; WelcomeFUBerlin Program. Berlin: Weißensee Verlag (Berliner Beiträge zur Ethnologie, Band 40).

Dippelhofer-Stiehm, Barbara (2008): Gesundheitssozialisation. Theoretische und empirische Analysen zur Genese des subjektiven Gesundheitsbildes. Weinheim, München: Juventa.

Dodson, Sarity; Good, Suvajee; Osborne, Richard H. (Hg.) (2015): Health literacy toolkit for low- and middle-income countries. A series of information sheets to empower communities and strengthen health systems. New Dehli: WHO Regional Office for South-East-Asia. Retrieved from https://apps.searo.who.int/PDS_DOCS/B5148.pdf, last checked on 07.03.2019.

Dolby, Nadine; Dimitriadis, Greg (Hg.) (2004): Learning to Labor in New Times. with Paul Willis. London: Routledge.

Duong, Tuyen V.; Aringazina, Altyn; Baisunova, Gaukhar; Nurjanah; Pham, Thuc V.; Pham, Khue M. et al. (2017): Measuring health literacy in Asia: Validation of the HLS-EU-Q47 survey tool in six Asian countries. In: *Journal of epidemiology* 27 (2), S. 80–86. DOI: https://doi.org/10.1016/j.je.2016.09.005.

Ecarius, Jutta; Köbel, Nils; Wahl, Katrin (2011): Familie, Erziehung und Sozialisation. Wiesbaden: VS.

Eichler, Katja Johanna (2008): Migration, transnationale Lebenswelten und Gesundheit. Eine qualitative Studie über das Gesundheitshandeln von Migrantinnen. Zugl.: Hamburg, Univ., Diss., 2006 u.d.T.: Eichler, Katja Johanna: Gesundheit und Transnationalität. 1. Aufl. Wiesbaden: VS Verl. für Sozialwiss. Retrieved from https://gbv.eblib.com/patron/FullRecord.aspx?p=748368.

Elkeles, Thomas; Mielck, Andreas (1997): Entwicklung eines Modells zur Erklärung gesundheitlicher Ungleichheit. In: *Das Gesundheitswesen* 59 (3), S. 137–143.

Emerson, Robert M.; Fretz, Rachel I.; Shaw, Linda L. (2011): Writing ethnographic fieldnotes. Chicago, IL: The University of Chicago press.

Emirbayer, Mustafa; Mische, Ann (1998): What is agency? In: *American Journal of Sociology* 103 (4), S. 962–1023.

Emmerich, Markus; Hormel, Ulrike (2013): Heterogenität – Diversity – Intersektionalität. Zur Logik sozialer Unterscheidungen in pädagogischen Semantiken der Differenz. Wiesbaden: VS Verlag für Sozialwissenschaften.

Eng, T. R. (2001): The e-Health Landscape: A Terrain Map of Emerging Information and Communication Technologies in Healthand Health Care. Princeton, NJ: The Robert Wood Johnson Foundation.

Erhart, Michael; Hurrelmann, Klaus; Ravens-Sieberer, Ulrike (2008a): Sozialisation und Gesundheit. In: Klaus Hurrelmann, Matthias Grundmann und Sabine Walper (Hg.): Handbuch Sozialisationsforschung. Weinheim und Basel: Beltz, S. 424–442.

Erhart, Michael; Schenk, Liane; Ravens-Sieberer, Ulrike (2008b): Migration und gesundheitliche Ungleichheit im Kindes- und Jugendalter. In: Matthias Richter, Klaus Hurrelmann, Andreas Klocke, Wolfgang Melzer und Ulrike Ravens-Sieberer (Hg.): Gesundheit, Ungleichheit und jugendliche Lebenswelten. Ergebnisse der zweiten internationalen Vergleichsstudie im Auftrag der Weltgesundheitsorganistaion WHO. Weinheim, München: Juventa, S. 141–159.

Eriksson, Monica; Mittelmark, Maurice B. (2017): The Sense of Coherence and Its Measurement. In: Maurice B. Mittelmark, Shifra Sagy, Monica Eriksson, Georg F. Bauer, Jürgen M. Pelikan, Bengt Lindström und Geir Arild Espnes (Hg.): The Handbook of Salutogenesis. Cham (CH), S. 97–106.

Etzold, Benjamin (2019): Auf der Flucht – (Im)Mobilisierung und (Im)Mobilität von Schutzsuchenden. State-of-Research Papier 04, Verbundprojekt ‚Flucht: Forschung und Transfer'. IMIS. Osnabrück. Retrieved from https://flucht-forschung-transfer.de/wp-content/uploads/2019/06/SoR-04-Benjamin-Etzold-WEB.pdf, last checked on 08.10.2019.

EuroStat; Statista (2014): Verdienstunterschiede zwischen Männern und Frauen 2014 in Prozent. Retrieved from https://www.tagesschau.de/faktenfinder/inland/genderpaygap-103~magnifier_pos-1.html; 12.03.2020, last checked on 06.04.2020.

Evans-Pritchard, Edward E. (1988): Hexerei, Orakel und Magie bei den Zande. 1. Aufl. Frankfurt am Main: Suhrkamp (Suhrkamp-Taschenbuch Wissenschaft, 721).

Eysenbach, Gunter (2001): What is e-health? In: *Journal of medical Internet research* 3 (2). https://doi.org/10.2196/jmir.3.2.e20.

Faltermaier, Toni (2001): Migration und Gesundheit: Fragen und Konzepte aus einer salutogenetischen und gesundheitspsychologischen Perspektive. In: Peter Marschalck (Hg.): Migration und Krankheit. 1. Aufl. Osnabrück: Rasch (Schriften des Instituts für Migrationsforschung und Interkulturelle Studien (IMIS) der Universität Osnabrück, 10), S. 93–112.

Faltermaier, Toni; Kühnlein, Irene; Burda-Vierig, Martina (1998a): Subjektive Gesundheitstheorien: Inhalt, Dynamik ud ihre Bedeutung für das Gesundheitshandeln im Alltag. In: *Zeitschrift für Gesundheitswissenschaften* 6 (4), S. 309–325.

Faltermaier, Toni; Kühnlein, Irene; Burda-Viering, Martina (1998b): Gesundheit im Alltag. Laienkompetenz in Gesundheitshandeln und Gesundheitsförderung. Weinheim: Juventa-Verl. (Juventa-Materialien).

Faltermaier, Toni; Kühnlein, Irene; Burda-Viering, Martina (1998c): Gesundheit. Laienkompetenz in Gesundheitshandeln und Gesundheitsförderung. Weinheim, München: Juventa.

Federal Statistical Office (2018a): Bevölkerung - Einwohnerzahl in Deutschland nach Geschlecht von 1995 bis 2016 (in 1.000). Online available: https://statista.com/statistik/daten/studie/161868/umfrage/entwicklung-der-gesamtbevoelkerung-nach-geschlecht-seit-1995/ (last check 2023/11/26.

Fennelly, Katherine (2007): Health and well-being of immigrants: The healthy migrant phenomenon. In: Patricia Frye Walker und Elizabeth D. Barnett (Hg.): Immigrant medicine. St. Louis, MO: Saunders Elsevier, S. 19–26.

Feuser, Georg (2017): Inklusion – Das Mögliche, das im Wirklichen noch nicht sichtbar ist. In: Georg Feuser (Hg.): Inkluision – ein leeres Versprechen. Zum Verkommen eines Gesellschaftsprojekts. Gießen: Psychosozial-Verlag, S. 183–285.

Fischer, Karl (2014): Pakistan und Afghanistan nach 2014. In: Hubert Thielicke (Hg.): Am Ende nichts? Krieg in Afghanistan – Bilanz und Ausblick. Potsdam: WeltTrends, S. 61–67.

Fleisher, J. E.; Minger, J.; Fitts, W.; Dahodwala, N. (2014): Low health literacy: An under-recognized obstacle in Parkinson's disease. In: *Movement disorders: official journal of the Movement Disorder Society* 29, S. 158–159.

Flick, Uwe (1998): Subjektive Vorstellungen von Gesundheit und Krankheit. Überblick und Einleitung. In: Uwe Flick (Hg.): Wann fühlen wir uns gesund? Subjektive Vorstellungen von Gesundheit und Krankheit. Weinheim: Juventa, S. 9–30.

Flick, Uwe (2014): Der qualitative Forschungsprozess. In: Uwe Flick (Hg.): Qualitative Sozialforschung. Eine Einführung. Reinbek bei Hamburg: Rowohlt, S. 122–130.

Fok May S M, Wong Thomas KS (2002). What does health literacy mean to children? Contemp Nurse, 13:249–58.

Forbis, Shalini G.; Aligne, C. A.; Auinger, P.; Byrd, Robert S. (2002): The association between maternal literacy and birth weight. In: *E-PAS (Pediatric Academic Societies)* 51, S. 1046.

Foucault, Michel (1983): Der Wille zum Wissen. Sexualität und Wahrheit, Band 1. 14., durchges., korrig. Aufl. Frankfurt a.M.: Suhrkamp (Suhrkamp-Taschenbuch Wissenschaft, 716).

Foucault, Michel (1988): Die Geburt der Klinik. Eine Archäologie des ärztlichen Blicks. Frankfurt a.M.: Fischer.

Franke, Alexa (2016): Modelle von Gesundheit und Krankheit. Bern: Hans Huber/Hogrefe.

Freedman, Darcy A., Bess, Kimberly D., Tucker, Holly A., Boyd, David L, Tuchman, Arleen M. & Wallston, Kenneth A. (2009): Public Health Literacy defined. In: American Journal of Preventive Medicine, 36 (5), 446–451.

Frisch, Anne-Linda; Camerini, Luca; Diviani, Nicola; Schulz, Peter J. (2012): Defining and measuring health literacy: how can we profit from other literacy domains? In: *Health promotion international* 27 (1), S. 117–126. DOI: https://doi.org/10.1093/heapro/dar043.

Frisch, Max (1965): Vorwort. In: Alexander J. Seiler: Siamo Italiani. Die Italiener. Gespräche mit italienischen Arbeitern in der Schweiz. Zürich: EVZ-Verlag.

Fuchs-Heinritz, Werner (Hg.) (2013): Lexikon zur Soziologie. 5., überarb. Aufl. 2011. Wiesbaden: Springer VS.

Furuya, Yoko; Kondo, Naoki; Yamagata, Zentaro; Hashimoto, Hideki (2013): Health literacy, socioeconomic status and self-rated health in Japan. In: *Health promotion international* 30 (3), S. 505–513. DOI: https://doi.org/10.1093/heapro/dat071.

Ganser, Daniele (2016): Illegale Kriege. Wie die Nato-Länder die UNO sabotieren. Eine Chronik von Kuba bis Syrien. Zürich: Orell Füssli Verlag.

Garfinkel, Herold (1967): Studies in Ethnomethodogy. Englewood Cliffs, N.J.: Prentice Hall.

Gayle, Damien (2016): EU-Turkey refugee plan could be illegal, says UN official. Retrieved from https://www.theguardian.com/world/2016/apr/02/eu-turkey-refugee-plan-could-be-illegal-says-un-official.

Geene, Raimund (2018): Familiäre Gesundheitsförderung. In: Klaus Hurrelmann, Matthias Richter, Theodor Klotz und Stephanie Stock (Hg.): Referenzwerk Prävention und Gesundheitsförderung. Grundlagen, Konzepte und Umsetzungsstrategien. 5., vollst. überarb. Aufl. Göttingen: Hogrefe, S. 371–389.

Geertz, Clifford (1973): Thick description: Toward an interpretive theory of culture. In: Clifford Geertz (Hg.): The interpretation of cultures. Selected essays. New York, NY: Basic Books, S. 3–30.

Geertz, Clifford (2003): Dichte Beschreibung. Beiträge zum Verstehen kultureller Systeme. Frankfurt: Suhrkamp.

Geertz, Clifford (2015): Dichte Beschreibung. Beiträge zum Verstehen kultureller Systeme. Unter Mitarbeit von Brigitte Luchesi und Rolf Bindemann. 13. Auflage. Frankfurt am Main: Suhrkamp (Suhrkamp-Taschenbuch Wissenschaft, 696).

Gerdes, Jürgen (1996): Autonomie und Kultur. Philosophischer Liberalismus und Minderheitenrechte bei Will Kymlicka. In: *Peripherie. Zeitschrift für Politik und Ökonomie in der Dritten Welt* 16 (64), S. 46–69.

Gerdes, Jürgen; Bittlingmayer, Uwe H.; Osipov, Igor; Okcu, Gözde (2016): Die Verteilung von Life Skills nach sozialstrukturellen Merkmalen und Aspekten der Schulperformanz. Eine Auswertung der 1. Erhebung im Projekt „Zur Evidenzbasierung in der schulischen Gesundheitsförderung, Primärprävention und inklusiven Beschulung" (EGePriB). 1. Zwischenbericht im Rahmen der Wirksamkeits- und Akzeptanz-Evaluation des schulischen Unterrichtsprogramms „Erwachsen werden" von Lions-Quest (4. Ausgabe) in 5. Klassen verschiedener Schul-formen in sechs Bundesländern. Freiburg: Institut für Soziologie.

Gerdes, Jürgen; Osipov, Igor; Okcu, Gözde; Bittlingmayer, Uwe H. (2018): Die Entwicklung von Life Skills in eineinhalb Schuljahren. Wirksamkeitsevaluation des schulischen Life Skills-Förderprogramms Lions Quest „Erwachsen werden". Endbericht. Freiburg.

Gerny, Daniel (2016): Muslime werden zum Handschlag gezwungen. In: *Neue Zürcher Zeitung*, 25.05.2016. Retrieved from https://www.nzz.ch/schweiz/aktuelle-themen/religionsfreiheit-haendedruck-wird-in-baselland-zur-pflicht-ld.84599, last checked on 30.03.2020.

Gieler, Wolfgang (2017): Die deutsch-türkische Beziehungen- Vom Anwerbeabkommen bis zur Gegenwart. In: Wolfgang Gieler, Burak Gümüş und Yunus Yoldaş (Hg.): Deutsch-türkische Beziehungen. Historische, sektorale und migrationsspezifische Aspekte. 1st, New ed. Frankfurt a.M: Peter Lang GmbH Internationaler Verlag der Wissenschaften, S. 43–56.

Giesecke, Johannes; Müters, Stephan (2009): Strukturelle und verhaltensbezogene Faktoren gesundheitlicher Ungleichheit: Methodische Überlegungen zur Ermittlung der Erklärungsanteile. In: Klaus Hurrelmann und Matthias Richter (Hg.): Gesundheitliche Ungleichheit. Grundlagen, Probleme, Perspektiven. 2., aktualisierte Aufl. Wiesbaden: VS Verlag für Sozialwissenschaften/GWV Fachverlage GmbH Wiesbaden, S. 353–366.

Gilstad, Heidi (2014): Toward a comprehensive model of eHealth literacy. Retrieved from https://doi.org/10.13140/2.1.4569.0247.

Girtler, Roland (2001): Methoden der Feldforschung. Wien u.a.: Böhlau.

Glaser, Barney G.; Strauss, Anselm L. (2010): Grounded Theory. Strategien qualitativer Forschung. Bern: Hogrefe.

Goffman, Alice. (2014): On the run. Fugitive life in an American city. Chicago etc.: The University of Chicago press (Fieldwork encounters and discoveries).

Goffman, Erving (1980): Rahmen-Analyse. Ein Versuch über die Organisation von Alltagserfahrungen. Frankfurt a.M.: Suhrkamp.

Goffman, Erving (1996): Interaktionsrituale. Über Verhalten in direkter Kommunikation. 4. Aufl. Frankfurt am Main: Suhrkamp (Suhrkamp-Taschenbuch Wissenschaft, 594).

Goffman, Erving (2008): Wir alle spielen theater. Die Selbstdarstellung im Alltag. Unter Mitarbeit von Ralf Dahrendorf. 6. Aufl. München: Piper (Serie Piper, 3891).

Goguikian Ratcliff, Betty; Bolzman, Claudio; Gakuba, Théogène Octave (2015): Déqualification des femmes migrantes en Suisse: mécanismes sous-jacents et effets psychologiques. In: *2015* 4, S. 14.

Goldberg, Andreas; Sauer, Martina (2003): Perspektiven der Integration der türkischstämmigen Migranten in Nordrhein-Westfalen. Ergebnisse der vierten Mehrthemenbefragung 2002. Münster: Lit Verlag

Gomolla, Mechtild; Radkte, Frank-Olaf (2009): Institutionelle Diskriminierung. Die Herstellung ethnischer Differenz in der Schule. 3. Aufl. Wiesbaden: VS Verlag für Sozialwissenschaften.

Gomolla, Methild; Radtke, Frank-Olaf (2000): Mechanismen institutionalisierter Diskriminierung in der Schule. In: Ingrid Gogolin und Bernhard Nauck (Hg.): Migration, gesellschaftliche Differenzierung und Bildung. Resultate des Forschungsschwerpunktprogramms FABER. Wiesbaden, s.l.: VS Verlag für Sozialwissenschaften.

Gordon Shirley C, Barry Charlotte D, Dunn Dorothy J, King Beth (2011). Clarifying a vision for health literacy: a holistic school-based community approach. Holist Nurs Pract, 25:120–6. https://doi.org/10.1097/HNP.0b013e3182157c34.

Graneheim, Ulla H.; Norberg, Astrid; Jansson, Lilian (2001): Interaction relating to privacy, identity, autonomy and security. An observational study focusing on a woman with dementia and 'behavioural disturbances', and on her care providers. In: *Journal of advanced nursing* 36, S. 256–265. DOI: https://doi.org/10.1046/j.1365-2648.2001.01966.x.

Griffey, Richard T.; Kennedy, Sarah K.; McGownan, Lucy; Goodman, Melody; Kaphings, Kimberly A. (2014): Is low health literacy associated with increased emergency department utilization and recidivism? In: *Academic Emergency Medicine* 21 (10), S. 1109–1115.

Grotlüschen, Anke; Buddeberg, Klaus (Hg.) (2020): LEO 2018. Leben mit geringer Literalität. 1. Auflage. Bielefeld: wbv Media.

Grotlüschen, Anke; Riekmann, Wibke (Hg.) (2012): Funktionaler Analphabetismus in Deutschland. Ergebnisse der ersten leo, Level-One Studie. Münster: Waxmann (Alphabetisierung und Grundbildung, 10). Retrieved from https://www.content-select.com/index.php?id=bib_view&ean=9783830977759.

Grundmann, Matthias (2006): Handlungsbefähigung und Milieu: zur Analyse milieuspezifischer Alltagspraktiken und ihrer Ungleichheitsrelevanz. Münster: LIT Verlag (2).

Grundmann, Matthias (2011): Sozialisation – Erziehung – Bildung: Eine kritische Begriffsbestimmung. In: Rolf Becker (Hg.): Lehrbuch der Bildungssoziologie. Wiesbaden: VS Verlag für Sozialwissenschaften, S. 63–85.

Grundmann, Matthias; Dravenau, Daniel; Bittlingmayer, Uwe H.; Edelstein, Wolfgang (2006): Handlungsbefähigung und Milieu. Zur Analyse milieuspezifischer Alltagspraktiken und ihrer Ungleichheitsrelevanz. Münster: LIT-Verl.

Grundmann, Matthias; Groh-Samberg, Olaf; Bittlingmayer, Uwe H.; Bauer; Ullrich Bauer (2003): Milieuspezifische Handlungsbefähigungen in Familie und Gleichaltrigengruppe. In: *Zeitschrift für Erziehungswissenschaft* 6 (1), S. 25.

Grundmann, Matthias; Wernberger Angela (2015): Familie und Sozialisation. In: Paul B. Hill und Johannes Kopp (Hg.): Handbuch Familiensoziologie. Wiesbaden: Springer VS (Handbuch), S. 413–436.

Guggisberg, Jürg; Gardiol, Lucien; Graf, Iris; Oesch, Thomas; Künzi, Kilian; Volken, Thomas et al. (2011): Gesundheitsmonitoring der Migrationsbevölkerung (GMM) in der Schweiz – Schlussbericht. Bundesamt für Gesundheit & Bundesamt für Migration. Bern.

Gugutzer, Robert (2004): Soziologie des Körpers. Bielefeld: transcript Verlag.

Habich, Roland (2013): Pressekonferenz „Datenreport 2013“ am 26. November in Berlin. Statement von Dr. Roland Habich (WZB). Retrieved from https://www.wzb.eu/sites/default/files/u6/datenreport_statement_habich.pdf, last checked on 25.10.2014.

Häfner, H.; Moschel, G.; Özek, M. (1977): Psychische Störungen bei türkischen Gastarbeitern. Eine prospektiv-epidemiologische Studie zur Untersuchung der Reaktion auf Einwanderung und partielle Anpassung. In: *Der Nervenarzt* 48, S. 268–275.

Haghdoost, Ali Akbar; Rakhshani, Fatemeh; Aarabi, Mohsen; Montazeri, Ali; Tavousi, Mahmoud; Solimanian, Atoosa et al. (2015): Iranian Health Literacy Questionnaire (IHLQ): An Instrument for Measuring Health Literacy in Iran. In: *Iranian Red Crescent Medical Journal* 17 (6). https://doi.org/10.5812/ircmj.17(5)2015.25831.

Hall, Stuart (1994a): Der Westen und der Rest: Diskurs und Macht. In: Stuart Hall (Hg.): Rassismus und kulturelle Identität. Ausgewählte Schriften 2. Hamburg: Argument, S. 137–179.

Hall, Stuart (Hg.) (1994b): Rassismus und kulturelle Identität. Ausgewählte Schriften 2. Hamburg: Argument.

Halm, Dirk (2009): Der transnationale Raum Deutschland-Türkei. Hg. v. Bundeszentrale für politische Bildung. Retrieved from https://www.bpb.de/apuz/31736/der-transnationale-raum-deutschland-tuerkei?p=all.

Hammersley, Martyn; Atkinson, Paul (2007): Ethnography. Principles in practice. 3rd ed. London: Routledge.

Han, Petrus (2016): Soziologie der Migration. Erklärungsmodelle, Fakten, politische Konsequenzen, Perspektiven. 4., unveränderte Auflage. Konstanz, München: UVK

Verlagsgesellschaft mbH; UVK Lucius (UTB Soziologie, 2118). Retrieved from https://www.utb-studi-e-book.de/9783838546858.

Harsch, S., Jawid, A., Jawid, M. E., Saboga-Nunes, L. A., Bittlingmayer, U. H., Sahrai, D., & Sørensen, K. (2021): Health without formal Education? Health Literacy, Quality of Life and Health Behavior Among Male Heads of the Household in Four Districts of the Ghazni Province, Afghanistan. *New Approaches to Health Literacy: Linking Different Perspectives*, 223–246.

Hartl, O.; Pürgyi, P. (1975): Die Ulkuskrankheit bei Gastarbeitern. In: *Wiender Medizinische Wochenschrift* (11), S. 169–171.

Hartung, Susanne (2011): Was hält uns gesund? Gesundheitsressourcen. Von der Salutogenese zum Sozialkapital. In: Thomas Schott und Claudia Hornberg (Hg.): Die Gesellschaft und ihre Gesundheit. 20 Jahre Public Health in Deutschland; Bilanz und Ausblick einer Wissenschaft. 1. Aufl. Wiesbaden: VS Verl. für Sozialwiss (Gesundheit und Gesellschaft), S. 235–255.

Hartung, Susanne (2014): Sozialkapital und gesundheitliche Ungleichheit. Wiesbaden: Springer Fachmedien Wiesbaden.

Hartung, Susanne; Kluwe, Sabine; Sahrai, Diana (2009): Elternbildung und Elternpartizipation in Settings. Eine programmspezifische und vergleichende Analyse von Interventionsprogrammen in Kita, Schule und Kommune. Universität Bielefeld, Fakultär für Gesundheitswissenschaften. Bielefeld.

Hartung, Susanne; Kluwe, Sabine; Sahrai, Diana (2010): „Es geht nur mit den Eltern!" – Kriterien erfolgreicher Präventionsprogramme. In: *Public Health Forum* 18, 15.e1–15.e3. DOI: https://doi.org/10.1016/j.phf.2010.09.007.

Hartung, Susanne; Kluwe, Sabine; Sahrai, Diana (2011): Gesundheitsförderung und Prävention in Settings: Elternarbeit in Kitas, Schule und Familienhilfe. In: Thomas Schott und Claudia Hornberg (Hg.): Die Gesellschaft und ihre Gesundheit: 20 Jahre Public Health in Deutschland: Bilanz und Ausblick einer Wissenschaft. Wiesbaden: VS Verlag für Sozialwissenschaften, S. 599–617.

Haug, Sonja; Müssig, Stephanie; Stichs, Anja (2009): Muslim life in Germany. A study conducted on behalf of the German Conference on Islam. 1. ed. Nürnberg, Germany: Federal Office for Migration and Refugees (Research report, 6).

haz/kle (afp, dpa) Pressemitteilung (2018): Neues Burka-Verbot in der Schweiz. Hg. v. dw.com. Retrieved from https://www.dw.com/de/neues-burka-verbot-in-der-schweiz/a-45608198, last checked on 30.03.2020.

Hefti, René (2010): Spiritualität-die vierte Dimensionoder der vergessene faktor im biopsychosozialen Modell. In: *PrimaryCare* 10 (14). Retrieved from https://www.rish.ch/mm/Hefti_(2010)_Spiritualitat-die_vierte_Dimension_oder_vergessener_Faktor_PrimaryCare.pdf.

Hehlmann, Thomas; Schmidt-Semisch, Henning; Schorb, Friedrich (2018): Soziologie der Gesundheit. München: UVK – UTB.

Helfferich, Cornelia (2019): Leitfaden- und Expterinterviews. In: Nina Baur und Jörg Blasius (Hg.): Handbuch Methoden der empirischen Sozialforschung. 2., vollständig überarbeitete und erweiterte Auflage. Wiesbaden: Springer VS (Handbuch), S. 559–574.

Helmert, Uwe (2003): Soziale Ungleichheit und Krankheitsrisiken. Augsburg: Maro Verlag.

Helmert, Uwe; Schorb, Friedrich (2006): Die Bedeutung verhaltensbezogener Faktoren im Kontext der sozialen Ungleichheit von Gesundheit. In: Matthias Richter und Klaus

Hurrelmann (Hg.): Gesundheitliche Ungleichheit. Grundlagen, Probleme, Perpektiven. Wiesbaden: Springer VS, S. 125–139.

Herburger, Silivia (2010): „Er hat alles vergessen, er hat einfach sein Leben gelebt". Arbeitsmigration und Alter am Beispiel ehemaliger türkischer Gastarbeiter und Gastarbeiterinnen. Universität Wien. Retrieved from https://othes.univie.ac.at/10224/1/2010-06-09_0348428.pdf.

Hesse, Christine; Steinbach, Udo (2002): Informationen zur politischen Bildung. Türkei.

Hoffmann, Rasmus; Borsboom, Gerard; Saez, Marc; Mari Dell'Olmo, Marc; Burström, Bo; Corman, Diana et al. (2014): Social differences in avoidable mortality between small areas of 15 European cities: an ecological study. In: *International journal of health geographics* 13, S. 8. https://doi.org/10.1186/1476-072X-13-8.

Hoffmeister, Dieter (2012): Der Wandel der Familie und dessen Effekte auf Erziehungs- und Bildungsprozesse. In: Ullrich Bauer, Uwe H. Bittlingmayer und Albert Scherr (Hg.): Handbuch Bildungs- und Erziehungssoziologie. Wiesbaden: Springer VS, S. 901–927.

Holly, Werner (2000): Was sind ‚Neue Medien' – was sollen ‚Neue Medien' sein? In: G. Günter Voß, Werner Holly und Klaus Boehnke (Hg.): Neue Medien im Alltag. Begriffsbestimmungen eines interdisziplinären Forschungsfeldes, Bd. 23. Wiesbaden, s. l.: VS Verlag für Sozialwissenschaften, S. 79–106.

Holzer, Daniela (2019): Kritisches Denken mit negativer Dialektik. In: Uwe H. Bittlingmayer, Alex Demirović und Tatjana Freytag (Hg.): Handbuch Kritische Theorie, Bd. 1. Wiesbaden: Springer VS.

Honneth, Axel (Hg.) (1994): Kommunitarismus. Eine Debatte. Frankfurt am Main, New York: Campus Verlag.

Hormel, Ulrike (2012): Intersektionalität als forschungsleitende Beobachtungsperspektive. In: Ullrich Bauer, Uwe H. Bittlingmayer und Albert Scherr (Hg.): Handbuch Bildungs- und Erziehungssoziologie. Wiesbaden: Springer VS, S. 491–506.

Hormel, Ulrike; Scherr, Albert (2004): Bildung für die Einwanderungsgesellschaft. Wiesbaden: VS Verlag für Sozialwissenschaften.

Horn, Annett; Vogt, Dominique; Messer, Melanie; Schaeffer, Doris (2015): Health Literacy von Menschen mit Migrationshintergrund in der Patientenberatung stärken. In: *Bundesgesundheitsblatt – Gesundheitsforschung – Gesundheitsschutz* 58 (6), S. 577–583. DOI: https://doi.org/10.1007/s00103-015-2147-0.

Horn, J.; Herfarth, C. (1978): Das Gastarbeiterulkus. In: *Medizinische Klinik* 73 (41), S. 1417–1421.

Horrigan, John; Rainie, Lee (2006): The Internet's Growing Role in Life's Major Moments. Retrieved from https://www.pewinternet.org/2006/04/19/the-internets-growing-role-in-lifes-major-moments/.

Hradil, Stefan (2006): Was prägt das Krankheitsrisiko: Schicht, Lage, Lebensstil? In: Matthias Richter und Klaus Hurrelmann (Hg.): Gesundheitliche Ungleichheit. Grundlagen, Probleme, Perpektiven. Wiesbaden: Springer VS, S. 33–52.

Hradil, Stefan (2012): Deutsche Verhältnisse. Eine Sozialkunde. Grundbegriffe. Bundeszentrale für politische Bildung. Retrieved from https://www.bpb.de/politik/grundfragen/deutsche-verhaeltnisse-eine-sozialkunde/138437/grundbegriffe.

Huber, Machteld; Knottnerus, J. André; Green, Lawrence; van der Horst, Henriëtte; Jadad, Alejandro R.; Kromhout, Daan et al. (2011): How should we define health? In: *BMJ (Clinical research ed.)* 343, d4163. https://doi.org/10.1136/bmj.d4163.

Hunn, Karin (2005): „Nächstes Jahr kehren wir zurück . . .". Die Geschichte der türkischen „Gastarbeiter" in der Bundesrepublik. Göttingen: Wallstein Verlag (Moderne Zeit, Band 11). Retrieved from https://gbv.eblib.com/patron/FullRecord.aspx?p=995273.

Hunt, Linda M. (2005): Health research: what's culture got to do with it? In: *The Lancet* 366, S. 617–618. DOI: https://doi.org/10.1016/S0140-6736(05)67118-8.

Hunt, Linda M.; Schneider, Suzanne; Comer, Brendon (2004): Should "acculturation" be a variable in health research? A critical review of research on US Hispanics. In: *Social Science & Medicine* 59, S. 973–986. DOI: https://doi.org/10.1016/j.socscimed.2003.12.009.

Huntington, Samuel P. (2002): Kampf der Kulturen. Die Neugestaltung der Weltpolitik im 21. Jahrhundert. Vollst. Taschenbuch-Ausg., 7. Aufl. München: Goldmann (Goldmann, 15190).

Hurrelmann, K.; Hartung, S.; Kluwe, S.; Sahrai, D. (2013): Gesundheitsförderung durch Elternbildung in „Settings". In: *Präv Gesundheitsf* 8 (4), S. 267–275. DOI: https://doi.org/10.1007/s11553-013-0402-5.

Hurrelmann, Klaus (2006): Einführung in die Sozialisationstheorie. 9. Aufl. Weinheim und Basel: Beltz.

Hurrelmann, Klaus; Bauer, Ullrich (2015): Einführung in die Sozialisationstheorie. Das Modell der produktiven Realitätsverarbeitung. 11. vollständig überarbeitete Auflage. Weinheim, Basel: Beltz (Pädagogik). Retrieved from https://eres.lb-oldenburg.de/redirect.php?url=https://content-select.com/index.php?id=bib_view&ean=9783407294333.

Hurrelmann, Klaus; Quenzel, Gudrun (2012): Lebensphase Jugend. Eine systematische Einführung in die sozialwissenschaftliche Jugendforschung. 11., vollständig überarb. Auflage. Weinheim, München: Beltz Juventa.

Hurrelmann, Klaus; Richter, Matthias (2013): Gesundheits- und Medizinsoziologie. Eine Einführung in sozialwissenschaftliche Gesundheitsforschung. 8., überarb. Aufl. Weinheim: Juventa Verlag (Grundlagentexte Soziologie).

Huschke, Susann (2013): Kranksein in der Illegalität. Undokumentierte Lateinamerikaner/-innen in Berlin. Eine medizinethnologische Studie. Bielefeld: transcript.

Huschke, Susann (2015): Giving back: Activist research with undocumented migrants in Berlin. In: *Medical Anthropology* 34, S. 54–69. DOI: https://doi.org/10.1080/01459740.2014.949375.

Incesu, Günal (2014): Ankara – Bonn – Brüssel. Die deutsch-türkischen Beziehungen und die Beitrittsbemühungen der Türkei in die Europäische Gemeinschaft, 1959–1987. Zugl.: Bielefeld, Univ., Diss., 2012–2013. Bielefeld: Transcript-Verl. (Histoire, 47).

Inchley, Joanna Catherine; Currie, Dorothy Bruce; Young, Taryn; Samdal, Oddrun; Torsheim, Torbjørn; Augustson, Lise et al. (Hg.) (2016): Growing up unequal: gender and socioeconomic differences in young people's health and well-being: Health Behaviour in School-aged Children (HBSC) study. International report from the 2013/2014 survey. Copenhagen: WHO Regional Office for Europe.

Ingleby, David (2012): Acquiring health literacy as a moral task. In: *Intl J of Migration, H and SC* 8 (1), S. 22–31. DOI: https://doi.org/10.1108/17479891211231383.

Irwin, Lori G.; Siddiqi, Arjumand; Hertzman, Clyde (2007): Early child development: A powerful equalizer. Final report for the World Health organizsation's Commission on the Social Determinants of Health. University of British Columbia. Vancouver.
Islertas, Zeynep (28.06.2016). Interview mit Leyla.
Islertas, Zeynep (10.07.2016). Interview mit Meryem.
Islertas, Zeynep (16.07.2016). Interview mit Leyla.
Islertas, Zeynep (05.08.2016). Interview mit Leyla.
Islertas, Zeynep (22.08.2016). Interview mit Meryem.
Islertas, Zeynep (23.08.2016). Interview mit Meryem.
Islertas, Zeynep (23.08.2016). Interview mit Leyla.
Islertas, Zeynep (27.08.2016). Interview mit Leylas Mutter.
Islertas, Zeynep (08.10.2016). Interview mit Meryem.
Jahrbuch Kritische Medizin und Gesundheitswissenschaften (Hg.) (2013): Divergentes Altern. Hamburg: Argument.
Jalilvand, David Ramin (2014): Strategische Tiefe. Irans Afghanistanpolitik. In: Hubert Thielicke (Hg.): Am Ende nichts? Krieg in Afghanistan – Bilanz und Ausblick, 69–75. Potsdam: WeltTrends.
Jaspert, Nikolas (2013): Die Kreuzzüge. 6., unveränd. Aufl. Darmstadt: WBG (Geschichte kompakt).
Joas, Hans (1996): Die Kreativität des Handelns. Frankfurt am Main: Suhrkamp.
Johnson, Sarah E.; Baur, Cynthia; Meissner, Helen I. (2011): Back to basics: why basic research is needed to create effective health literacy interventions. In: *Journal of health communication* 16 Suppl 3, S. 22–29. DOI: https://doi.org/10.1080/10810730.2011.604707.
Jordan, Joanne E.; Buchbinder, Rachelle; Osborne, Richard H. (2010): Conceptualising health literacy from the patient perspective. In: *Patient Education and Counseling* 79 (1), S. 36–42. DOI: https://doi.org/10.1016/j.pec.2009.10.001.
Jordan, Susanne; Hoebel, Jens (2015): Gesundheitskompetenz von Erwachsenen in Deutschland: Robert Koch-Institut, Epidemiologie und Gesundheitsberichterstattung. Retrieved from https://edoc.rki.de/bitstream/176904/2526/1/28uA47TXhHsT2.pdf.
Jungbauer-Gans, Monika; Gross, Christiane (2006): Erklärungsansätze sozial differenzierter Gesundheitschancen. In: Matthias Richter und Klaus Hurrelmann (Hg.): Gesundheitliche Ungleichheit. Grundlagen, Probleme, Perpektiven. Wiesbaden: Springer VS, S. 73–89.
Jungbauer-Gans, Monika; Kriwy, Peter (Hg.) (2004): Soziale Benachteiligung und Gesundheit bei Kindern und Jugendlichen. Wiesbaden: VS.
Kähnert, Heike (2003): Evaluation des schulischen Lebenskompetenzförderprogramms „Erwachsen werden". unveröff. Dissertation an der Fakultät für Gesundheitswissenschaften. Bielefeld: Universität Bielefeld.
Kassam, Azaad; Nanji, Anar. (2006): Mental health of Afghan refugees in Pakistan. A qualitative rapid reconnaissance field study. In: *Intervention: the international journal of mental health, psychosocial work and counselling in areas of armed conflict.*
Katz, Marra G.; Jacobson, Terry A.; Veledar, Emir; Kripalani, Sunil (2007): Patient literacy and question-asking behavior during the medical encounter: a mixed-methods analysis. In: *Journal of General Internal Medicine* 22 (6), S. 782–786. DOI: https://doi.org/10.1007/s11606-007-0184-6.

Kawachi, Ichiro; Kennedy, Bruce P.; Lochner, Kimberly; Prothrow-Stith, Deborah (1997): Social Capital, Income Inequality and Mortality. In: *American journal of public health* 87 (9), S. 1491–1498.

Kaya, Bülent; Efionayi-Mäder, Denise (2007): Grundlagendokument „Migration und Gesundheit". Entwicklung von Grundlagen zur Berücksichtigung der Migrationsdimension in der Prävention und Gesundheitsförderung. Swiss Forum for Migration and Population Studies. Neuchâtel.

Kazim, Hasnain (2014): Türke werfen Deutschland Heuchelei vor. Retrieved from https://www.spiegel.de/politik/ausland/bnd-spionage-in-der-tuerkei-ankara-veraergert-ueber-deutschland-a-986528.html.

Keskin, Hakkı (2017): Neue Entwicklungen in den deutsch-türkischen Beziehungen. In: Wolfgang Gieler, Burak Gümüş und Yunus Yoldaş (Hg.): Deutsch-türkische Beziehungen. Historische, sektorale und migrationsspezifische Aspekte. 1st, New ed. Frankfurt a.M: Peter Lang GmbH Internationaler Verlag der Wissenschaften, S. 273–307.

Keupp, Heiner (2012): Capability. Verwirklichungschancen zur positiven Jugendentwicklung. Freiburg: Centaurus.

Kickbusch, I. (2002): Health literacy: a search for new categories. In: *Health Promot Int* 17 (1), S. 1–2. DOI: https://doi.org/10.1093/heapro/17.1.1.

Kickbusch, Ilona (2009): Health literacy: engaging in a political debate. In: *International journal of public health* 54 (3), S. 131–132. DOI: https://doi.org/10.1007/s00038-009-7073-1.

Kickbusch, Ilona; Hartung, Susanne (2014): Die Gesundheitsgesellschaft. Konzepte für eine gesundheitsförderliche Politik. 2., vollständig überarbeitete Auflage. Bern: Huber. Retrieved from https://elibrary.hogrefe.de/9783456946757/.

Kickbusch, Ilona S. (2001): Health literacy: addressing the health and education divide. In: *Health Promot Int* 16 (3), S. 289–297. DOI: https://doi.org/10.1093/heapro/16.3.289.

Kiechle, Eric S.; Bailey, Stacy Cooper; Hedlund, Laurie A.; Viera, Anthony J.; Sheridan, Stacey L. (2015): Different Measures, Different Outcomes? A Systematic Review of Performance-Based versus Self-Reported Measures of Health Literacy and Numeracy. In: *Journal of General Internal Medicine* 30 (10), S. 1538–1546. DOI: https://doi.org/10.1007/s11606-015-3288-4.

Kim, Henna; Xie, Bo (2017): Health literacy in the eHealth era: A systematic review of the literature. In: *Patient Education and Counseling* 100 (6), S. 1073–1082. DOI: https://doi.org/10.1016/j.pec.2017.01.015.

Kizilhan, Jan Ilhan (2009): Subjektive Krankheitswahrnehmung bei MigrantInnen aus familienorientieren Gesellschaften. In: Heinrich-Böll-Stiftung (Hg.): DOSSIER Migration & Gesundheit, S. 69–79.

Klein, Alexandra (2008): Soziales Kapital Online. Soziale Unterstützung im Internet. Eine Rekonstruktion virtualisierter Formen sozialer Ungleichheit. Universität Bielefeld, Bielefeld. Fakultät für Pädagogik. Retrieved from https://bieson.ub.uni-bielefeld.de/volltexte/2008/1260/.

Klein, Alexandra (2016): Zero-Level Digital Divide: Neues Netz und neue Ungleichheiten. In: *SI:SO. Analysen – Berichte – Kontroversen* (21), S. 50–55.

Klein, Constantin; Albani, Cornelia (2007): Religiösität und psychische Gesundheit. Eine Übersicht über Befunde, Erklärungssätze und Konsequenzen für die klinische Praxis. In:

Psychiatrische Praxis (34), e2–e12. Retrieved from https://www.uni-bielefeld.de/theologie/forschung/religionsforschung/personen/dateien/klein/Klein%20Albani%202007%20-%20Religiosit%C3%A4t%20und%20psychische%20Gesundheit%5b1%5d.pdf.

Klocke, Andreas (2006): Gesundheitsrelevante Verhaltensweisen im Jugendalter. Sozioökonomische, kulturelle und geschlechtsspezifische Einflussfaktoren im internationalen Vergleich. In: Claus Wendt und Christof Wolf (Hg.): Soziologie der Gesundheit. Kölner Zeitschrift für Soziologie und Sozialpsychologie. Wiesbaden: VS Verl. für Sozialwiss (Kölner Zeitschrift für Soziologie und Sozialpsychologie Sonderhefte, 46), S. 198–223.

Klocke, Andreas; Lipsmeier, Gero (2008): Soziale Determinanten der Gesundheit im Kindes- und Jugendalter: Eine Mehrebenenanalyse. In: Matthias Richter, Klaus Hurrelmann, Andreas Klocke, Wolfgang Melzer und Ulrike Ravens-Sieberer (Hg.): Gesundheit, Ungleichheit und jugendliche Lebenswelten. Ergebnisse der zweiten internationalen Vergleichsstudie im Auftrag der Weltgesundheitsorganistaion WHO. Weinheim, München: Juventa, S. 231–254.

Knipper, Michael; Bilgin, Yasar (2009): Migration und Gesundheit. Sankt Augustin: Konrad-Adenauer-Stiftung (Eine Veröffentlichung der Konrad-Adenauer-Stiftung e.V. und der Türkisch-Deutschen Gesundheitsstiftung e.V.).

Knipper, Michael; Bilgin, Yasar (2010): Medizin und Ethnisch-Kulturelle Vielfalt. Migration und andere Hintergründe. In: *Deutsches Ärzteblatt* 107 (3), S. 76–79.

Kolip, Petra (1997): Geschlecht und Gesundheit im Jugendalter. Die Konstruktion von Geschlechtlichkeit über somatische Kulturen. Opladen: Leske + Budrich.

Kolip, Petra (Hg.) (2000): Weiblichkeit ist keine Krankheit. Die Medikalisierung körperlicher Umbruchphasen im Leben von Frauen. Weinheim, München: Juventa.

Kolip, Petra; Klocke, Andreas; Melzer, Wolfgang; Ravens-Sieberer, Ulrike (Hg.) (2013): Gesundheit und Gesundeitsverhalten im Geschlechtervergleich. Ergebnisse des WHO-Jugendgesundheitssurvey „Health Behavior in School-Aged-Children". Weinheim, Basel: Juventa.

Kowalski, Christoph; Loss, Julika; Kölsch, Florian; Janssen, Christian (2014): Utilization of Prevention Services by Gender, Age, Socioeconomic Status, and Migration Status in Germany: An Overview and a Systematic Review. In: Christian Janssen, Enno Swart und Thomas von Lengerke (Hg.): Health Care Utilization in Germany, Bd. 74. New York, NY: Springer New York, S. 293–320.

Krais, Beate; Gebauer, Gunter (2002): Habitus. Bielefeld: transcript Verlag.

Kreckel, Reinhart (1993): Politische Soziologie sozialer Ungleichheit. Frankfurt am Main, New York: Campus.

Kristen, Cornelia; Dollmann, Jörg (2012): Migration und SChulerfolg: Zur Erklärung ungleicher Bildungsmuster. In: Michael Matzner (Hg.): Handbuch Migration und Bildung. Weinheim, München: Juventa, S. 102–117.

Kroll, Lars E. (2010): Sozialer Wandel, soziale Ungleichheit und Gesundheit. Die Entwicklung sozialer und gesundheitlicher Ungleichheiten in Deutschland zwischen 1984 und 2006. Wiesbaden: Springer VS.

Krönert-Othman, Susanne; Lenz, Ilse (2002): Geschlecht und Ethnizität bei Pierre Bourdieu. Kämpfe um Anerkennung und symbolische Regulation. In: Uwe H. Bittlingmayer, Rolf Eickelpasch, Jens Kastner und Claudia Rademacher (Hg.): Theorie als Kampf? Zur politischen Soziologie Pierre Bourdieus. Opladen: Leske + Budrich, S. 159–178.

Kronzer, Vanessa L. (2016): Screening for health literacy is not the answer. It's quicker and less stigmatizing to make all communication clearer. In: *BMJ (British Medical Journal)*, S. 1–2. https://doi.org/10.1136/bmj.i3699.

Krug, Susanne; Finger, Jonas D.; Lange, Cornelia; Richter, Almut; Mensink, Gert B. M. (2018): Sport- und Ernährungsverhalten bei Kindern und Jugendlichen in Deutschland. Querschnittsergebnisse aus KiGGS Welle 2 und Trends. In: *Journal of Health Monitoring* 3 (2), S. 3–22.

Krummenacher, Jörg (2017): Kanton St. Gallen verbietet Burka. In: *Neue Zürcher Zeitung*, 18.09.2017.

Kryspin-Exner, Ilse; Stetina, Sofianopoulou (Hg.) (2009): Gesundheit und Neue Medien. Psychologische Aspekte der Interaktion mit Informations- und Kommunikationstechnologien. 1. Aufl. s.l.: Springer Verlag Wien. Retrieved from https://site.ebrary.com/lib/alltitles/docDetail.action?docID=10355888.

Kuhlmann, Ellen (2016): Gendersensible Perspektiven auf Gesundheit und Gesundheitsversorgung. In: Matthias Richter und Klaus Hurrelmann (Hg.): Soziologie von Gesundheit und Krankheit. 1. Auflage. Wiesbaden: Springer VS (Lehrbuch), S. 183–196.

Kuhlmann, Ellen; Kolip, Petra (2008): Die „gemachten" Unterschiede – Geschlecht als Dimension gesundheitlicher Ungleichheit. In: Ullrich Bauer, Uwe H. Bittlingmayer und Matthias Richter (Hg.): Health Inequalities. Determinanten und Mechanismen gesundheitlicher Ungleichheit. 1. Aufl. Wiesbaden: VS Verl. für Sozialwiss (Gesundheit und Gesellschaft), S. 191–219.

Kühn, Hagen (1993): Healthismus. Eine Analyse der Präventionspolitik und Gesundheitsförderung in den U.S.A. Berlin: edition sigma.

Kuntz, Benjamin; Waldhauer, Julia; Zeiher, Johannes; Finger, Jonas D.; Lampert, Thomas (2018): Soziale Unterschiede im Gesundheitsverhalten von Kindern und Jugendlichen in Deutschland – Querschnittsergebnisse aus KiGGS Welle 2. In: *Journal of Health Monitoring* 3 (2), S. 45–63. DOI: https://doi.org/10.17886/RKI-GBE-2018-067.

Kutner, Mark; Greenberg, Elizabeth; Jin, Ying; Boyle, Bridget; Hsu, Yungchen; Eric Dunleavy (2007): Literacy in everyday life: Results from the 2003 National Assessment of Adult Literacy. National Center for Education Statistics. Washington (DC).

Kutscher, Nadia; Otto, Hans-Uwe (2010): Digitale Ungleichheit – Implikationen für die Betrachtung digitaler Jugendkulturen. In: Karl-Ulrich Hugger (Hg.): Digitale Jugendkulturen. Wiesbaden: Springer VS, S. 73–87.

Kymlicka, Will (Hg.) (2000): Multikulturalismus und Demokratie. Über Minderheiten in Staaten und Nationen. Frankfurt am Main, Wien: Büchergilde Gutenberg.

Kymlicka, Will (2013, cop. 2007): Multicultural odysseys. Navigating the new international politics of diversity. Repr. Oxford: Oxford University Press.

Laine, Marlene de (2000): Fieldwork, participation and practice. Ethics and dilemmas in qualitative research. London: Sage.

Lamnek, Siegfried (2005): Qualitative Sozialforschung. Weinheim/Basel: Beltz.

Lampert, T.; Koch-Gromus, U. (2016): Soziale Ungleichheit und Gesundheit. In: *Bundesgesundheitsblatt, Gesundheitsforschung, Gesundheitsschutz*, S. 151–152. Retrieved from https://link.springer.com/content/pdf/10.1007%2Fs00103-015-2306-3.pdf.

Lampert, T.; Kroll, Lars Eric (2010): Armut und Gesundheit. Robert Koch Institut. Retrieved from https://edoc.rki.de/bitstream/handle/176904/3090/29wYJ9AaKy3gU.pdf?sequence=1&isAllowed=y.

Lampert, Thomas (2016): Soziale Ungleichheit und Gesundheit. In: Matthias Richter und Klaus Hurrelmann (Hg.): Soziologie von Gesundheit und Krankheit. 1. Auflage. Wiesbaden: Springer VS (Lehrbuch), S. 121–138.

Lampert, Thomas; Hagen, Christine; Heizmann, Boris (2010): Gesundheitliche Ungleichheit bei Kindern und Jugendlichen in Deutschland. Berlin (Beiträge zur Gesundheitsberichterstattung des Bundes).

Lampert, Thomas; Kroll, Lars E.; Dunkelberg, Annalena (2007): Soziale Ungleichheit in der Lebenserwartung in Deutschland. In: *Aus Politik und Zeitgeschichte* B42/2007, S. 11–18.

Lampert, Thomas; Kuntz, Benjamin; KiGGS-Study Group (2015): Gesund aufwachsen – Welche Bedeutung kommt dem sozialen Status zu? Hg. v. Robert Koch-Institut (GBE kompakt 6 (1)).

Lampert, Thomas; Schenk, Liane (2004): Gesundheitliche Konsequenzen des Aufwachsens in Armut und sozialer Benachteiligung. In: Monika Jungbauer-Gans und Peter Kriwy (Hg.): Soziale Benachteiligung und Gesundheit bei Kindern und Jugendlichen. Wiesbaden: VS, S. 57–83.

Lange, Dirk; Polat, Ayça (Hg.) (2010): Migration und Alltag. Unsere Wirklichkeit ist anders. Schwalbach/Ts.: Wochenschau-Verl. (Reihe Politik und Bildung, 61). Retrieved from https://www.socialnet.de/rezensionen/isbn.php?isbn=978-3-89974-659-4.

Lareau, Annette (2003): Unequal Childhood. Class, Race, and Family Life. Berkeley, Los Angeles, London: University of Califormia Press.

Lareau, Annette (2006): Social Class Differences in Family-School Relationships: The Importance of Cultural Capital, last checked on 03.02.2018.

Lareau, Annette (2011): Unequal childhoods: class, race, and family life. 2nd edition, with an update a decade later. Berkeley/Los Angeles: University of California Press.

Lauterbach, K.; Lüngen, M.; Stollenwerk, B.; Gerber, A.; Klever-Deichert, G. (2006): Zum Zusammenhang zwischen Einkommen und Lebenserwartung. Forschungsberichte des Instituts für Gesundheitsökonomie und klinische Epidemiologie der Universität zu Köln. Köln (Studien zu Gesundheit, Medizin und Gesellschaft, 01/2006). Retrieved from https://gesundheitsoekonomie.uk-koeln.de/forschung/schriftenreihe-sgmg/2006-01_einkommen_und_rentenbezugsdauer.pdf, last checked on 04.09.2019.

Lawson, Clive (2010): Technology and the Extension of Human Capabilities. In: *Journal for the Theory of Social Behaviour* 40 (2), S. 207–223.

Lee, Shoou-Yih D.; Tsai, Tzu-I; Tsai, Yi-Wen; Kuo, Ken N. (2010): Health literacy, health status, and healthcare utilization of Taiwanese adults: results from a national survey. In: *BMC public health* 10, S. 614. https://doi.org/10.1186/1471-2458-10-614.

Leiß, Ottmar (2001): Ärztliche Weltbilder: Helicobaterisierung psychosomatischer Konzepte? In: *Deutsches Ärzteblatt*, S. 886–889.

Lenger, Alexander; Schneickert, Christian; Schumacher, Florian (Hg.) (2013): Pierre Bourdieus Konzept des Habitus. Grundlagen, Zugänge, Forschungsperspektiven. Wiesbaden: Springer VS.

Lessenich, Stephan (2013): Die Neuerfindung des Sozialen. Der Sozialstaat im flexiblen Kapitalismus. 3. Aufl. Bielefeld: transcript Verlag.

Levin-Zamir, Diane; Lemish, Dafna; Gofin, Rosa (2011): Media Health Literacy (MHL): development and measurement of the concept among adolescents. In: *Health Education Research* 26 (2), S. 323–335. DOI: https://doi.org/10.1093/her/cyr007.

Levin-Zamir, Diane; Leung, Angela Yee Man; Dodson, Sarity; Rowlands, Gillian (2017): Health literacy in selected populations: Individuals, families, and communities from the international and cultural perspective. In: *ISU* 37 (2), S. 131–151. DOI: https://doi.org/10.3233/ISU-170834.

Lin, H.; Sawyer, P.; Allman, R. P.; Kennedy, R. E.; Williams, C. P. (2014): he association between health literacy and medication selfmanagement in community-dwelling older adults. In: *Journal of the American Geriatrics Society* 62, S. 271.

Lin, Nan (1999): Building a network theory of social capital. In: *Connections* 22 (1), S. 28–51.

Lin, Nan (2017): Building a Network Theory of Social Capital. In: Nancy Lin, Karen Cook und Ronald S. Burt (Hg.): Social Capital. London: Routledge, S. 3–28.

Lincoln, Alisa; Paasche-Orlow, Michael K.; Cheng, Debbie M.; Lloyd-Travaglini, Christine; Caruso, Christine; Saitz, Richard; Samet, Jeffrey H. (2006): Impact of health literacy on depressive symptoms and mental health-related Quality of Life among adults with addiction. In: *Journal of General Internal Medicine* 21 (8), S. 818–822.

Liu, C.-H.; Liao, L.-L.; Shih, S.-F.; Chang, T.-C.; Osborne, R. H. (2014): Development and Implementation of Taiwan's child health literacy test. In: *Taiwan Journal of Public Health* 33 (3), S. 251–270. DOI: https://doi.org/10.6288/TJPH201433102105.

Lokhande, Mohini (2016): Doppelt benachteiligt? Kinder und Jugendliche mit Migrationshintergrund im deutschen Bildnugssystem. Eine expertise im Auftrag der Stuftung Mercator. Hg. v. Sachverständigenrat deutscher Stiftungen für Integration und Migration. Retrieved from https://www.stiftung-mercator.de/media/downloads/3_Publikationen/Expertise_Doppelt_benachteiligt.pdf.

Lüdke, Tilman (2017): Die deutsch-türkischen Beziehungen in historischer Perspektive. In: Wolfgang Gieler, Burak Gümüş und Yunus Yoldaş (Hg.): Deutsch-türkische Beziehungen. Historische, sektorale und migrationsspezifische Aspekte. 1st, New ed. Frankfurt a.M: Peter Lang GmbH Internationaler Verlag der Wissenschaften, S. 15–43.

Luft, Stefan (2014): Die Anwerbung türkischer Arbeitnehmer und ihre Folgen. Retrieved from https://www.bpb.de/internationales/europa/tuerkei/184981/gastarbeit.

Lyles, Courtney; Schillinger, Dean; Sarkar, Urmimala (2015): Cennecting the Dots: Health Information Technology Expansion and Health Disparities /Connecting the Dots: Health Information Technology Expansion and Health Disparities. In: *PLOS Medicine* 12 (7), S. 1–5. DOI: https://doi.org/10.1371/journal.pmed.1001852.

Mackert, Michael; Champlin, Sara; Su, Zhaohui; Guadagno, Marie (2015): The Many Health Literacies: Advancing Research or Fragmentation? In: *Health communication* 30 (12), S. 1161–1165. DOI: https://doi.org/10.1080/10410236.2015.1037422.

Mackert, Michael; Champlin, Sara E.; Holton, Avery; Muñoz, Isaac I.; Damásio, Manuel José (2014): eHealth and Health Literacy: A Research Methodology Review. In: *J Comput-Mediat Comm* 19 (3), S. 516–528. DOI: https://doi.org/10.1111/jcc4.12044.

Maier, Gunter; Felder-Puig, Rosemarie (2017): Gesundheitskompetenzen von Kindern und Jugendlichen. Herausforderungen und Überblick zum aktuellen Stand der Forschung.

Wien. Retrieved from https://www.ifgp.at/cdscontent/load?contentid=10008.649229&version=1518160812, last checked on 17.09.2019.

Maier, Ulrich (2012): Türkische „Gastarbeiterkinder" in den 1970er-Jahren. Verein türkischer Arbeitnehmer in Heilbronn forndern Schulklasssen für türkische Gastarbeiterkinder. Retrieved from https://www.landesarchiv-bw.de/sixcms/media.php/120/53803/Archivnachrichten_44_Quellen_43.pdf.

Mancuso, Carol A.; Rincon, Melina (2006): Impact of health literacy on longitudinal asthma outcomes. In: *Journal of General Internal Medicine* 21 (8), S. 813–817. DOI: https://doi.org/10.1111/j.1525-1497.2006.00528.x.

Mancuso, Josephine M. (2009): Assessment and measurement of health literacy: An integrative review of the literature. In: *Nursing and Health Sciences* 11 (1), S. 77–89. DOI: https://doi.org/10.1111/j.1442-2018.2008.00408.x.

Maneze, D., Salamonson, Y., Poudel, C., DiGiacomo, M., Everett, B., & Davidson, P. M. (2016). Health-Seeking Behaviors of Filipino Migrants in Australia: The Influence of Persisting Acculturative Stress and Depression. Journal of immigrant and minority health, 18(4), 779–786. https://doi.org/10.1007/s10903-015-0233-x

Manganello, Jennifer A. (2008): Health literacy and adolescents: a framework and agenda for future research. In: *Health Education Research* 23 (5), S. 840–847. DOI: https://doi.org/10.1093/her/cym069.

Mansel, Jürgen; Klocke, Andreas (Hg.) (1996): Die Jugend von heute e Selbstanspruch, Stigma und Wirklichkeit. Weinheim: Juventa (Jugendforschung).

Mantwill, Sarah; Monestel-Umaña, Silvia; Schulz, Peter J. (2015): The relationship between health literacy and health disparities: a systematic review. In: *PloS one* 10, S. 1–22. DOI: https://doi.org/10.1371/journal.pone.0145455.

Marcuse, Herbert (1968): Aggressivität in der gegenwärtigen Industriegesellschaft. In: Herbert Marcuse, Anatol Rapoport, Klaus Horn, Alexander Mitscherlich, Dieter Senghaas und Mihailo Marković (Hg.): Agression und Anpassung in der Industriegesellschaft. Frankfurt am Main: Suhrkamp, S. 7–29.

Marmot, Michael (2005): Social determinants of health inequalities. In: *The Lancet* 365, S. 1099–1104. DOI: https://doi.org/10.1016/S0140-6736(05)71146-6.

Marmot, Michael; Wilkinson, Richard G. (Hg.) (2006): Social determinants of health. Oxford: Oxford University Press.

Massey Philip M, Prelip Michael, Calimlim Brian M, Quiter Elaine S, Glik D Deborah C (2012). Contextualizing an expanded definition of health literacy among adolescents in the health care setting. Health Educ Res., 27:961–74. https://doi.org/10.1093/her/cys054.

Matischek-Jauk, Marlies; Krammer, Georg; Reicher, Hannelore (2017): The life-skills program Lions Quest in Austrian schools: implementation and outcomes. In: *Health promotion international* 33 (6), S. 1022–1032. DOI: https://doi.org/10.1093/heapro/dax050.

McCormack, Lauren; Bann, Carla; Squiers, Linda; Berkman, Nancy D.; Squire, Claudia; Schillinger, Dean et al. (2010): Measuring health literacy: a pilot study of a new skills-based instrument. In: *Journal of health communication* 15 Suppl 2, S. 51–71. DOI: https://doi.org/10.1080/10810730.2010.499987.

Mediendienst Integration (2018): Religion an Schulen. Islamischer Religionsunterricht in Deutschland; online available https://mediendienstintegration.de/fileadmin/Dateien/MDI_Informationspapier_islamischer_Religionsunterricht_April_2018.pdf

Megerlin, David Friedrich (1772): Die türkische Bibel, oder des Korans allererste teutsche Uebersetzung aus der Arabischen Urschrift selbst verfertiget welcher Nothwendigkeit und Nutzbarkeit in einer besondern Ankündigung hier erwiesen. Franckfurt am Mayn.

Mensing, Monika (2012): HLS-EU: Ergebnisse für Nordrhein-Westfalen. Landeszentrum Gesundheit Nordrhein-Westfalen. Bielefeld.

Merbach, Martin; Wittig, Ulla; Brähler, Elmar (2008): Angst und Depression polnischer und vietnamesischer MigrantInnen in Leipzig unter besonderer Berücksichtigung ihres Eingliederungsprozesses. In: *Psychotherapie, Psychosomatik, medizinische Psychologie* 58 (3–4), S. 146–154. DOI: https://doi.org/10.1055/s-2008-1067351.

Mergenthal, Karola (2014): Migrantinnen empowern! In: *Präv Gesundheitsf* 9 (1), S. 52–59. DOI: https://doi.org/10.1007/s11553-013-0415-0.

Merten, Sonja; Gari, Sara (2013): Die reproduktive Gesundheit der Migrationsbevölkerung in der Schweiz und anderen ausgewählten Aufnahmeländern. Basel: Swiss Tropical and Public Health Institute.

Messer, Melanie; Vogt, Dominique; Quenzel, Gudrun; Schaeffer, Doris (2015): Health Literacy bei Menschen mit Migrationshintergrund. In: *Public Health Forum* 23 (2), S. 71. https://doi.org/10.1515/pubhef-2015-0044.

Mielck, Andreas (2000): Soziale Ungleichheit und Gesundheit. Empirische Ergebnisse, Erklärungsansätze, Interventionsmöglichkeiten. Bern: Huber.

Mielck, Andreas (2005): Soziale Ungleichheit und Gesundheit. Eine Einführung in die aktuelle Diskussion. Bern: Huber.

Miller, Elizabeth; Lee, Jessica Y.; DeWalt, Darren A.; Vann, William F. (2010): Impact of caregiver literacy on children's oral health outcomes. In: *Pediatrics* 126 (1), S. 107–114. DOI: https://doi.org/10.1542/peds.2009-2887.

Milz, Kristina; Tuckermann, Anja (Hg.) (2018): Todesursache: Flucht. Eine unvollständige Liste. Berlin: Hirnkost.

Ministerium für Arbeit, Soziales, Gesundheit, Frauen und Familie Brandenburg (2018): Gender und Gesundheit. Retrieved from https://masgf.brandenburg.de/sixcms/detail.php/bb1.c.187234.de.

Mittelmark, Maurice B.; Bull, Torill; Bouwman, Laura (2017): The Handbook of Salutogenesis. Emerging Ideas Relevant to the Salutogenic Model of Health. Hg. v. Maurice B. Mittelmark, Shifra Sagy, Monica Eriksson, Georg F. Bauer, Jürgen M. Pelikan, Bengt Lindström und Geir Arild Espnes. Cham (CH).

Montesinos, Amanda Heredia; Bromand, Z.; Aichberger, M. C.; Temur-Erman, S.; Yesil, R.; Rapp, M. et al. (2010): Suizid und suizidales Verhalten bei Frauen mit türkischem Migrationshintergrund. In: *Zeitschrift für Psychiatrie, Psychologie und Psychotherapie*, S. 173–179. Retrieved from https://econtent.hogrefe.com/doi/pdf/10.1024/1661-4747.a000025.

Moussa, Jehane; Pecoraro, Marco (2013): Ecarts de genre dans l'état de santé des migrants et des migrantes en Suisse: Analyse sur la base d'une analyse des données du monitoring de santé des migrants GMM II. Swiss Forum for Migration and Population Studies. Neuchâtel.

mpfs – Medienpädagogischer Forschungsverbund Südwest (2018): JIM-Studie 2018. Jugend, Information, Medien. Basisuntersuchung zur Medienumgang 12- bis 19-Jähriger. Retrieved from https://www.mpfs.de/fileadmin/files/Studien/JIM/2018/Studie/JIM_2018_Gesamt.pdf, last checked on 31.07.2019.

Müller, Stefan (2011): Logik, Widerspruch und Vermittlung. Aspekte der Dialektik in den Sozialwissenschaften. Wiesbaden: VS Verlag für Sozialwissenschaften.

Mullins, Nicholas C. (1981): Ethnomethodologie: Das Spezialgebiet, das aus der Kälte kam. In: Wolf Lepenies (Hg.): Geschiche der Soziologie. 4 Bände. Frankfurt a.M.: Suhrkamp, S. 97–136.

Mürner, Christian; Sierck, Udo (2013): Behinderung. Chronik eines Jahrhunderts. Bonn: Bundeszentrale für politische Bildung.

Murphy, Peggy W.; Davis, Terry C.; Long, Sandra W.; Jackson, Robert H.; Decker, Barbara C. (1993): Rapid Estimate of Adult Literacy in Medicine (REALM): A quick reading test for patients. In: *Journal of Reading* 37 (2), S. 124–130. DOI: https://doi.org/10.2307/40033408.

Murray, T. Scott; Kirsch, Irwin S.; Jenkins, Lynn B. (1998): Adult literacy in OECD countries: Technical report on the first International Adult Literacy Survey. U.-S. Department of Education, National Center for Education Statistics. Washington (DC).

Nagel, Thomas (1990): Was bedeutet das alles? Eine ganz kurze Einführung in die Philosophie. Stuttgart: Reclam.

Navarra, Ann-Margaret; Neu, Natalie; Toussi, Sima; Nelson, John; Larson, Elaine L. (2014): Health literacy and adherence to antiretroviral therapy among HIV-infected youth. In: *The Journal of the Association of Nurses in AIDS Care: JANAC* 25 (3), S. 203–213. DOI: https://doi.org/10.1016/j.jana.2012.11.003.

Netzwerk Bildung + Gesundheit Schweiz (2019): Begriffsdefinitionen. Retrieved from https://www.bildungundgesundheit.ch/app/download/13280548824/Begriffsdefinitionen_psychische+Gesundheit.pdf?t=1503655498, zuletzt aktualisiert am 04.09.2019, last checked on 04.09.2019.

Neubauer, Jochen (2011): Türkische Deutsche, Kanakster und Deutschländer. Dissertation.

Ng, Edward; Omariba, Walter R. (2010): Health Literacy and immigrants in Canada: Determinants and effects on health outcomes. Retrieved from https://pdfs.semanticscholar.org/7f7d/78e6f2f0e183a02adee41ce1989a3fc2c714.pdf.

Nguyen, Tam H.; Paasche-Orlow, Michael K.; Kim, Miyong T.; Han, Hae-Ra; Chan, Kitty S. (2015): Modern Measurement Approaches to Health Literacy Scale Development and Refinement: Overview, Current Uses, and Next Steps. In: *Journal of health communication* 20 Suppl 2, S. 112–115. DOI: https://doi.org/10.1080/10810730.2015.1073408.

Nguyen, Tam H.; Paasche-Orlow, Michael K.; McCormack, Lauren A. (2017): The state of the science of health literacy measurement. In: *Information Services & Use* 37 (2), S. 189–203. DOI: https://doi.org/10.3233/ISU-170827.

Nideröst, Sibylle (2007): Männer, Körper und Gesundheit. Somatische Kultur und soziale Milieus bei Männern. Bern: Huber.

Nielsen-Bohlman, Lynn; Panzer, Allison M.; Kindig, David A. (Hg.) (2004a): Health Literacy: A Prescription to End Confusion. National Academies Press (US). Washington (DC), last checked on 14.04.2018.

Nielsen-Bohlman, Lynn; Panzer, Allison M.; Kindig, David A. (Hg.) (2004b): Health Literacy: A Prescription to End Confusion. National Academies Press (US). Washington (DC).

Nold, Daniela (2010): Sozioökonomischer Status von Schülerinnen und Schülern 2008. Ergebnisse des Mikrozensus. In: *Wirtschaft und Statistik*. Retrieved from https://www.destatis.de/DE/Publikationen/WirtschaftStatistik/BildungForschungKultur/StatusSchueler_22010.pdf?__blob=publicationFile.

Norman, Cameron D.; Skinner, Harvey A. (2006): eHealth Literacy: Essential Skills for Consumer Health in a Networked World. In: *Journal of medical Internet research* 8 (2), e9. DOI: https://doi.org/10.2196/jmir.8.2.e9.

Norman, Cameron D.; Skinner, Harvey A.; Jaffery, Jonathan; O'Boyle, Irene (2006): eHEALS: The eHealth Literacy Scale. In: *Journal of medical Internet research* 8 (4). https://doi.org/10.2196/jmir.8.4.e27.

Nussbaum, Martha C. (1999): Gerechtigkeit oder Das gute Leben. Frankfurt am Main: Suhrkamp (Gender Studies).

Nutbeam, Don (1998): Health promotion glossary. In: *Health promotion international* 13, S. 349–364.

Nutbeam D (2000). Health literacy as a public health goal: A challenge for contemporary health education and communication strategies into the 21st century. Health Promot Int., 15:259–67. https://doi.org/10.1093/heapro/15.3.259.

Nutbeam, Don (2008): The evolving concept of health literacy. In: *Social science & medicine (1982)* 67 (12), S. 2072–2078. https://doi.org/10.1016/j.socscimed.2008.09.050.

Nutbeam, Don (2009): Defining and measuring health literacy: what can we learn from literacy studies? In: *International journal of public health* 54, S. 303–305.

NZZ (2009): Zunehmende Empörung über Minarett-Verbot. In: *Neue Zürcher Zeitung*, 01.12.2009. Retrieved from https://www.nzz.ch/zunehmende_empoerung_ueber_minarett-verbot-1.4089840#register, last checked on 30.03.2020.

O Neill, Braden; Gonçalves, Daniela; Ricci-Cabello, Ignacio; Ziebland, Sue; Valderas, Jose (2014): An overview of self-administered health literacy instruments. In: *PloS one* 9 (12), e109110. DOI: https://doi.org/10.1371/journal.pone.0109110.

Obrist, Brigit; Büchi, Silvia (2008): Stress as an idiom for resilience: health and migration among sub-Saharan Africans in Switzerland. In: *Anthropology & medicine* 15 (3), S. 251–261. DOI: https://doi.org/10.1080/13648470802357596.

OECD (2018): International migration outlook 2018. Paris: OECD.

Oevermann, Ulrich (1983): Zur Sache. Die Bedeutung von Adornos methodologischem Selbstverständnis für die Begründung einer materialen soziologischen Strukturanalyse. In: Ludwig von Friedeburg und Jürgen Habermas (Hg.): Adorno-Konferenz 1983. Frankfurt a.M.: Suhrkamp, S. 234–289.

Oevermann, Ulrich (2010): Strukurprobleme supervisorischer Praxis. Eine objektiv hermeneutische Sequenzanalyse zur Überprüfung der Professionalisierungsthese. 3. Aufl. Frankfurt a.M.: Humanities Online.

Oeye, Christine; Bjelland, Anne Karen; Skorpen, Aina (2007): Doing participant observation in a psychiatric hospital -Research ethics resumed. In: *Social Science & Medicine* 65, S. 2296–2306. DOI: https://doi.org/10.1016/j.socscimed.2007.07.016.

Ohlbrecht, Heike; Schönberger, Christine (Hg.) (2010): Gesundheit als Familienaufgabe. Zum Verhältnis von Autonomie und staatlicher Intervention. Weinheim/München: Juventa.

Okan, O.; Bollweg, T. M.; Bröder, J.; Pinheiro, P.; Bauer, U. (2017a): Qualitative methods in health literacy research in young children. In: *The European Journal of Public Health* 27 (suppl_3). https://doi.org/10.1093/eurpub/ckx187.139.

Okan, Orkan (2019a): From Saranac Lake to Shanghai: A brief history of health literacy. In: Orkan Okan, Ullrich Bauer, Diane Levin-Zamir, Paulo Pinheiro und Kristine Sørensen

(Hg.): International Handbook of Health Literacy. Research, practice and policy across the lifespan. Bristol: POLICY Press, S. 21–37.

Okan, Orkan (2019b): The importance of early childhood in addressing equity and health literacy development in the life-course. In: *Public Health Panorama* 5 (2–3), S. 170–176.

Okan, Orkan; Bauer, Ullrich; Levin-Zamir, Diane; Pinheiro, Paulo; Sørensen, Kristine (Hg.) (2019a): International Handbook of Health Literacy. Research, practice and policy across the lifespan. Bristol: POLICY Press, last checked on 03.09.2019.

Okan, Orkan; Bröder, Janine; Pinheiro, Paulo; Bauer, Ullrich (2017b): Gesundheitsförderung und Health Literacy. In: Andreas Lange, Christine Steiner, Sabina Schutter und Herwig Reiter (Hg.): Handbuch Kindheits- und Jugendsoziologie. Living reference work, continuously updated edition. Wiesbaden: Springer (Springer Reference Sozialwissenschaften), S. 1–21.

Okan, Orkan; Pinheiro, P.; Zamora, P.; Bauer, U. (2015): Health Literacy bei Kindern und Jugendlichen. In: *Bundesgesundheitsblatt – Gesundheitsforschung – Gesundheitsschutz* 58 (9), S. 930–941. DOI: https://doi.org/10.1007/s00103-015-2199-1.

Okan, Orkan; Pinheiro, Paulo; Bauer, Ullrich (2019b): Gesundheit, gesundheitliche Ungleichheiten und die Rolle der Gesundheitskompetenz: Der Blick auf Kinder und Jugendliche. In: Pundt, Johanne: Cacace, Mirella und Gerd G. Wagner (Hg.): Diversität und gesundheitliche Chancengleichheit. Bremen: Appollon University Press, S. 61–98.

Önder, Tunay (2018): Wenn "unsere Türken" wählen gehen. Deutschlandfunk Kultur; online available https://www.deutschlandfunkkultur.de/parlamentswahl-inder-tuerkei-wenn-unsere-tuerken-waehlen.1005.de.html?dram:article_id=420864

Organisation for Economic Co-operation and Development (2018): The Resilience of Students with an Immigrant Background. Factors that Shape Well-being. Paris: OECD Publishing.

Orkan, Okan; Lopes, Ester; Bollweg, Torsten M.; Bröder, Janine; Messer, Melanie; Bruland, Dirk et al. (2018): Generic health literacy measurement instruments for children and adolescents: a systematic review of the literature. In: *BMC public health* 18 (1), S. 166. https://doi.org/10.1186/s12889-018-5054-0.

Ormshaw, Michael J.; Paakkari, Leena T.; Kannas, Lasse K. (2013): Measuring child and adolescent health literacy: a systematic review of literature. In: *Health Education* 113 (5), S. 433–455. DOI: https://doi.org/10.1108/HE-07-2012-0039.

Osipov, Igor; Gerdes, Jürgen; Bittlingmayer, Uwe H.; Okcu, Gözde (2017): Die Entwicklung von Life Skills im Schuljahresverlauf. Wirksamkeitsevaluation des schulischen Life Skills-Förderungsprogramms Lions-Quest „Erwachsen werden“ in der 5. Klassenstufe allgemeinbildender Schulen. Eine Auswertung der ersten beiden Erhebungswellen im Projekt „Zur Evidenzbasierung in der schulischen Gesundheitsförderung, Primärprävention und inklusiven Beschulung“ (EGePriB). Institut für Soziologie. Freiburg.

Otyakmaz, Berrin Özlem; Karakaşoğlu, Yasemin (Hg.) (2015): Frühe Kindheit in der Migrationsgesellschaft. Wiesbaden: Springer Fachmedien Wiesbaden.

Paakkari Lena, Paakkari Olli (2012). Health literacy as a learning outcome in schools. Health Educ. 2012;112:133–52. https://doi.org/10.1108/09654281211203411.

Paakkari, Leena (2015): Three Approaches to School Health Education as a Means to Higher Levels of Health Literacy. In: Venka Simovska und Patricia Mannix McNamara (Hg.): Schools for Health and Sustainability. Dordrecht: Springer Netherlands, S. 275–289.

Paakkari, Leena T.; George, Shanti (2018): Ethical underpinnings for the development of health literacy in schools: ethical premises ('why'), orientations ('what') BMC. In: *BMC public health*, S. 1–10. https://doi.org/10.1186/s12889-018-5224-0.

Paakkari, Leena T.; Torppa, Minna P.; Paakkari, Olli-Pekka; Välimaa, Raili S.; Ojala, Kristiina S.A.; Tynjälä, Jorma A. (2019a): Does health literacy explain the link between structural stratifiers and adolescent health? In: *European Journal of Public Health*, S. 1–6. https://doi.org/10.1093/eurpub/ckz011.

Paakkari, Leena T.; Torppa, Minna P.; Paakkari, Olli-Pekka; Välimaa, Raili S.; Ojala, Kristiina S.A.; Tynjälä, Jorma A. (2019b): Does health literacy explain the link between structural stratifiers and edolescent health? In: *European Journal of Public Health*, S. 1–6. https://doi.org/10.1093/eurpub/ckz011.

Paakkari, Olli; Torppa, Minna; Villberg, Jari; Kannas, Lasse; Paakkari, Leena (2018): Subjective health literacy among school-aged children. In: *Health Education* 118 (2), S. 182–195. DOI: https://doi.org/10.1108/HE-02-2017-0014.

Paakkari, Olli-Pekka; Torppa, Minna; Kannas, Lasse K.; Paakkari, Leena (2016): Subjective health literacy: Development of a brief instrument for school-aged children. In: *Scandinavian journal of public health* 44, S. 751–757.

Papen, Uta (2005): Adult Literacy as Social Practice: More Than Skills: Taylor & Francis. Retrieved from https://books.google.de/books?id=y5XpAGcFweoC.

Papen, Uta (2008): Literature review: Understanding literacy and health, last checked on 14.06.2018.

Papen, Uta (2009): Literacy, Learning and Health – A social practices view of health literacy. In: *Literacy & Numeracy Studies* 16/17 (2/1), S. 19–34.

Parikh, Nina S.; Parker, Ruth M.; Nurss, Joanne R.; Baker, David W.; Williams, Mark V. (1996): Shame and health literacy: the unspoken connection. In: *Patient Education and Counseling* 27 (1), S. 33–39. DOI: https://doi.org/10.1016/0738-3991(95)00787-3.

Parker, Melissa; Harper, Ian (2006): The anthropology of public health. In: *Journal of biosocial science* 38 (1), S. 1–5. DOI: https://doi.org/10.1017/S0021932005001148.

Parker, R. M.; Ratzan, S. C.; Lurie, N. (2003): Health Literacy. A Policy Challenge For Advancing High-Quality Health Care. In: *Health Affairs* 22 (4), S. 147–153. https://doi.org/10.1377/hlthaff.22.4.147.

Parker, Ruth M.; Baker, David W.; Williams, Mark V.; Nurss, Joanne R. (1995): The test of functional health literacy in adults. In: *J GEN INTERN MED* 10 (10), S. 537–541. DOI: https://doi.org/10.1007/BF02640361.

Pauer-Studer, Herlinde (1999): Einleitung. In: Nussbaum, Martha C. Gerechtigkeit oder Das gute Leben. Frankfurt a.M.: Suhrkamp, S. 7–23.

Pecoraro, Marco; Fibbi, Rosita (2010): Highly skilled migrants in the Swiss labour market, with a special focus on migrants from developing countries. In: Gabriela Tejada und Jean-Claude Bolay (Hg.): Scientific diasporas as development partners. Skilled migrants from Colombia, India and South Africa in Switzerland: empirical evidence and policy responses. Bern: Peter Lang, S. 179–195.

Pelikan, J. M.; Röthlin, Florian; Ganahl, Kristin (2012a): Anhang: Die Gesundheitskompetenz der österreichischen Bevölkerung – nach Bundesländern und im internationalen Vergleich. Abschlussbericht der Österreichischen Gesundheitskompetenz (Health Literacy) Bundesländer-Studie. LBIHPR Forschungsbericht. PBIHR. Wien.

Retrieved from https://www.hauptverband.at/cdscontent/load?contentid=10008.597349&version=1395738801.

Pelikan, Jürgen; Röthlin, Florian; Ganahl, Kristin (2012b): Comparative report of health literacy in eigth EU member states. The European Health Literacy Survey HLS-EU. Retrieved from https://ec.europa.eu/chafea/documents/news/Comparative_report_on_health_literacy_in_eight_EU_member_states.pdf.

Pelikan, Jürgen M.; Ganahl, Kristin; van den Broucke, Stephan; Sørensen, Kristine (2019): Measuring health literacy in Europe: Introducing the European Health Literacy Survey Questionnaire (HLS-EU-Q). In: Orkan Okan, Ullrich Bauer, Diane Levin-Zamir, Paulo Pinheiro und Kristine Sørensen (Hg.): International Handbook of Health Literacy. Research, practice and policy across the lifespan. Bristol: POLICY Press, S. 115–138.

Perren-Klingler, Gisela (2000): Refugees: Assistance in a world full of dilemmas: some Swiss experience, last checked on 03.05.2018.

Perrig-Chiello, Pasqualina; Höpflinger, François (Hg.) (2003): Gesundheitsbiographien. Variationen und Hintergründe. Bern: Huber.

Peters, Bernhard (1993): Die Integration moderner Gesellschaften. Frankfurt am Main: Suhrkamp.

Peters, E.; Pritzkuleit, R.; Beske, F.; Katalinic, A. (2010): Demografischer Wandel und Krankheitshäufigkeiten. Eine Projektion bis 2050. In: *Bundesgesundheitsblatt, Gesundheitsforschung, Gesundheitsschutz* 53 (5), S. 417–426. Retrieved from https://link.springer.com/article/10.1007%2Fs00103-010-1050-y.

Peterson, Pamela N.; Shetterly, Susan M.; Clarke, Christina L.; Bekelman, David B.; Chan, Paul S.; Allen, Larry A.; Daniel D. Matlock, David J. Magid, and Frederick A. Masoudi (2011): Health literacy and outcomes among patients with heart failure. In: *JAMA: The Journal of the American Medical Association* 305 (16), S. 1665–1701.

Pickett, Kate E.; Wilkinson, Richard G. (2015): Income inequality and health: a causal review. In: *Social science & medicine (1982)* 128, S. 316–326. DOI: https://doi.org/10.1016/j.socscimed.2014.12.031.

Pinheiro, Paulo (2019): Future avenues for health literacy: Learning from literacy and literacy learning. In: Orkan Okan, Ullrich Bauer, Diane Levin-Zamir, Paulo Pinheiro und Kristine Sørensen (Hg.): International Handbook of Health Literacy. Research, practice and policy across the lifespan. Bristol: POLICY Press, S. 555–571.

Pinheiro, P, George S, Okan O, Sijthoff E, Bittlingmayer UH, Kahlert R, Merchant A, Bruland D, Bröder J, Bauer U (2021): Towards new perspectives on health literacy for children: From 'health information' to recognizing young citizens' capacities for meaning-making (Debate from a 'liquid network'). In: Saboga-Nunes, L.A., Bittlingmayer, U.H., Okan, O., Sahrai, D. (eds) New Approaches to Health Literacy. Gesundheit und Gesellschaft. Springer VS, Wiesbaden. New Approaches to Health Literacy: Linking Different Perspectives, 145–166. https://doi.org/10.1007/978-3-658-30909-1_8

Pitt, Ruth; Davis, Terry; Manganello, Jennifer; Massey, Phillip; Okan, Orkan; McFarlane, Elizabeth et al. (2019): Health literacy in a social context: A meta-narrative review. In: Orkan Okan, Ullrich Bauer, Diane Levin-Zamir, Paulo Pinheiro und Kristine Sørensen (Hg.): International Handbook of Health Literacy. Research, practice and policy across the lifespan. Bristol: POLICY Press, S. 665–703.

Pleasant, Andrew (2014): Advancing health literacy measurement: a pathway to better health and health system performance. In: *Journal of health communication* 19 (12), S. 1481–1496. DOI: https://doi.org/10.1080/10810730.2014.954083.

Pleasant, Andrew; Maish, Caitlin; O'Leary, Catina; Carmona, Richard H. (2018): A theory-based self-report measure of health literacy: The Calgary Charter of Health Literacy Scale. In: *Methodological Innovations* (1–9). https://doi.org/10.1177/2059799118814394.

Pleasant, Andrew; McKinney, Julie (2011): Coming to consensus on health literacy measurement: an online discussion and consensus-gauging process. In: *Nursing outlook* 59 (2), 95–106.e1. DOI: https://doi.org/10.1016/j.outlook.2010.12.006.

Pleasant, Andrew; Rikard, R. V. (2013): A Prescription Is Not Enough- Improving Public Health with Health Literacy, last checked on 31.08.2018.

Polaschegg, Andrea (2005): Der andere Orientalismus. Regeln deutsch-morgenländischer Imagination im 19. Jahrhundert. Berlin: W. De Gruyter (Quellen und Forschungen zur Literatur- und Kulturgeschichte, 35 (269)). Retrieved from https://site.ebrary.com/lib/uniregensburg/Doc?id=10597715.

Popp, Maximilian; Schmitz, Charlotte (2016): Flüchtlingsdeal mit der Türkei. Europas Türsteher. Retrieved from https://www.spiegel.de/politik/ausland/fluechtlinge-in-der-tuerkei-gescheitert-an-europas-tuersteher-a-1074744.html.

Powell, Caroline K.; Hill, Elizabeth G.; Clancy, Dawn E. (2007): The relationship between health literacy and diabetes knowledge and readiness to take health actions. In: *The Diabetes educator* 33 (1), S. 144–151. DOI: https://doi.org/10.1177/0145721706297452.

Prüss-Üstün, Annette; Stein, Claudia; Zeeb, Hajo (2006): Globale Krankheitslast: Daten, Trends und Methoden. In: Razum. Oliver, Hajo Zeeb und Ulrich Laaser (Hg.): Globalisierung – Gerechtigkeit – Gesundheit. Einführung in International Public Health. Bern: Huber, S. 27–42.

Quenzel, G.; Vogt, D.; Schaeffer, D. (2016a): Unterschiede der Gesundheitskompetenz von Jugendlichen mit niedriger Bildung, Älteren und Menschen mit Migrationshintergrund. In: *Gesundheitswesen (Bundesverband der Arzte des Offentlichen Gesundheitsdienstes (Germany))* 78 (11), S. 708–710. https://doi.org/10.1055/s-0042-113605.

Quenzel, Gudrun; Schaeffer, Doris; Messer, Melanie; Vogt, Dominique (2015): Gesundheitskompetenz bildungsferner Jugendlicher. Einflussfaktoren und Folgen. In: *Bundesgesundheitsblatt*, S. 951–957.

Quenzel, Gudrun; Schaeffer, Doris; Messer, Melanie; Vogt, Dominique (2016b): Health Literacy – Gesundheitskompetenz vulnerabler Bevölkerungsgruppen. Ergebnisbericht. Retrieved from https://www.uni-bielefeld.de/gesundhw/ag6/publikationen/QuenzelSchaeffer_GesundheitskompetenzVulnerablerGruppen_Ergebnisbericht_2016.pdf, last checked on 21.03.2018.

Rademacher, Claudia; Wiechens, Peter (Hg.) (2001): Geschlecht – Ethnizität – Klasse. Zur sozialen Konstruktion von Hierarchie und Differenz. Opladen: Leske + Budrich.

Rager, Günther; Sehl, Annika (2008): Chats, Videos und Communities. Wie Jugendliche das Internet nutzen. Berlin: Friedrich Ebert Stiftung., Stabsabt (Medien digital, 8).

Rashid, Ahmed (2010): Taliban. Afghanistans Gotteskämpfer und der neue Krieg am Hindukusch. Bonn: Bundeszentrale für politische Bildung.

Rathmann, Katharina (2015): Bildungssystem, Wohlfahrtsstaat und gesundheitliche Ungleichheit. Ein internationaler Vergleich für das Jugendalter. Wiesbaden: Springer VS.

Ravens-Sieberer, Ulrike; Ehrhart, Michael; Ottová-Jordan, Veronika (2018): Prävention und Gesundheitsförderung im Kinderalter. In: Klaus Hurrelmann, Matthias Richter, Theodor Klotz und Stephanie Stock (Hg.): Referenzwerk Prävention und Gesundheitsförderung. Grundlagen, Konzepte und Umsetzungsstrategien. 5., vollst. überarb. Aufl. Göttingen: Hogrefe, S. 75–88.

Ravens-Sieberer, Ulrike; Erhart, Michael (2008): Die Beziehung zwischen sozialer Ungleichheit und Gesundheit im Kindes- und Jugendalter. In: Matthias Richter, Klaus Hurrelmann, Andreas Klocke, Wolfgang Melzer und Ulrike Ravens-Sieberer (Hg.): Gesundheit, Ungleichheit und jugendliche Lebenswelten. Ergebnisse der zweiten internationalen Vergleichsstudie im Auftrag der Weltgesundheitsorganistaion WHO. Weinheim, München: Juventa, S. 38–62.

Rawls, John (1979): Eine Theorie der Gerechtigkeit. Frankfurt am Main: Suhrkamp.

Razum, Oliver (2006): Migration, Mortalität und der Healthy-migrant-Effekt. In: Matthias Richter und Klaus Hurrelmann (Hg.): Gesundheitliche Ungleichheit. Grundlagen, Probleme, Perpektiven. Wiesbaden: Springer VS, S. 255–270.

Razum, Oliver; Spallek, Jacob (2009): Wie gesund sind Migranten? Retrieved from https://focus-migration.hwwi.de/typo3_upload/groups/3/focus_Migration_Publikationen/Kurzdossiers/KD_12_Migranten_Gesundheit.pdf, last checked on 03.02.2018.

Razum, Oliver; Spallek, Jacob; Zeeb, Hajo (2011): Migration und Gesundheit. In: Thomas Schott und Claudia Hornberg (Hg.): Die Gesellschaft und ihre Gesundheit. Wiesbaden: VS Verlag für Sozialwissenschaften, S. 555–574.

Razum, Oliver; Zeeb, Hajo; Meesmann Uta; Schenk Liana; Bredehorst Maren; Brzoska Patrick et al. (2008): Schwerpunktbericht der Gesundheitsberichtserstattung des Bundes. Migration und Gesundheit. Retrieved from https://www.rki.de/DE/Content/Gesundheitsmonitoring/Gesundheitsberichterstattung/GBEDownloadsT/migration.pdf;jsessionid=2043830C46BF97A8FD32E2D2B7B96389.2_cid372?__blob=publicationFile.

Reckwitz, Andrea (2003): Grundelemente einer Theorie sozialer Praktiken. Eine sozialtheoretische Perspektive. In: *Zeitschrift für Soziologie* 32 (4), S. 282–301. Retrieved from https://www.zfs-online.org/index.php/zfs/article/viewFile/1137/674.

Regitz-Zagrosek, Vera (2018): Gesundheit, Krankheit und Geschlecht. Bundeszentrale für politische Bildung. Retrieved from https://www.bpb.de/apuz/270310/gesundheit-krankheit-und-geschlecht?p=all.

Reichmayr, J. (2003). Ethnopsychoanalyse: Geschichte, Konzepte, Anwendungen. Psychosozial-Verlag.

Reich, Helmut (2003): Spiritualität, Religiösität und Gesundheit. In: *Forsch Komplementärmed Klass Naturheilkd* (10), S. 269–275. Retrieved from https://www.karger.com/Article/Pdf/74782.

Riaño, Yvonne (2003): Migration of skilled Latin American women to Switzerland and their struggle for integration. In: Mutsuo Yamada (Hg.): Emigración latinoamericana: Comparación interregional entre América del Norte, Europa y Japón. Osaka: The Japan Centre for Area Studies.

Riaño, Yvonne (2007): Migración de mujeres latinoamericanas universitarias a Suiza. Geografías migratorias, motivos de migración y cuestiones de género. In: Claudio

Bolzman, Myrian Carbajal und Giuditta Mainardi (Hg.): La Suisse au rythme latino. Dynamiques migratoires des Latino-américains: logiques d'action, vie quotidienne, pistes d'intervention sociales et de santé. Genève: Editions IES.

Riaño, Yvonne (2011a): Barrieren aufbrechen: Erfahrungen und Strategien von qualifizierten Migrantinnen beim Zugang zum Schweizer Arbeitsmark. In: Deutsche Akademie für Landeskunde e.V (Hg.): Berichte zur deutschen Landeskunde. Leipzig, S. 25–48.

Riaño, Yvonne (2011b): Drawing new boundaries of participation: experiences and strategies of economic citizenship among skilled migrant women in Switzerland. In: *Environment and Planning A* 43, S. 1530–1546. DOI: https://doi.org/10.1068/a4374.

Riaño, Yvonne (2012): The invisibility of family in studies of skilled migration and brain drain. In: *Diversities* 14, S. 25–44.

Riaño, Yvonne; Baghdadi, Nadia (2007): Je pensais que je pourrais avoir une relation plus égalitaire avec un Européen. Le rôle du genre et des imaginaires géographiques dans la migration des femmes. In: *Nouvelles Questions Féministes* 26, S. 38–53. DOI: https://doi.org/10.3917/nqf.261.0038.

Richter, Matthias (2005): Gesundheit und Gesundheitsverhalten im Jugendalter. Der Einfluss sozialer Ungleichheit. Wiesbaden: VS Verlag für Sozialwissenschaften.

Richter, Matthias (2008): Soziale Determinanten der Gesundheit im Spannungsfeld zwischen Ungleichheit und jugendlichen Lebenswelten: Der WHO-Jugendgesundheitssurvey. In: Matthias Richter, Klaus Hurrelmann, Andreas Klocke, Wolfgang Melzer und Ulrike Ravens-Sieberer (Hg.): Gesundheit, Ungleichheit und jugendliche Lebenswelten. Ergebnisse der zweiten internationalen Vergleichsstudie im Auftrag der Weltgesundheitsorganistaion WHO. Weinheim, München: Juventa, S. 9–37.

Richter, Matthias; Hurrelmann, Klaus (Hg.) (2006a): Gesundheitliche Ungleichheit. Grundlagen, Probleme, Perpektiven. Wiesbaden: Springer VS.

Richter, Matthias; Hurrelmann, Klaus (2006b): Gesundheitliche Ungleichheit: Ausgangsfragen und Herausforderungen. In: Matthias Richter und Klaus Hurrelmann (Hg.): Gesundheitliche Ungleichheit. Grundlagen, Probleme, Perpektiven. Wiesbaden: Springer VS, S. 11–31.

Richter, Matthias; Hurrelmann, Klaus; Klocke, Andreas; Melzer, Wolfgang; Ravens-Sieberer, Ulrike (Hg.) (2008): Gesundheit, Ungleichheit und jugendliche Lebenswelten. Ergebnisse der zweiten internationalen Vergleichsstudie im Auftrag der Weltgesundheitsorganistaion WHO. Weinheim, München: Juventa.

Riedesser, P. (1973): Psychische Störungen bei ausländischen Arbeitern in der Bundesrepublik Deutschland. In: *Medizinische Klinik* 70 (21), S. 954–959.

Riegel, Christine (2012): Intersektionalität und Jugendforschung.

Riegel, Christine; Scherr, Albert; Stauber, Barbara (Hg.) (2010): Transdisziplinäre Jugendforschung. Grundlagen und Forschungskonzepte. 1. Aufl. Wiesbaden: VS Verlag für Sozialwissenschaften.

Rieger-Ladich, Markus; Grabau, Christian (Hg.) (2017): Pierre Bourdieu: Pädagogische Lektüren. Wiesbaden: Springer VS.

Ritsert, Jürgen (1997): Kleines Lehrbuch der Dialektik. Darmstadt: Wissenschaftliche Buchgesellschaft.

Ritsert, Jürgen (2017): Summa Dialectica. Ein Lehrbuch zur Dialektik. Weinheim, Basel: Beltz Juventa.

RKI (2008): Migration und Gesundheit. Berlin (Gesundheitsberichterstattung des Bundes). Retrieved from https://www.rki.de/DE/Content/Gesundheitsmonitoring/Gesundheitsberichterstattung/GBEDownloadsT/migration.pdf?__blob=publicationFile, last checked on 03.09.2019.

RKI (2009): Lebensphasenspezifische Gesundheit von Kindern und Jugendlichen in Deutschland. Retrieved from https://www.rki.de/DE/Content/Gesundheitsmonitoring/Gesundheitsberichterstattung/GBEDownloadsB/KiGGS_SVR.pdf?__blob=publicationFile.

RKI (2016): Schwerpunktthema Gesundheit von Migranten und Geflüchteten. Retrieved from https://www.rki.de/DE/Content/Service/Presse/Pressemitteilungen/2016/08_2016.html, zuletzt aktualisiert am 03.02.2018, last checked on 03.02.2018.

Robards, Fiona; Kang, Melissa; Usherwood, Tim; Sanci, Lena (2018): How Marginalized Young People Access, Engage With, and Navigate Health-Care Systems in the Digital Age: Systematic Review. In: *Journal of Adolescent Health* 62, S. 365–381. DOI: https://doi.org/10.1016/j.jadohealth.2017.10.018.

Robert Koch-Institut (RKI) (2015): GBE kompakt 1–2015 Gesund aufwachsen – Welche Bedeutung kommt dem sozialen Status zu – PDF UA. Retrieved from https://www.rki.de/DE/Content/Gesundheitsmonitoring/Gesundheitsberichterstattung/GBEDownloadsK/2015_1_gesund_aufwachsen.pdf?__blob=publicationFile, last checked on 08.03.2019.

Robinson, Christie; Graham, Joy (2010): Perceived Internet health literacy of HIV-positive people through the provision of a computer and Internet health education intervention. In: *Health information and libraries journal* 27 (4), S. 295–303. DOI: https://doi.org/10.1111/j.1471-1842.2010.00898.x.

Rosenbaum, Sara; Shin, Peter; DeBuono, Barbara (2007): Achieving Family Health Literacy: The Case for Insuring Children. Retrieved from https://hsrc.himmelfarb.gwu.edu/cgi/viewcontent.cgi?referer=https://scholar.google.de/&httpsredir=1&article=1232&context=sphhs_policy_facpubs.

Rosenbrock, Rolf (2005): Public Health – Politische Anforderungen zur Überwindung sozial bedingter Ungleichheit von Gesundheitschancen bei Kindern und Jugendlichen. Berlin.

Rosenbrock, Rolf (2015a): Prävention in Lebenswelten – der Setting-Ansatz. In: *Zeitschrift für Allgemeinmedizin* 91, S. 213–219. DOI: https://doi.org/10.3238/zfa.2015.0213-0219.

Rosenbrock, Rolf (2015b): Stellungnahme in der Podiumsdiskussion: Gesundheitspolitik für gesunde Wahrmöglichkeiten – Partnerschaften für die Gesundheitsbildung. European Health Forum Gastein, 08.10.2015.

Rosenthal, Gabriele; Loch, Ulrike (2002): Das narrative Interview. In: Doris Schaeffer und Gabriele Müller-Mundt (Hg.): Qualitative Gesundheits- und Pflegeforschung. Bern: Huber, S. 221–232.

Ross, R. D. (2001): Medical management of chronic heart failure in children 1 (1), S. 37–44.

Rother, Nina; Brücker, Herbert; Schupp, Jürgen (Hg.) (2016): IAB-BAMF-SOEP-Befragung von Geflüchteten: Überblick und erste Ergebnisse. Stand: 15.11.2016. Nürnberg: Bundesamt für Migration und Flüchtlinge (Forschungsbericht, 29).

Röthlin, Florian; Pelikan, Jürgen M.; Ganahl, Kristin (2013): Die Gesundheitskompetenz von 15-jährigen Jugendlichen in Österreich. Abschlussbericht der österreichischen Gesundheitskompetenz Jugendstudie im Auftrag des Hauptverbands der österreichischen Sozialversicherungsträger. Wien. Retrieved from https://www.hauptverband.at/

cdscontent/load?contentid=10008.597350&version=1395738807, last checked on 18.03.2019.

Rothman, Russell L.; Yin, H. Shonna; Mulvaney, Shelagh; Co, John Patrick T.; Homer, Charles; Lannon, Carole (2009): Health literacy and quality: focus on chronic illness care and patient safety. In: *Pediatrics* 124 Suppl 3, S 315–26. DOI: https://doi.org/10.1542/peds.2009-1163H.

Rubene, Zanda; Stars, Inese; Goba, Liva (2015): Health Literate Child: Transforming Teaching in School Health Education. In: *Society. Integration. Education* 1. https://doi.org/10.17770/sie2015voll.314.

Rudd, Rima; Epstein Anderson, Jennie; Oppenheimer Sarah; Nath, Charlotte (2007): Health Literacy: An Update of Medical and Public Health Literature. Retrieved from https://cdn1.sph.harvard.edu/wp-content/uploads/sites/135/2012/09/rudd_et_al_2007_hl_literature_review.pdf, last checked on 05.04.2018.

Rudd, Rima; Kirsch, Irwin S.; Yamamoto, Kentaro (2004): Literacy and Health in America. Policy Information Report. Educational Testing Service. Princeton, NJ.

Saboga-Nunes, Luis; Bittlingmayer, Uwe H.; Okan, Orkan (2019): Salutogenesis and health literacy: The health promotion simplex! In: Orkan Okan, Ullrich Bauer, Diane Levin-Zamir, Paulo Pinheiro und Kristine Sørensen (Hg.): International Handbook of Health Literacy. Research, practice and policy across the lifespan. Bristol: POLICY Press, S. 649–664.

Sahrai, Diana (2009): Healthy Migrants oder besondere Risikogruppe? Zur Schwierigkeit des Verhältnisses von Ethnizität, Migration, Sozialstruktur und Gesundheit*. In: *Jahrbuch für Kritische Medizin und Gesundheitswissenschaften* Bd. 45, S. 70–94.

Sahrai, Diana (2010a): Differenz in der Wahrnehmung präventiver Angebote und von Elternpartizipation im Setting Kita. Eine Analyse der Wechselwirkung schicht-und migrationsspezifischer Einflüsse. Retrieved from https://pub.uni-bielefeld.de/download/2304725/2304728.

Sahrai, Diana (2010b): Differenzen in der Wahrnehmung präventiver Angebote und von Elternpartizipation im Setting Kita. Eine Analyse der Wechselwirkung schicht- und migrationsspezifischer Einflüsse. Unveröffentlichte Dissertation an der Fakultät für Gesundheitswissenschaften der Universität Bielefeld. Bielefeld: Fakultät für Gesundheitswissenschaften.

Sahrai, Diana (2010c): Differenzen in der Wahrnehmung präventiver Angebote und von Elternpartizipation im Setting Kita. Eine Analyse der Wechselwirkung schicht- und migrationsspezifischer Einflüsse. Universität Bielefeld.

Sahrai, Diana; Gerdes, Jürgen; Drucks, Stephan; Tuncer, Hidayet (2011): Eine Typologie des funktionalen Analphabetismus. Strukturelle Bestimmungen und notwendige Differenzierungen zur Analyse einer schwer greifbaren und heterogenen Zielgruppe. In: Projektträger im DLR e.V. (Hg.): Zielgruppen in Alphabetisierung und Grundbildung Erwachsener. Bestimmung, Verortung, Ansprache. Bielefeld: Bertelsmann, S. 33–58.

Sahrai, Omar Khaled (2018): Ethnizität, Widerstand und politische Legitimation in pashtunischen Stammesgebieten Afghanistans und Pakistans. Berlin: Peter Lang.

Saito, Mamiko (2009): Searching For My Homeland: Dilemmas Between Borders. Experiences of youung Afghans returning "home" from Pakistan and Iran. AREU Synthesis Paper. Kabul. Retrieved from https://pdfs.semanticscholar.org/38fd/

48932bd6b2f5093fccacfdb1322dea99dc7d.pdf?_ga=2.265662155.57688066.1570330542-1788618260.1567589305, last checked on 06.10.2019.

Samerski, Silja (2019): Health Literacy as a social practice: Social and empirical dimensions of knowledge on health and healthcare. in press. In: *Social Science & Medicine* 81, S. 1–26.

Sanders, Lee M.; Robinson, Thomas N.; Forster, Lourdes Q.; Plax, Katie; Brosco, Jeffrey P.; Brito, Arturo (2005): Evidence-based community pediatrics: building a bridge from bedside to neighborhood. In: *Pediatrics* 115 (4 Suppl), S. 1142–1147. DOI: https://doi.org/10.1542/peds.2004-2825H.

Sanders, Lee M.; Shaw, Judith S.; Guez, Ghislaine; Baur, Cynthia; Rudd, Rima (2009): Health literacy and child health promotion: implications for research, clinical care, and public policy. In: *Pediatrics* 124 Suppl 3, S306–14. DOI: https://doi.org/10.1542/peds.2009-1162G.

Sarkar, Urmimala; Fisher, L.; SCHILLINGER, DEAN (2006): Is self-efficacy associated with diabetes self-management across race/ethnicity and health literacy? In: *Diabetes Care* 29 (4), S. 823–829.

Sauer, Martina (2007): Perspektiven des Zusammenlebens: die Integration türkischstämmiger Migrantinnen und Migranten in Nordrhein-westfalen. Ergebnisse der vierten Mehrthemenbefragung. Essen (Materialien und Berichte des Zentrums für Türkeistudien). Retrieved from https://www.ssoar.info/ssoar/bitstream/handle/document/34974/ssoar-2007-sauer-Perspektiven_des_Zusammenlebens__die.pdf?sequence=1.

Schaeffer, Doris; Hurrelmann, Klaus; Bauer, Ullrich; Kolpatzik, Kai (2019): Nationaler Aktionsplan Gesundheitskompetenz. Retrieved from https://www.nap-gesundheitskompetenz.de/, zuletzt aktualisiert am 04.03.2019.

Schaeffer, Doris; Hurrelmann, Klaus; Bauer, Ullrich; Kolpatzk, Kai (2018): Nationaler%20Aktionsplan%20Gesundheitskompetenz, last checked on 30.03.2018.

Schaeffer, Doris; Vogt, Dominique; Berens, Eva-Maria; Messer, Melanie; Quenzel, Gudrun; Hurrelmann, Klaus (2016): Health Literacy in Deutschland. Retrieved from https://www.aok-bv.de/imperia/md/aokbv/presse/pressemitteilungen/archiv/2016/08_pk_buchauszugweb.pdf.

Schäfers, Bernhard (1998): Soziologie des Jugendalters. Eine Einführung. 6. aktualisierte und überarb. Aufl. Opladen: Leske und Budrich (Uni-Taschenbücher, 1131).

Schatzman, Leonard; Strauss, Anselm L. (2005): Strategy for analyzing. In: Christopher Pole (Hg.): Fieldwork, Bd. 4. London: Sage, S. 3–21.

Scheffer, Thomas (2002): Das Beobachten als sozialwissenschaftliche Methode – von den Grenzen der Beobachtbarkeit und ihrer methodischen Bearbeitung. In: Doris Schaeffer und Gabriele Müller-Mundt (Hg.): Qualitative Gesundheits- und Pflegeforschung. Bern: Huber, S. 351–374.

Schenk, Liane (2007): Migration und Gesundheit--Entwicklung eines Erklärungs- und Analysemodells für epidemiologische Studien. In: *International journal of public health* 52 (2), S. 87–96. DOI: https://doi.org/10.1007/s00038-007-6002-4.

Scherr, Albert; Niermann, Debora (2012): Migration und Kultur im schulischen Kontext. In: Ullrich Bauer, Uwe H. Bittlingmayer und Albert Scherr (Hg.): Handbuch Bildungs- und Erziehungssoziologie. Wiesbaden: Springer VS, S. 863–882.

Schillinger, Dean; Bindman, Andrew; Wang, Frances; Stewart, Anita; Piette, John (2004): Functional health literacy and the quality of physician – patient communication among diabetes patients. In: *Patient Education and Counseling* 52 (3), S. 315–323.

Schillinger, Dean; Grumbach, Kevin; Piette, John; Wang, Frances; Osmond, Dennis; Daher, Carolyn et al. (2002): Association of health literacy with diabetes outcomes. In: *JAMA: The Journal of the American Medical Association* 288 (4), S. 475–482.

Schmidt, Bettina (2008): Eigenverantwortung haben immer die Anderen. Der Verantwortungsdiskurs im Gesundheitswesen. Bern: Huber.

Schmidt, Bettina (Hg.) (2014): Akzeptierende Gesundheitsförderung. Unterstützung zwischen Einmischung und Vernachläsigung. Weinheim, Basel: Beltz Juventa.

Schmidt, Bettina (2017): Exklusive Gesundheit. Gesundheit als Instrument zur Sicherstellung sozialer Ordnung. Wiesbaden: Springer VS.

Schmidt, Robert; Woltersdorff, Volker (Hg.) (2008): Symbolische Gewalt. Herrschaftsanalyse nach Pierre Bourdieu. Konstanz: UVK.

Schnabel, Peter-Ernst (1988): Krankheit und Sozialisation. Vergesellschaftung als pathogener Prozeß. Opladen: Westdeutscher Verlag.

Schnabel, Peter-Ernst (2001a): Familie und Gesundheit. Bedingungen, Möglichkeiten und Konzepet der Gesundheitsförderung. Weinheim, München: Juventa.

Schnabel, Peter-Ernst (2001b): Familie und Gesundheit. Bedingungen, Möglichkeiten und Konzepte der Gesundheitsförderung. Weinheim/München: Juventa.

Schnabel, Peter-Ernst (2007a): Gesundheit fördern und Krankheit prävenieren. Besonderheiten, Leistungen und Potentiale aktueller Konzepte vorbeugenden Versorgungshandelns. Weinheim, München: Juventa.

Schnabel, Peter-Ernst (2007b): Gesundheit fördern und Krankheit prävenieren. Besonderheiten, Leistungen und Potenziale aktueller Konzepte vorbeugenden Gesundheitshandelns. Weinheim und München: Juventa.

Schnegg, Michael; Pauli, Julia; Beer, Bettina; Alber, Erdmute (2010): Verwandschaft heute: Positionen, Ergebnisse und Perspektiven. In: Erdmute Alber (Hg.): Verwandtschaft heute. Positionen, Ergebnisse und Perspektiven. Berlin: Reimer, S. 7–44.

Schneiderheinze, Klaus (2004): Politische und wirtschaftliche Begegnung: „Nur in gewissen Kreisen". In: *Zeitschrift der Ausländerbeauftragten des Landes Niedersachsen* (3), S. 4.

Schouler-Ocak, Meryam; Aichberger, M.C; Penka, S.; Klugee, U.; Heinz, A. (2015): Psychische Störungen bei Menschen mit Migrationshintergrund in Deutschland. In: *Bundesgesundheitsblatt, Gesundheitsforschung, Gesundheitsschutz*, S. 527–532. Retrieved from https://link.springer.com/content/pdf/10.1007%2Fs00103-015-2143-4.pdf.

Schultheis, Kathirn (2014): Die drei Sektoren der beruflichen Bildung- Übergangssystem. Bundeszentrale für politische Bildung. Retrieved from https://www.bpb.de/politik/innenpolitik/arbeitsmarktpolitik/187852/uebergangssystem?p=all.

Schulze, Alexander; Preisendörfer, Peter (2013): Bildungserfolg von Kindern in Abhängigkeit von der Stellung in der Geschwisterreihe. In: *Köln Z Soziol* 65 (2), S. 339–356. DOI: https://doi.org/10.1007/s11577-013-0205-x.

Schütz, Alfred (1971): Das Problem der Relevanz. Frankfurt a.M.: Suhrkamp.

Schütz, Alfred; Luckmann, Thomas (2003): Strukruren der Lebenswelt. Konstanz: UVK – UTB.

Schweizerische Akademie der Medizinischen Wissenschaften (2015): Gesundheitskompetenz in der Schweiz – Stand und Perspektiven. In: *Swiss Academics Report* 10 (4), last checked on 05.03.2019.

Schweizerische Eidgenossenschaft (2016): Gesundheitskompetenz in der Schweiz, last checked on 06.06.2018.

Schweizerische Eidgenossenschaft – Bundesamt für Statistik (2019a): Armutsgefährungsquote. Retrieved from https://www.bfs.admin.ch/bfs/de/home/statistiken/bevoelkerung/migration-integration/integrationindikatoren/indikatoren/armutsgefaehrdungsquote.html, last checked on 30.03.2020.

Schweizerische Eidgenossenschaft – Bundesamt für Statistik (2019b): Ausländische Bevölkerung. Retrieved from https://www.bfs.admin.ch/bfs/de/home/statistiken/bevoelkerung/migration-integration/nach-migrationsstatuts.html#accordion_3822535761585575076707, last checked on 30.03.2020.

Schwinn, Thomas (2015): Soziale Ungleichheit. Bielefeld: transcript Verlag.

Sebo, Paul; Jackson, Yves; Haller, Dagmar M.; Gaspoz, Jean-Michel; Wolff, Hans (2011): Sexual and reproductive health behaviors of undocumented migrants in Geneva: a cross sectional study. In: *Journal of immigrant and minority health* 13 (3), S. 510–517. DOI: https://doi.org/10.1007/s10903-010-9367-z.

Seçkin, Gül; Yeatts, Dale; Hughes, Susan; Hudson, Cassie; Bell, Valarie (2016): Being an Informed Consumer of Health Information and Assessment of Electronic Health Literacy in a National Sample of Internet Users: Validity and Reliability of the e-HLS Instrument. In: *Journal of medical Internet research* 18 (7), e161. DOI: https://doi.org/10.2196/jmir.5496.

Seifert, Wolfganf (2012): Geschichte der Zuwanderung nach Deutschland nach 1950. Retrieved from https://www.bpb.de/politik/grundfragen/deutsche-verhaeltnisse-eine-sozialkunde/138012/geschichte-der-zuwanderung-nach-deutschland-nach-1950?p=all.

Sen, Amartya (2010): Die Idee der Gerechtigkeit. München: C.H.Beck.

Sentell, Tetine; Pitt, Ruth; Buchthal, Opal Vanessa (2017): Health Literacy in a Social Context: Review of Quantitative Evidence. In: *HLRP: Health Literacy Research and Practice* 1 (2), e41–e70. https://doi.org/10.3928/24748307-20170427-01.

Seurer, Andrea C.; Vogt, H. Bruce (2013): Low health literacy: a barrier to effective patient care. In: *South Dakota Medicine* 66 (2), S. 51–53.

Sharif, Iman; Blank, Arthur E. (2010): Relationship between child health literacy and body mass index in overweight children. In: *Patient Education and Counseling* 79 (1), S. 43–48. DOI: https://doi.org/10.1016/j.pec.2009.07.035.

Shaw, Susan J.; Huebner, Cristina; Armin, Julie; Orzech, Kathryn; Orzech, Katherine; Vivian, James (2009): The role of culture in health literacy and chronic disease screening and management. In: *Journal of immigrant and minority health* 11 (6), S. 460–467. DOI: https://doi.org/10.1007/s10903-008-9135-5.

Shih, Shu-Fang; Liu, Chieh Hsing; Liao, Li-Ling; Osborne, Richard H. (2016): Health literacy and the determinants of obesity: a population-based survey of sixth grade school children in Taiwan. In: *BMC public health* 16, S. 1–8. DOI: https://doi.org/10.1186/s12889-016-2879-2.

Siegrist, Johannes; Dragano, Nico; dem Knesebeck, Olaf von (2006): Soziales Kapital, soziale Ungleichheit und Gesundheit. In: Matthias Richter und Klaus Hurrelmann (Hg.):

Gesundheitliche Ungleichheit. Grundlagen, Probleme, Perpektiven. Wiesbaden: Springer VS, S. 157–170.

Sijthoff, Elise (2014): Mevement, learning and wellbeing in and outside the classroom: The Class Moves! in various European countries. In: Goof Buijs, Kevin Dadaczynski und Schulz, Anette, Vilaça, Teresa (Hg.): Equity, education and health: learning from practice. Case studies of practice presented during the 4th European Conference on Health Promoting Schools, Odense, Denmark. Utrecht: CBO, S. 71–76.

Simon, Michael (2011): Von der Koalitionsvereinbarung bis Ende 2010: Eine Zwischenbilanz schwarz-gelber Gesundheitspolitik. In: *Jahrbuch für Kritische Medizin und Gesundheitswissenschaften* Bd. 47, S. 9–28.

Simon, Michael (2016): Die ökonomischen und strukturellen Veränderungen des Krankenhausbereichs seit den 1970er Jahren. In: Inge Bode und Werner Vogd (Hg.): Mutationen des Krankenhauses. Soziologische Diagnosen in organisations- und gesellschaftstheoretischer Perspektive. Wiesbaden: Springer VS, S. 29–45.

Simovska, Venka; Paakkari, Leena; Paakkari, Olli (2012): Health literacy as a learning outcome in schools. In: *Health Education* 112 (2), S. 133–152. DOI: https://doi.org/10.1108/09654281211203411.

Slewa-Younan, Shameran; Guajardo, Maria; Yaser, Anisa; Mond, Jonathan; Smith, Mitchell; Milosevic, Diana et al. (2017): Causes of and risk factors for posttraumatic stress disorder. The beliefs of Iraqi and Afghan refugees resettled in Australia. Retrieved from https://www.ijmhs.com/content/11/1/4.

Slotala, Lukas (2011): Ökonomisierung in der ambulanten Pflege. Eine Analyse der wirtschaftlichen Bedingungen und deren Folgen für die Versorgungspraxis ambulanter Dienste. Wiesbaden: Springer VS.

Soellner, Renate; Huber, Stefan; Reder, Maren (2014): The Concept of eHealth Literacy and Its Measurement. In: *Journal of Media Psychology* 26 (1), S. 29–38. DOI: https://doi.org/10.1027/1864-1105/a000104.

Song, Lixin; Mishel, Merle; Bensen, Jeannette T.; Chen, Ronald C.; Knafl, George J.; Blackard, Bonny et al. (2012): How does health literacy affect quality of life among men with newly diagnosed clinically localized prostate cancer? Findings from the North Carolina-Louisiana Prostate Cancer Project (PCaP). In: *Cancer* 118 (15), S. 3842–3851. DOI: https://doi.org/10.1002/cncr.26713.

Sørensen, Kristine (2016): Health literacy is a political choice. A... (PDF Download Available). Retrieved from https://www.researchgate.net/publication/311455482_Health_literacy_is_a_political_choice_A_health_literacy_guide_for_politicians, last checked on 03.05.2018.

Sørensen, K. (2021). Health Literacy Champions. In: Saboga-Nunes, L.A., Bittlingmayer, U.H., Okan, O., Sahrai, D. (eds) New Approaches to Health Literacy. Gesundheit und Gesellschaft. Springer VS, Wiesbaden. https://doi.org/10.1007/978-3-658-30909-1_15

Sørensen, Kristine; Pleasant, Andrew (2017): Health literacy. New directions in research, theory and practice. Washington DC: IOS Press (Studies in health technology and informatics, 240), last checked on 06.06.2018.

Sørensen, Kristine; van den Broucke, Stephan; Fullam, James; Doyle, Gerardine; Pelikan, Jürgen; Slonska, Zofia; Brand, Helmut (2012a): Health literacy and public health: a systematic review and integration of definitions and models. In: *BMC public health* 12, S. 80. https://doi.org/10.1186/1471-2458-12-80.

Sørensen, Kristine; van den Broucke, Stephan; Fullam, James; Doyle, Gerardine; Pelikan, Jürgen; Slonska, Zofia; Brand, Helmut (2012b): Health literacy and public health: a systematic review and integration of definitions and models. In: *BMC public health* 12, S. 80. https://doi.org/10.1186/1471-2458-12-80.

Soricone, Lisa; Rudd, Rima; Santos, Marciel; Capistrant, Ben (2007): Health Literacy in Adult Basic Educaiton. Designing Lessons, Units, and Evaluation Plans for an Integrated Curriculum, last checked on 26.03.2018.

Souza, Jessé (2008): Die Naturalisierung der Ungleichheit. Ein neues Paradigma zum Verständnis peripherer Gesellschaften. Mit einem Vorwort von Axel Honneth. Wiesbaden: VS Verlag für Sozialwissenschaften.

Spahn, Jens (2019): „Wir werden das Feld nicht Dr. Google und Co. überlassen!". Spezial 7–8/2019. In: *Gesundheit und Gesellschaft. Das AOK-Forum für Politik, Praxis und Wissenschaft* 22 (7–8), S. 3.

Spallek, Jacob; Razum, Oliver (2008a): Einflussgrößen auf die Gesundheit von Migranten aus Sicht der Lifecourse Epidemology. Retrieved from https://focus-migration.hwwi.de/typo3_upload/groups/3/focus_Migration_Publikationen/Kurzdossiers/bilder/KD-12-gesundheit/Abbildung1_gr.gif, zuletzt aktualisiert am 29.04.2009, last checked on 27.01.2018.

Spallek, Jacob; Razum, Oliver (2008b): Erklärungsmodelle für die gesundheitliche Situation von Migrantinnen und Migranten. In: Ullrich Bauer, Uwe H. Bittlingmayer und Matthias Richter (Hg.): Health Inequalities. Determinanten und Mechanismen gesundheitlicher Ungleichheit. Wiesbaden: VS Verlag für Sozialwissenschaften, S. 271–290.

Speer, Michael E. (2017): Health Literacy and Child Health Outcomes: From Parental to Birth and Infant Stages. In: Rosina Avila Connelly und Teri Turner (Hg.): Health Literacy and Child Health Outcomes. Cham: Springer International Publishing, S. 15–18.

Sperlich, Stefanie (2016): Handlungsorientierte Perspektiven auf Gesundheit und Krankheit. In: Matthias Richter und Klaus Hurrelmann (Hg.): Soziologie von Gesundheit und Krankheit. 1. Auflage. Wiesbaden: Springer VS (Lehrbuch), S. 41–54.

Sperlich, Stefanie; Mielck, Andreas (2003): Sozialepidemiologische Erklärungsansätze im Spannungsfeld zwischen Schicht- und Lebensstilkonzeptionen. In: *Zeitschrift für Gesundheitswissenschaften* 11 (2), S. 165–179.

St Leger, Lawrence (2001): Schools, health literacy and public health: possibilities and challenges. In: *Health Promot Int* 16 (2), S. 197–205.

Statista (2017): Gender Pay Gap in der Schweiz von 2008 bis 2017. In Prozent des durchschnittlichen Bruttostundenverdienstes der Männer. Retrieved from https://de.statista.com/statistik/daten/studie/292066/umfrage/verdienstabstand-zwischen-maennern-und-frauen-gender-pay-gap-in-der-schweiz/, last checked on 06.04.2020.

Statista (2018): Ausländeranteil in den OECD-Mitgliedsstaaten im Jahr 2017. Retrieved from https://de.statista.com/statistik/daten/studie/2032/umfrage/auslaenderanteil-der-oecd-mitgliedsstaaten-in-2005/, last checked on 30.003.2020.

Statistics Canada; OECD (2005): Learning a living: First results of the Adult Literacy and Life Skills Survey. OECD. Ottawa, Paris.

Statistisches Bundesamt (2007): Bevölkerung mit Migrationshintergrund. Ergebnisse des Mikrozensus 2005. Retrieved from https://www.destatis.de/DE/Publikationen/Thematisch/Bevoelkerung/MigrationIntegration/Migrationshintergrund2010220057004.pdf?__blob=publicationFile.

Statistisches Bundesamt (2010): Bevölkerung und Erwerbstätigkeit. Bevölkerung mit Migrationhintergrund- Ergebnisse des Mikrozensus 2009-. Retrieved from https://www.destatis.de/DE/Publikationen/Thematisch/Bevoelkerung/MigrationIntegration/Migrationshintergrund2010220097004.pdf?__blob=publicationFile.

Statistisches Bundesamt (2016): Bildung der Eltern beeinflusst die Schulwahl für Kinder. Retrieved from https://www.destatis.de/DE/PresseService/Presse/Pressemitteilungen/2016/09/PD16_312_122pdf.pdf?__blob=publicationFile.

Statistisches Bundesamt (2018a): Bevölkerung- Einwohnerzahl in Deutschland nach Geschlecht von 1995 bis 2016 (in 1.000). Retrieved from https://de.statista.com/statistik/daten/studie/161868/umfrage/entwicklung-der-gesamtbevoelkerung-nach-geschlecht-seit-1995/.

Statistisches Bundesamt (2018b): Bevölkerung in Deutschland nach Alter und Geschlecht. Retrieved from https://www.govdata.de/daten/-/details/de-bmbf-datenportal-tabelle-0_14.

Statistisches Bundesamt (2018c): Bildungsstand: verteilung der türkischstämmigen bevölkerung in Deutschland nach höchstem Abschluss (Stand 2016). Retrieved from https://de.statista.com/statistik/daten/studie/165263/umfrage/verteilung-der-tuerkischstaemmigen-bevoelkerung-in-deutschland-nach-schulbildung/.

Statistisches Bundesamt (2018d): Bildungsstand: Verteilung der Bevölkerung mit und ohne Migrationshintergrund in Deutschland nach höchstem Schulabschluss (Stand 2016). Retrieved from https://de.statista.com/statistik/daten/studie/245651/umfrage/bildungsstand%2D%2Dverteilung-der-bevoelkerung-nach-migrationshintergrund-und-schulabschluss/.

Statistisches Bundesamt (2018e): Monatliches persönliches Nettoeinkommen im Jahr 2006 nach jeweiligem Migrationshintergrund. Retrieved from https://de.statista.com/statistik/daten/studie/150623/umfrage/monatliches-persoenliches-einkommen-nach-jeweiligem-migrationshintergrund/.

Statistisches Bundesamt (2019): Anzahl der minderjährigen Kinder in Familien in Deutschland von 2000 bis 2017 (in 1.000). Retrieved from https://de.statista.com/statistik/daten/studie/197783/umfrage/minderjaehrige-kinder-in-deutschland/.

Stavemann, H. H. (2008): Sokratische Gesprächsführung. In: Michael Linden und Martin Hautzinger (Hg.): Verhaltenstherapiemanual. 6. Aufl. s.l.: Springer-Verlag, S. 280–286.

Stichs, Anja (2016): Wie viele Muslime leben in Deutschland? Bundesamt für Migration und Flüchtlinge. Retrieved from https://www.bamf.de/SharedDocs/Anlagen/DE/Publikationen/WorkingPapers/wp71-zahl-muslime-deutschland.pdf?__blob=publicationFile.

Sting, Stephan (2007): Gesundheit. In: Jutta Ecarius (Hg.): Handbuch Familie. Wiesbaden: VS Verlag für Sozialwissenschaften, S. 480–499.

Stollberg, Gunnar (2001): Medizinsoziologie. Bielefeld: transcript (Einsichten).

Stutz Steiger, Therese (2011): Gesundheitskompetenz – ein Thema auch für die Weiterbildung. In: *Education Permanente* 4, S. 4–6.

Sudore, Rebecca L.; Yaffe, Kristine; Satterfield, Suzanne; Harris, Tamara B.; Mehta, Kala M.; Simonsick, Eleanor M. et al. (2006): Limited literacy and mortality in the elderly: the health, aging, and body composition study. In: *Journal of General Internal Medicine* 21 (8), S. 806–812. DOI: https://doi.org/10.1111/j.1525-1497.2006.00539.x.

Sukys, Saulius; Trinkuniene, Laima; Tilindiene, Ilona (2019): Subjective Health Literacy among School-Aged Children: First Evidence from Lithuania. In: *International journal of environmental research and public health*, S. 1–11. https://doi.org/10.3390/ijerph16183397.

Sundmacher, Leonie (2016): Regionale Variationen in der Gesundheit und Gesundheitsversorgung. In: Matthias Richter und Klaus Hurrelmann (Hg.): Soziologie von Gesundheit und Krankheit. 1. Auflage. Wiesbaden: Springer VS (Lehrbuch), S. 197–209.

Susan Caplan (2007): Latinos, acculturation, and acculturative stress: A dimensional concept analysis. In: *Policy, Politics, & Nursing Practice* 8, S. 93–106. DOI: https://doi.org/10.1177/1527154407301751.

Suter, Lilian; Waller, Gregor; Bernath, Jael; Külling, Céline; Willemse, Isabel; Süß, Daniel (2018): JAMES – Jugend, Aktivitäten, Medien – Erhebung Schweiz. Zürcher Hochschule für Angewandte Wissenschaften. Zürich.

Tagesschau.de (2018): Deutschtürkische Wähler. Zwei Drittel der Stimmen für Erdogan. Retrieved from https://www.tagesschau.de/inland/tuerkei-wahl-deutschland-107.html.

Taylor, Charles (1995): Atomismus. In: Bert van den Brink und Willem van Reijen (Hg.): Bürgergesellschaft, Recht und Demokratie. Frankfurt am Main: Suhrkamp, S. 73–106.

Taylor, Charles (1996): Quellen des Selbst. Die Entstehung der neuzeitlichen Identität. Frankfurt am Main: Suhrkamp.

Tejada, Gabriela (2010): The Colombian scientific diaspora in Switzerland. In: Gabriela Tejada und Jean-Claude Bolay (Hg.): Scientific diasporas as development partners. Skilled migrants from Colombia, India and South Africa in Switzerland: empirical evidence and policy responses. Bern: Peter Lang, S. 199–313.

Tejada, Gabriela; Kwankam, Francelle (2007): Preliminary findings of South African and Colombian scientific diasporas in Switzerland: A qualitative overview.

Telama, R.; Yang, X.; Laakso, L.; Viikari, J. (1997): Physical activity in childhood and adolescence as predictor of physical activity in young adulthood. In: *American journal of preventive medicine* 13 (4), S. 317–323.

The Scottish Government (2014): Making it Easier: A Health Literacy Action Plan for Scotland. The Scottish Governement. Edinburgh. Retrieved from www.gov.scot, last checked on 06.06.2018.

Thiersch, Hans (2012): Lebensweltorientierte Soziale Arbeit. Aufgaben der Praxis im sozialen Wandel. 8. Aufl. Weinheim: Beltz Juventa (Edition Soziale Arbeit).

Tiesmeyer, Karin; Brause, Michaela; Lierse, Meike; Lukas-Nülle, Martina; Hehlmann, Thomas (Hg.) (2008): Der blinde Fleck. Ungleichheiten in der Gsundheitsversorgung. Bern: Huber.

Tokuda, Yasuharu; Doba, Nobutaka; Butler, James P.; Paasche-Orlow, Michael K. (2009): Health literacy and physical and psychological wellbeing in Japanese adults. In: *Patient Education and Counseling* 75 (3), S. 411–417. DOI: https://doi.org/10.1016/j.pec.2009.03.031.

Tones, K. (2002): Health literacy. New wine in old bottles? In: *Health Education Research* 17 (3), S. 287–290. https://doi.org/10.1093/her/17.3.287.

Trebbe, Joachim; Heft, Annett; Weiß, Hans-Jürgen (2010): Mediennutzung junger Menschen mit Migrationshintergrund. Umfragen und Gruppendiskussion mit Personen türkischer Herkunft und russischen Aussiedlern im Alter zwischen 12 und 29 Jahren in Nordrhein-

Westfalen. Retrieved from publikationen.medienanstalt-nrw.de/modules/pdf_download.php?products_id=238.

Treibel, Annette (2003): Migration in modernen Gesellschaften. Soziale Folgen von Einwanderung, Gastarbeit und Flucht. 3. Aufl. Weinheim: Juventa-Verl. (Grundlagentexte Soziologie).

Trezona, Anita; Fitzsimon, Emma; Dodson, Sarity (2019): Health literacy policy in Australia: Past, present and future directions. In: Orkan Okan, Ullrich Bauer, Diane Levin-Zamir, Paulo Pinheiro und Kristine Sørensen (Hg.): International Handbook of Health Literacy. Research, practice and policy across the lifespan. Bristol: POLICY Press, S. 471–488.

Trout, Alexandra L.; Hoffman, Steven; Epstein, Michael H.; Nelson, Timothy D.; Thompson, Ronald W. (2014): Health Literacy in High-Risk Youth: A Descriptive Study of Children in Residential Care. In: *Child & Youth Services* 35 (1), S. 35–45. DOI: https://doi.org/10.1080/0145935X.2014.893744.

TRT Deutsch (2018): Maas vor Gedenkfeier: Türkische Zuwanderer sind Teil Deutschlands. Retrieved from https://www.trt.net.tr/deutsch/europa/2018/05/29/maas-vor-gedenkfeier-turkische-zuwanderer-sind-teil-deutschlands-981035.

Turra, Cassio M.; Elo, Irma T. (2009): The Impact of Salmon Bias on the Hispanic Mortality Advantage. New Evidence from Social Security Data. In: *Popul Res Policy Rev* 27 (5), S. 515–530.

Ulbricht, Christian (2017): Ein- und Ausgrenzungen von Migranten. Zur sozialen Konstruktion (un-)erwünschter Zuwanderung. Bielefeld: transcript (Kultur und soziale Praxis).

UN Secretary-General (UNSG) (2016): The situation in Afghanistan and its implications for international peace and security. A/71/682–S/2016/1049. Retrieved from https://www.refworld.org/docid/5a2566824.html, last checked on 06.10.2018.

Unger, Hella von (Hg.) (2017): Junge Geflüchtete, Bildung und Arbeitsmarkt – Ein Lehrforschungsprojekt in München. LMU. Retrieved from https://epub.ub.uni-muenchen.de/41306/1/Unger_2017_Junge_Gefluechtete_Bildung_Arbeitmarkt_Lehrforschung_LMU.pdf, last checked on 27.01.2018.

UNHCR (2017a): Figures at a Glance. Retrieved from https://www.unhcr.org/figures-at-a-glance.html, last checked on 12.06.2018.

UNHCR (2017b): UNHCR Statistical Yearbook 2016, 16th edition, last checked on 05.04.2018.

UNHCR – The UN Refugee Agency (2019): Figues at a glance. Statistical Yeabook. Retrieved from https://www.unhcr.org/figures-at-a-glance.html, last checked on 05.10.2019.

United Nations High Commissioner for Refugees (UNHCR) (2018): Desperate Journeys. Refugees and migrants arriving in Europe and at Europe's borders. Retrieved from https://www.unhcr.org/desperatejourneys, last checked on 29.06.2019.

United Nations, General Assembly Security Council (UNGASC) (2019): The situation in Afghanistan and its implications for international peace and security. Report of the Secretary-General. A/73/902–S/2019/493. Retrieved from https://unama.unmissions.org/sites/default/files/sg_report_on_afghanistan_-english-_3_september_2019.pdf, last checked on 05.10.2019.

Uygun-Altunbaş, Ayşe (2017): Religiöse Sozialisation in muslimischen Familien. Dissertation.

van der Heide, Iris; Heijmans, Monique; Rademakers, Jany (2019): Health Literacy Policies: Europeans Perspectives. In: Orkan Okan, Ullrich Bauer, Diane Levin-Zamir, Paulo Pinheiro und Kristine Sørensen (Hg.): International Handbook of Health Literacy. Research, practice and policy across the lifespan. Bristol: POLICY Press, S. 403–418.

van der Vaart, Rosalie; van Deursen, Alexander Jam; Drossaert, Constance Hc; Taal, Erik; van Dijk, Jan Amg; van de Laar, Mart Afj (2011): Does the eHealth Literacy Scale (eHEALS) measure what it intends to measure? Validation of a Dutch version of the eHEALS in two adult populations. In: *Journal of medical Internet research* 13 (4), e86. DOI: https://doi.org/10.2196/jmir.1840.

Vaz, Nafisa Fatima Maria (2017): Mobile Health Literacy to Improve Health Outcomes in Low-Middle Income Countries. In: *IJRQEH* 6 (4), S. 4–16. DOI: https://doi.org/10.4018/IJRQEH.2017100102.

Vereinte Nationen. Wirtschafts- und Sozialrat (2018): Abschließende Bemerkungen zum sechsten periodischen Berichts Deutschlands. Ausschuss für wirtschaftliche, soziale und kulturelle Rechte. Retrieved from https://www.institut-fuer-menschenrechte.de/fileadmin/user_upload/PDF-Dateien/Pakte_Konventionen/ICESCR/icescr_Staatenbericht_6_CoObs_de.pdf, last checked on 08.03.2019.

Vernon, John A.; Trujillo, Antonio; Rosenbaum, Sara; DeBuono, Barbara (2007): Low health literacy: Implications for national health policy. Retrieved from https://publichealth.gwu.edu/departments/healthpolicy/CHPR/downloads/LowHealthLiteracyReport10_4_07.pdf, last checked on 28.09.2019.

Vester, Michael (2009): Milieuspezifische Lebensführung und Gesundheit. In: *Jahrbuch für Kritische Medizin und Gesundheitswissenschaften* Bd. 45, S. 36–56.

Vester, Michael; Oertzen, Peter von; Geiling, Heiko; Hoffmann, Thomas; Müller, Dagmar (2001): Soziale Milieus im gesellschaftlichen Strukturwandel. Zwischen Integration und Ausgrenzung. Frankfurt am Main: Suhrkamp.

Viruell-Fuentes, Edna A.; Miranda, Patricia Y.; Abdulrahim, Sawsan (2012): More than culture: structural racism, intersectionality theory, and immigrant health. In: *Social science & medicine (1982)* 75 (12), S. 2099–2106. https://doi.org/10.1016/j.socscimed.2011.12.037.

Walford, Geoffrey (2009): The practice of writing ethnographic fieldnotes. In: *Ethnography and Education* 4, S. 117–130. DOI: https://doi.org/10.1080/17457820902972713.

Wallmann, Birgit; Gierschner, Susann; Froböse, Ingo (2012): Gesundheitskompetenz: was wissen unsere Schüler über Gesundheit? Eine empirische Erhebung. In: *Präv Gesundheitsf* 7 (1), S. 5–10. DOI: https://doi.org/10.1007/s11553-011-0322-1.

Wallston, Kenneth A.; Cawthon, Courtney; McNaughton, Candace D.; Rothman, Russell L.; Osborn, Chandra Y.; Kripalani, Sunil (2014): Psychometric properties of the brief health literacy screen in clinical practice. In: *Journal of General Internal Medicine* 29 (1), S. 119–126. DOI: https://doi.org/10.1007/s11606-013-2568-0.

Walter, Jochen (2008): Die Türkei – „das Ding auf der Schwelle“. (De-)Konstruktionen der Grenzen Europas. 1. Aufl. Wiesbaden: VS Verlag für Sozialwissenschaften/GWV Fachverlage GmbH Wiesbaden. Retrieved from https://doi.org/10.1007/978-3-531-91026-0.

Walter, U.; Krauth, C.; Kurtz, V.; Salman, R.; Machleidt, W. (2007): Gesundheit und gesundheitliche Versorgung von Migranten unter besonderer Berücksichtigung von Sucht. In: *Der Nervenarzt* 78 (9), S. 1058–1061. DOI: https://doi.org/10.1007/s00115-007-2295-z.

Walters, Sue; Papen, Uta (2008): Literacy, learning and health. Research report. London: National Research and Development Centre for adult literacy and numeracy.

Wångdahl, Josefin; Lytsy, Per; Mårtensson, Lena; Westerling, Ragnar (2015): Health literacy and refugees' experiences of the health examination for asylum seekers – a Swedish cross-sectional study. In: *BMC public health* 15, S. 1162. DOI: https://doi.org/10.1186/s12889-015-2513-8.

Wångdahl, Josefin; Lytsy, Per; Mårtensson, Lena; Westerling, Ragnar (2018): Poor health and refraining from seeking healthcare are associated with comprehensive health literacy among refugees: a Swedish cross-sectional study. In: *International journal of public health* 63 (3), S. 409–419. DOI: https://doi.org/10.1007/s00038-017-1074-2.

Wartella, Ellen; Rideout, Vicky; Montague, Heather; Beaudoin-Ryan, Leanne; Lauricella, Alexis (2016): Teens, Health and Technology: A National Survey. In: *MaC* 4 (3), S. 13. https://doi.org/10.17645/mac.v4i3.515.

Wartella, Ellen; Rideout, Vicky; Zupancic, Heather; Beaudoin-Ryan, Leanne; Lauricella, Alexis (2015): Teens, Health, and Technology. A National Survey. Northwestern University. Retrieved from https://cmhd.northwestern.edu/wp-content/uploads/2015/05/1886_1_SOC_ConfReport_TeensHealthTech_051115.pdf, last checked on 07.10.2019.

Weber, Max (1972): Wirtschaft und Gesellschaft. Grundriss der verstehenden Soziologie. 5. revidierte Auflage. Tübingen: J.C.B. Mohr.

Weiss, Barry D. (1999): 20 common problems in primary care. New York: McGraw-Hill Open Univ. Press.

Weiss, Barry D. (2005): The epidemiology of low health literacy. In: Joanne G. Schwartzberg, Jonathan VanGeest und Claire Wang (Hg.): Understanding health literacy. Implications for medicine and public health. Chicago Ill.: American Medical Association, S. 65–81.

Weiss, Barry D.; Mays, Mary Z.; Martz, William; Castro, Kelley Merriam; DeWalt, Darren A.; Pignone, Michael P. et al. (2005): Quick Assessment of Literacy in Primary Care: The Newest Vital Sign. In: *Annals of Family Medicine* 3 (6), S. 514–522. DOI: https://doi.org/10.1370/afm.405.

Weiss, Dieter (2008): Deutschland am Hindukusch (43), S. 6–14. Retrieved from https://www.bpb.de/apuz/30897/deutschland-am-hindukusch?p=all, last checked on 05.10.2019.

Wettstein, Felix (2018): Gesunder Schlaf ist eine soziale Frage. Beim Schlaf wird zu stark auf das Individuum fokussiert. In: *Psychoscope* (3), S. 21–23.

Wharf Higgins, Joan; Begoray, Deborah (2012): Exploring the Borderlands between Media and Health: Conceptualizing 'Critical Media Health Literacy'. In: *Journal of Media Literacy Education* 4 (2), S. 136–148.

Wharf Higgins, Joan; Begoray, Deborah L.; MacDonald, Marjorie (2009): A Social Ecological Conceptual Framework for Understanding Adolescent Health Literacy in the Health Education Classroom. In: *American journal of community psychology* 44, S. 350–362. DOI: https://doi.org/10.1007/s10464-009-9270-8.

WHO (1986): Ottawa-Charta zur Gesundheitsförderung. Retrieved from https://www.euro.who.int/__data/assets/pdf_file/0006/129534/Ottawa_Charter_G.pdf.

WHO (1998): Health Promoting School, last checked on 27.06.2018.

WHO (2009): Nairobi Call to Action. Retrieved from https://www.who.int/oral_health/events/2010_seventh_who_global_conference_health_promotion.pdf, last checked on 06.03.2019.

WHO (2016): Shanghai Declaration on promoting health in the 2030 Agenda for Sustainable Development, last checked on 02.05.2018.

WHO (2019): Sharpening the focus on gaming disorder. In: *Bulletin of the World Health Organization* 97 (6), S. 382–383. DOI: https://doi.org/10.2471/BLT.19.020619.

WHO Europe (1986): Ottawa Charter for Health Promotion, last checked on 05.02.2018.

WHO Europe (2013): Health Literacy. The solid facts. Edited by Ilona Kickbusch, Jürgen Pelikan, Franklin Apfel & Agis D. Tsouros. Copenhagen: WHO Regional Office for Europe.

Whyte, William Foote (2005): Focusing the study and analysing the data. In: Christopher Pole (Hg.): Fieldwork, Bd. 4. London: Sage, S. 57–79.

Wilkinson, Richard (2005): The Impact of Inequality. How to Make Sick Societies Healthier. New York: The New Press. Retrieved from https://ebookcentral.proquest.com/lib/gbv/detail.action?docID=579087.

Wilkinson, Richard G. (1996): Unhealthy Societies. The Affliction of Inequality. London: Routledge.

Wilkinson, Richard G.; Marmot, Michael (2003): Social Determinants of Health. The Solid Facts. 2nd edition. WHO. Retrieved from https://www.euro.who.int/__data/assets/pdf_file/0005/98438/e81384.pdf, last checked on 03.09.2017.

Wilkinson, Richard G.; Pickett, Kate E. (2010): The spirit level. Why equality is better for everyone. Publ. with rev. London: Penguin Books (Pinguin sociology).

Williams, M. V.; Parker, R. M.; Baker, D. W.; Parikh, N. S.; Pitkin, K.; Coates, W. C.; Nurss, J. R. (1995): Inadequate functional health literacy among patients at two public hospitals. In: *JAMA* 274 (21), S. 1677–1682.

Willis, Paul (1979): Spaß am Widerstand. Gegenkultur in der Arbeiterschule. Frankfurt a. M.: Syndikat.

Willis, Paul (2000): The ethnographic imagination. Cambridge: Blackwell.

Willis, Paul (2004): Twenty-Five Years On. Old Books, New Times. In: Nadine Dolby und Greg Dimitriadis (Hg.): Learning to Labor in New Times. with Paul Willis. London: Routledge, S. 167–196.

Wills, Jane (2009): Health literacy: new packaging for health education or radical movement? In: *International journal of public health* 54 (1), S. 3–4. DOI: https://doi.org/10.1007/s00038-008-8141-7.

Wilson, Petra (2002): How to find the good and avoid the bad or ugly: a short guide to tools for rating quality of health information on the internet. In: *BMJ: British Medical Journal* 324 (7337), S. 598–602.

Winker, Gabriele; Degele, Nina (2010): Intersektionalität. Zur Analyse sozialer Ungleichheiten. Bielefeld: transcript.

Woellert, Franziska; Klingholz, Reiner (2014): Neue Potenziale. Zur Lage der Integration in Deutschland. Berlin.

Wolf, Michael S.; Davis, Terry C.; Shrank, William; Rapp, David N.; Bass, Pat F.; Connor, Ulla M. et al. (2007): To err is human: patient misinterpretations of prescription drug label instructions. In: *Patient Education and Counseling* 67 (3), S. 293–300. DOI: https://doi.org/10.1016/j.pec.2007.03.024.

Wolf, Michael S.; Wilson, Elizabeth A. H.; Rapp, David N.; Waite, Katherine R.; Bocchini, Mary V.; Davis, Terry C.; Rudd, Rima E. (2009): Literacy and learning in health care. In: *Pediatrics* 124 Suppl 3, S275-81. DOI: https://doi.org/10.1542/peds.2009-1162C.

Wright, Michael (2016): Partizipative Gesundheitsforschung. In: BZgA (Hg.): Leitbegriff der Prävention und Gesundheitsförderung. Ergänzungsband 2016. Köln: BZgA, S. 157–165.

Wu Amery D, Begoray Deborah L, Macdonald Marjorie, Wharf Higgins Joan, Frankish Jim, Kwan Brenda, Fung, Winny, Rootman, Irvin (2010). Developing and evaluating a relevant and feasible instrument for measuring health literacy of Canadian high school students. Health Promot Int., 25:444–52. https://doi.org/10.1093/heapro/daq032.

Yee, Lynn M.; Simon, Melissa A. (2014): The role of health literacy and numeracy in contraceptive decision-making for urban Chicago women. In: *Journal of community health* 39 (2), S. 394–399. DOI: https://doi.org/10.1007/s10900-013-9777-7.

Yin, H. Shonna (2017): Health Literacy and Child Health Outcomes: Parental Health Literacy and Medication Errors. In: Rosina Avila Connelly und Teri Turner (Hg.): Health Literacy and Child Health Outcomes. Cham: Springer International Publishing, S. 19–38.

Yin, H. Shonna; Forbis, Shalini G.; Dreyer, Benard P. (2007): Health literacy and pediatric health. In: *Current problems in pediatric and adolescent health care* 37 (7), S. 258–286. DOI: https://doi.org/10.1016/j.cppeds.2007.04.002.

Young, Iris Marion (1996): Fünf Formen der Unterdrückung. In: Herta Nagl-Docekal und Herlinde Pauer-Studer (Hg.): Politische Theorie. Differenz und Lebensqualität. Frankfurt am Main: Suhrkamp, S. 99–139.

Zamora, Pablo; Pinheiro, Paulo; Okan, Orkan; Bitzer, Eva-Maria; Jordan, Susanne; Bittlingmayer, Uwe H. et al. (2015): „Health Literacy" im Kindes- und Jugendalter. In: *Präv Gesundheitsf* 10 (2), S. 167–172. DOI: https://doi.org/10.1007/s11553-015-0492-3.

Zarcadoolas, Christina; Pleasant, Andrew; Greer, David S. (2005): Understanding health literacy: an expanded model. In: *Health promotion international* 20 (2), S. 195–203. DOI: https://doi.org/10.1093/heapro/dah609.

Zarcadoolas, Christina; Pleasant, Andrew F.; Greer, David S. (2006): Advancing health literacy. A framework for understanding and action. 1st ed. San Francisco, CA: Jossey-Bass (J-B Public Health/Health Services Text, v.17). Retrieved from https://site.ebrary.com/lib/alltitles/docDetail.action?docID=10304017.

Zhang, Ning Jackie; Terry, Amanda; McHorney, Colleen A. (2014): Impact of health literacy on medication adherence: a systematic review and meta-analysis. In: *The Annals of pharmacotherapy* 48 (6), S. 741–751. DOI: https://doi.org/10.1177/1060028014526562.

Zimmermann, David (2012): Migration und Trauma. PaÈdagogisches Verstehen und Handeln in der Arbeit mit jungen FluÈchtlingen. Gießen: Psychosozial-Verlag (Psychoanalytische Paedagogik, Bd. 38).

Zinn, Jens O. (2008): Normativität in der Ungleichheitsforschung. In: Johannes Ahrens, Raphael Beer, Uwe H. Bittlingmayer und Jürgen Gerdes (Hg.): Beschreiben und/oder Bewerten I. Normativität in sozialwissenschaftlichen Forschungsfeldern. Münster: LIT-Verl., S. 159–183.

Zou, P.; Parry, M. (2012): Strategies for health education in North American immigrant populations. In: *International nursing review* 59 (4), S. 482–488. DOI: https://doi.org/10.1111/j.1466-7657.2012.01021.x.

Zschorlich, Beate; Gechter, Dorothea; Janßen, Inger M.; Swinehart, Thomas; Wiegard, Beate; Koch, Klaus (2015): Gesundheitsinformationen im Internet: wer sucht was, wann und wie? In: *Zeitschrift für Evidenz, Fortbildung und Qualität im Gesundheitswesen*, S. 144–152. Retrieved from https://zefq-journal.com/article/S1865-9217(15)00055-0/pdf.

Zwick, Michael M.; Deuschle, Jürgen; Renn, Ortwin (Hg.) (2011): Übergewicht und Adipositas bei Kindern und Jugendlichen. 1. Aufl. Wiesbaden: VS Verl. für Sozialwiss. Retrieved from https://doi.org/10.1007/978-3-531-93158-6.

MIX
Papier aus verantwortungsvollen Quellen
Paper from responsible sources
FSC® C105338

If you have any concerns about our products,
you can contact us on
ProductSafety@springernature.com

In case Publisher is established outside the EU,
the EU authorized representative is:
Springer Nature Customer Service Center GmbH
Europaplatz 3, 69115 Heidelberg, Germany

Printed by Libri Plureos GmbH
in Hamburg, Germany